PEAK PERFORMANCE

Radiant Health

Moving Beyond The Zone

By
Brian Peskin

with
Marcus Conyers

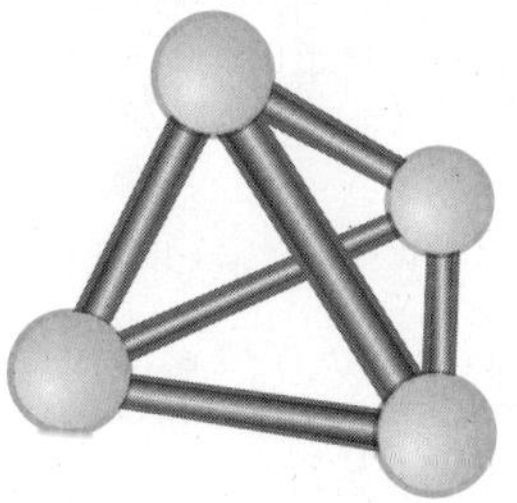

Noble Publishing

Dedicated to my loving wife, Debra.
The inspiration for my quest of knowledge whom without, Radiant Health would not be possible.

Copyright @ 2001 by Brian S. Peskin, Life-Systems Engineer

No part of this book may be reproduced or transmitted in any form or by any means, electronic or mechanical, including photocopying, recording, taping, or any information storage and retrieval mechanism presently known or to be invented, without permission, in writing, from the publisher, except by a reviewer who wishes to quote excerpts from this work in reference to a review written for publication in a magazine, newspaper, or broadcast.

Editing by Wayne McGinty and Stephen Ruback

Cover Design by
Bart Noble

Illustrations and layout by
Stephen Ruback and Digital Output

Third Edition

Published by

Noble Publishing

2020 Naomi Street, Houston, TX 77054

(713) 796-2431

Printed in the United States of America

Dedicated to bringing you the best nutrition information from the world's leading universities and Nobel Prize-winning research

Library of Congress Cataloging-in-Publication Data

Peak Performance, Radiant Health: Moving Beyond The Zone
Peskin, Brian Scott.
P. cm.
Includes bibliographical references and index.
1.Obesity—Nutritional aspects. 2. Obesity—Etiology. 3. Nutrition. 4. Diet therapy.
I. Title.
RC628.P47 1997 616.3'98 QBI96-40672
ISBN: 0-9651551-3-7 96-71593

Preface

This book is for information purposes only. No representations, either express or implied, are made or given regarding the medical consequences of opinions presented. This book contains only the opinions of the author, who is a Life-Systems Engineer, not a physician. This book is not intended to provide medical diagnosis or treatment advice, nor is this book intended as a substitute for medical advice for any condition requiring medical supervision. Statements made in this book are factual, based on credible and authoritative sciences or the opinions of the author. Comments, reviews, and criticisms of diets or writings by other people are solely the author's opinions and beliefs, and are intended only to review and discuss the opinions of the author in this book.

Most people eating **basic essence** tend to desire fewer carbohydrates. If you are **diabetic**, your insulin or other medication requirements may change. When you start eating basic essence, consult your physician about any needed changes in your medication as a result of changing insulin levels. Don't automatically take the same amount of insulin based on your previous carbohydrate consumption. Readers who are diabetic and take insulin must closely monitor their glucose levels. Also consult your physician if you aren't regularly checking blood glucose levels before each meal.

Women, because of your generally strong willpower in following what you thought was correct – the great 25-year carbohydrate eating experiment – you may require an additional 90 days (6 months total) of Radiant Health to re-balance your hormones. **Please be patient; your improved health is worth it!**

If you are **sick** or suspect that you are sick, you should consult a physician. If you are on any prescription medications, check with your physician when you start taking basic essence to see if the same levels of those medications are still required. You should not change your diet, even if for the better, without consulting your physician to determine the diet's effect on the medication, because dietary change can affect a prescription drug's action. The author and publisher expressly disclaim any responsibility or liability arising directly or indirectly from the application of this book or of any nutritional products mentioned herein without appropriate medical supervision.

The discoveries in this book will allow you to enjoy the pleasure of eating again. Your taste and appetite for certain foods will automatically change — expect a decrease in your craving for processed carbohydrates. **Americans have exceptional willpower, so don't stop eating all of them at once — just minimize them (for example, eat half the normal amount)**— otherwise, you change your system balance too rapidly.

The name **basic essence** and EFA/EFAs, are used throughout this book as shorthand for essential fatty acids, or healthy essential oils. The EFAs, linoleic acid and alpha-linolenic acid, are also known, respectively, as omega 6 and omega 3.

What is **Beyond The Zone?**

It is being lean for life and brimming with boundless energy. It is being able to accelerate through your workload with laser-sharp concentration and a steel-trap memory. It is maximizing protection for you and your loved ones against the assault of life-threatening diseases. It is supporting your body with the nutrition it needs and was designed to have. When you are living **Beyond The Zone**, peak performance and radiant health happen naturally.

Athletes refer to "*the zone*" as the moment when they achieve peak physical performance. *Radiant Health* takes you *beyond* the zone because:

1. Anyone can benefit – we go beyond athletes.

2. You can be in the Zone permanently – we go beyond temporary states.

3. You can enjoy peak mental performance – we go beyond just the body and physical performance.

4. You can begin eating for pleasure again – we go beyond diet plans.

5. You curb cravings naturally with the nutrition discovery of the century – we go beyond willpower.

6. We bring you established medical research from the world's leading institutions and Nobel Prize-winning discoveries. We go beyond commonly accepted assumptions about nutrition. We go beyond "studies" or reports, which are often subject to *mis*interpretation.

Can I rely on the Media to tell the Truth?

Certainly not from television! "A report on organic food televised on ABC's *20/20* (Feb. 4, 2000 and July 7, 2000) had **misrepresented tests** done on behalf of ABC." Ken Cook, president of The Environmental Working Group, stated, "...they lied and threatened an entire industry **by disseminating false and damaging information.**"

***Life-Systems* Engineering analysis:** rely on science – not reports or studies which may be misleading.

Source: *The New York Times*, August 10, 2000.

This book gives you a new perspective — a "second opinion" — based on Nobel Prize-winning research from world-leading authorities in medicine and health.

For years, many physicians and scientists have known the truth about what is required for radiant health, but their voices have not been heard by the public. This book is dedicated to all physicians who are committed to providing the very best of care, preventive medicine, and nutrition advice to their patients.

"I am grateful to find nutrition information based on established medical research. In my opinion, this book ranks amoung the most significant works on diet and nutrition published in the past 100 years."

Stephen Weiss, M.D. – Orthopedic Surgeon

"After you read Brian Peskin's book [Peak Performance, Radiant Health], he will challenge you to rethink everything you have learned... ."

Lorrie Medford – Certified Nutritionist

"This book is invaluable. No opinions or assumptions here: just the facts. Finally, a nutrition book not out to prove anything except to explain real-life results based on established medical science. We owe Mr. Peskin a big THANK YOU."

Max Motyka, M.S., R.Ph. – Registered Pharmacist

"We are honored to have a scientist of Professor Peskin's standing as a member of the faculty of Texas Southern University, College of Pharmacy and Health Science. His Scientific Medical Research has uncovered a great Nutrition Program with an effective approach to Health."

Dr. Doris Jackson – Associate Dean (1998)
College of Pharmacy and Health Science, Texas Southern University

"We are honored to have Professor Peskin as a member of the faculty. His nutritional discoveries and practical applications through Life-Systems Engineering are unprecedented."

Dr. James Douglas – President (1998)
Texas Southern University

Landmarks in Nutrition and Health – Timeline

1848 Dr. Semmelweis is fired for showing that sterilizing hands prior to surgery and child delivery stops infection.

1863 William Banting demonstrates that Dr. Harvey's program minimizing carbohydrates achieves weight loss (and excellent health).

1944 Dr. Blake Donaldson proves with radio isotope tagging that carbohydrates are immediately converted to bodyfat.

1955 Insulin found to convert carbohydrates to bodyfat.

1956 Drs. Parvan and Kekwick independently confirm that carbohydrates are immediately converted to bodyfat.

Lancet warns of hydrogenated oils (like margarine) causing massive heart disease.
Nutritional recommendations do not change.

1980 Carbohydrate producers start heavily promoting processed carbohydrates (cereals, breads, pastas, etc.) as nutritious.

1990 A flood of books published giving one-sided "half-truths" concerning cholesterol, carbohydrates, fats and proteins. (Confusion results.)

Obesity, chronic fatigue and diabetes start increasing dramatically.

1993 Life-Systems Engineering developed to explain nutritional requirements for humans.

Medical Journal *Circulation* urges food-processing industry to replace *un*natural man-made transfats with naturally occurring fats.
Nutritional recommendations do not change.

1994 *Journal of Cardiovascular Risk* reports that replacing fat with carbohydrates does not significantly reduce cholesterol levels.
Nutritional recommendations do not change.

1995 Diet drugs reach record sales.

1996 Massive advertising money increases sales of processed carbohydrates.

Chronic illness, obesity, and diabetes conditions worsen.

Massive money pumped into advertising cholesterol-lowering drugs.

Life-Systems Engineers discover solutions to widely misunderstood epidemic nutritional deficiencies – eliminating food cravings, increasing fat-burning and achieving much better over-all health.

1997 FDA recalls Phen-Fen and Redux – weight reducing drugs.

Major Harvard University study concludes: Heart Disease NOT caused by natural fats.
Nutritional recommendations do not change.

New England Journal of Medicine reports that diets high in polyunsaturated fats are more effective than low-fat, high-carbohydrate diets in reducing cholesterol and coronary disease.
Nutritional recommendations do not change.

1998 *Journal of Cardiovascular Risk* reports low-fat diets without lots of exercise worthless in decreasing cholesterol levels
Nutritional recommendations do not change.

Protein shown to help broken bones heal faster – not slower.
Nutritional recommendations do not change.

1999 Landmark book published, which in simple, readily understandable form, reveals critical life-systems.
It is titled: *Beyond The Zone*.

Major Harvard University study concludes:
Colon cancer risk NOT helped by fiber;
Colon cancer risk NOT caused by meat.

Major Harvard University study concludes:
Breast cancer risk NOT increased by fat.

Studies show it's safe to eat an egg a day. (More confusion results.)

Diet of 50% fat, 30% protein, and 20% carbohydrate improves weight-loss and lipid profile in more than 150 type II diabetics. Americans are not given the results. (*Abstract of presentation before the 1999 annual meeting of the Endocrine Society*, James Hayes, M.D., Endocrinologist.)

2000 *New England Journal of Medicine* reports major study showing vitamin E is worthless in preventing heart disease.
Significance is downplayed.

Journal of Cardiovascular Risk reports Stanford University study showing carbohydrates *raise* fasting triglycerides and fasting cholesterol, and *reduce* HDL - *the exact opposite of what we have been told carbohydrates do!* Carbohydrates found to *raise* the risk of cardiovascular disease! (Americans are not given the results.)

Newsflash: Vitamin C supplements appear to make arterial heart disease worse!

Cancer Institute admits 25 years of "fiber fiction." Lots of fruit and vegetables, and wheat bran worthless in decreasing colon cancer!
Americans are outraged over being mislead.

"Tofu (from soy) linked to mental decline" (*Journal of the American College of Nutrition*, 19:207-209, 242-255.)
More Confusion Results

Soy found worthless by Mayo Clinic in decreasing hot flashes.
Women aren't told.

American Heart Association Meeting (Presented June 2000):
- "Lowering total fat intake is probably not a very effective strategy for reducing CVD (heart disease) risk."
- "...place fats fairly low on the cancer [risk] list."
- The ideal diet for CVD (heart disease) prevention contains healthy essential oils (basic essence).

Why weren't you told?

Today

Discoveries of *Life-Systems* Engineering become available to everyone wanting science instead of opinion.

The solution is called *Radiant Health*.

Shocking Answers to Common Questions

Q: What exactly is insulin?

A: Insulin is that FAT STORAGE HORMONE everyone is talking about that treats the sugar, by turning it into fat. Carbohydrates stimulate insulin release, and **insulin stops fat-burning cold**, even when exercising. **Furthermore, insulin makes you hungry all of the time.** This is all in the *Textbook of Medical Physiology*.* Not accounting for this insulin function caused by carbohydrates is part of the reason the great 25-year carbohydrate eating *experiment* has caused the obesity epidemic! Has a physician or a nutritionist ever told you that **insulin** (a response to "low-fat" carbohydrates) **increases cholesterol** and **harmful triglycerides**? They should have: it's in *Basic Medical Biochemistry.*

Q: What is the body's preferred energy source?

A: Surprise; it's not carbohydrates. It **should be** your own **bodyfat**, but we have interfered with Mother Nature's system. Most of the time even your muscles, the largest calorie burners, can't use sugar, but we aren't told this. Did you know it? This, too, is in the *Textbook of Medical Physiology*.

Q: Because of the extra calories, does eating fat make you fat?

A: NO.* Most people miss this medical fact. Dietary fat and protein contribute to internal structures, including muscle and brain cells - or they are used to fuel the digestion process. This is published in *Basic Medical Biochemistry*. **Carbohydrates**, such as products made with flour, trigger more **insulin**, which **stores fat on your body**. The calorie theory applies to a lump of coal or maybe a cow - not to a human being.* If a nutritionist doesn't understand thermodynamics, then you'll probably miss this deduction, too. We've often been **grossly misled**. My Radiant Health Program gives you the science behind how a human being *really* works.

Q: Is it unhealthy to eat cholesterol and fat?

A: Not necessarily. *Peak Performance, Radiant Health* explains. For example, the *Journal of Cardiovascular Risk*, 1994; 1:3-8 (Sacks, F., "Dietary fats and coronary heart disease") was very clear on what helps. The *New England Journal of Medicine*, 1997; 337: 1491-1499 (Willett, Walter et. al., "Dietary fat intake and the risk of coronary heart disease in women"), reported that **"Diets high in polyunsaturated fats [basic essence]** have been **more effective** than low-fat, high-carbohydrate diets in lowering total serum cholesterol as well as the incidence of coronary heart disease." Most Americans never got this critical information. **Radiant Health** gives you the science about cholesterol, fat, protein, and carbohydrate so you can begin to protect yourself.

Q: I keep hearing how bad ketones are. The nutritionist scared me to death!

A: Staying lean requires ketone production, because ketones are produced naturally when you are running on your own bodyfat.* Ketones are the preferred energy source for your heart, muscles, and liver; they're brain-food, too* – This is all published in the *Textbook of Medical Physiology* and *(Stryer's) Biochemistry - 4th edition*. **Nutritionists need to go back to school and learn medical physiology and medical biochemistry.**

Q: American women are concerned about osteoporosis. Will more calcium help?

A: For most people, absolutely not. Remove the calcium from bone, and the bone becomes more flexible – like cartilage. If you add **more calcium**, bone becomes **more brittle and more likely to break**. So there is something wrong

* All references are fully discussed and documented in this book, *Peak Performance, Radiant Health*.

with this picture. There are 6 causes of osteoporosis listed in the *Textbook of Medical Physiology*, and lack of calcium **isn't one** of them!* Certain groups don't want you to know this. *Peak Performance, Radiant Health* gives more details on the true causes of osteoporosis.

***Q:** I don't understand! Why are eggs OK now, and for 20 years they weren't?*
A: Eggs were always OK; we were misled by false claims. **People's physiology doesn't change, but studies are often prejudiced.** Years ago, one or more "studies" were misinterpreted to mean that eating eggs was harmful. Cholesterol in eggs is now understood to be harmless.* Unfortunately, nutritionists and physicians often **refuse to admit that they've been wrong** – relying on faulty information and biased conclusions. I developed the Stat-Smart™ analysis so that you know whether or not to believe a study.

***Q:** Isn't just avoiding refined sugar enough? Nutritionists often say that we need lots of complex carbohydrates, not more refined sugar.*
***A:* No, just avoiding refined sugar is not sufficient.** *Peak Performance, Radiant Health* explains that the two most common sweeteners of foods (like soft drinks) are beets and corn syrup – both carbohydrates. You can look this up for yourself in any almanac. "Cane sugar" is not often used in commercial food processing, because other carbohydrate sweeteners are less expensive. Understand that a bagel, to your body, is the same as eating 4 teaspoons of sugar mixed in a glass of water. "Simple" carbohydrates, like table sugar, or so-called "complex carbohydrates," like brown organic rice, generate the same **total** overall insulin response to remove the sugar from the blood. Only the time lapse is different. **It's the same amount of sugar.** Shocking, but true!

***Q:** I recently heard that vitamin E doesn't protect against heart disease. Is this true?*
A: According to Dr. Yusuf's article, based on studying over 9,000 people, and published in the ***New England Journal of Medicine*** **(Jan. 2000),** it is true. There **was no protection against heart disease: "There is no reason to take vitamin E** as a means of **preventing heart disease**." This result is no surprise to *Life-systems* Engineers, who published, years ago, that there was no scientific reason to justify the claim that vitamin E supplements were "heart-healthy."

***Q:** Why am I getting opinion – not science?*
A:* Most likely, because the nutrition writers and editors themselves often don't understand the science! Nor will they often admit when they are wrong.** In 1999 Harvard University published a conclusion that fiber *doesn't protect* against colon cancer – **increased fiber actually <u>raised</u> the number of cases of colon cancer. Were you told of this new finding? Did you hear of the worthlessness of vitamin E? In college studies, nutrition is usually a humanities course, not a science degree. I'm tired of "experts" treating us as though we're stupid. I give you the science, so you can begin to judge for yourself what you are being told – instead of relying on someone who may be just guessing, but acting as though offering scientific fact.

***Q:** Isn't glucosamine sulfate, a popular anti-arthritis supplement, the best thing for joint pain relief?*
A: What you haven't been told is its effect on **inhibiting *hepatic glucokinase*,** the body's **glucose (sugar) sensor,** in the liver. If you are diabetic or concerned about becoming diabetic (insulin resistant) you need to be concerned over this supposedly "safe" supplement. The risk was known in 1996 (*Diabetes,* 45(10):1329-35, Oct 1996), but you probably haven't been warned of it.

* All references are fully discussed and documented in this book, *Peak Performance, Radiant Health.*

Q: For years, I've heard that reducing fat and cholesterol (replacing them with carbohydrates) was the only way to gain a healthy heart. This now appears to be unfounded.

A: **Yes, it is unfounded.** The *Journal of Cardiovascular Risk* (No. 1, June 1994) published a feature article, "Dietary Fats and Coronary Heart Disease." Here are some excerpts from the article: "All 3 classes of fatty acids [basic essence] raise HDL" ... "The HDL/LDL* **ratio does not change [does not improve] when saturated fat is replaced by carbohydrate**" ... "The low-fat diets have been **considerably less effective in lowering total or LDL cholesterol than predicted.**" "...the effect on decreasing CHD [Coronary Heart Disease] of decreasing saturated fat and cholesterol intake remains unanswered ...." **This is a far different story than most Americans have been given.**

Q: I have indigestion when taking the oils. Why?

A: As with a protein deficiency, correcting a healthy essential oil deficiency requires a few months for the body to function properly. The sugar overload caused by the great carbohydrate eating *experiment* has caused critical *Life-Systems* to virtually shut down. The good news is that, with Radiant Health supplements over a few months, these critical life-systems will begin to work properly again. Initially, just take less, so your body can re-adapt to what was proper for it in the first place.

Q: Do women take longer than men to get results from Radiant Health?

A: Yes. In general, and unfortunately, women's willpower has enabled them to improperly "adapt" to diets high in carbohydrates. **Over many years, women have unknowingly forced their bodies to "re-wire."** As you will learn in *Peak Performance, Radiant Health*, women's hormonal systems have been highly disrupted by this. **Fortunately, these negative effects of the 25-year carbohydrate eating *experiment* can be reversed.** Women: It took time for your body to adapt to eating *un*naturally, and it will take time for your body to realize it can work naturally again. **Please be patient; your health is worth it!**

Q: Can the "external aggressive" symptoms of (students and children) with ADD and ADHD be reduced by supplementing basic essence essential oils?

A: **YES.** As reported in *Journal of Clinical Investigation* (1996, 97:1129-1134), in just 5 months, a group of college students displayed **significantly less aggression.**

Q: Is Radiant Health good for children?

A: Absolutely! Attention Deficit Disorder as well as ADHD can often be **significantly improved by children taking Radiant Health.** Children's immunity to common colds, flus, and ear infections will increase and respiratory problems will decrease.

* HDL is what people erroneously call "good cholesterol." LDL is referred to as "bad cholesterol."

Q: Why do so many people look so sickly when they start losing weight?

A: **Bodyfat contains stored toxins. Fat-burning releases them.** Did your weight-loss clinic tell you this? That's why you need a *daily detoxifier*. **Radiant Health addresses this important issue.**

Q: Do nutrition writers understand science?

A: **Apparently not.** In *Men's Health*, (Dec. 1999, page 80), Nancy Clark, M.S., R.D., states in an article that when exercising, "a 180-lb. man should consume 540 to 900 grams of carbohydrates per day." This is the equivalent of **108 to 180 teaspoons of sugar! Do you think that she could understand this scientific fact yet still recommend it?**

Q: Isn't the "aspirin-a-day" that my physician prescribes the best defense against heart disease?

A: Absolutely not. **He needs to *understand* more current information.** *British Medical Journal* (2000; 321:13-17) concludes from their analysis: "Men with higher blood pressures may be exposed to the risk of bleeding **while deriving no benefit [aspirin increased the stroke rate].** ... For lower blood pressure there is still a **serious risk of (noncerebral) bleeding that outweigh any possible cardiovascular benefit** [at best, a mere 0.5%!]. **Surprised?**

> ***Total fat and saturated fatty acid intakes as a percentage of total energy have been declining over the past 30 years in the United States.***
>
> **Alice Litchenstein D.Sc., Tufts University, Boston**
> ***Muscular Development*, January 2000, page 47**

We are **decreasing** fat consumption [making Americans fatter than ever] leading us to ...

... increasing sugar [carbohydrate] and additives consumption [making children dumber].

> ***Study* with one million New York City students: Scholastic averages moved from 11% below, to 5% above the national mean (a significant 16% improvement – with less carbohydrates and less food additives).***
>
> ***Dr. Alexander Schauss' research suggests reducing sucrose and additives raised test scores in 803 schools based on California Achievement Tests from the 41 percentile to the 51 percentile in 4 years.***
>
> ****Reclaiming Our Health*, 1998**

You Weren't Getting the Most Important Information in 1981...

In 1981, these important findings were published. Did any educator, school administrator, or nutritionist tell you about this?

- **Lack of EFAs contributes to *hyperactivity* in children.**

- **Boys are much more affected** (by hyperactivity) than girls, and males are known to have much **higher requirements for EFAs** than females.

- Some children are **badly affected** by wheat and milk (**carbohydrates**) which are known to give rise to *exorphins* which block conversion of EFAs to PGE1 (a critical prostaglandin*).

- Many of our children are **deficient in zinc** – which is required for conversion of EFAs to PGs (prostaglandins*).

- Many of our children have **eczema, allergies, and asthma** – which some reports suggest **can be alleviated by EFAs.**

Source: Medical Hypotheses 1981 May;7(5):673-9

How much other critical peak performance and health information has been withheld? Isn't it time to learn what really works? It's called Radiant Health – and it's here today!

*Prostaglandins are made by the body from healthy essential oils (EFAs).

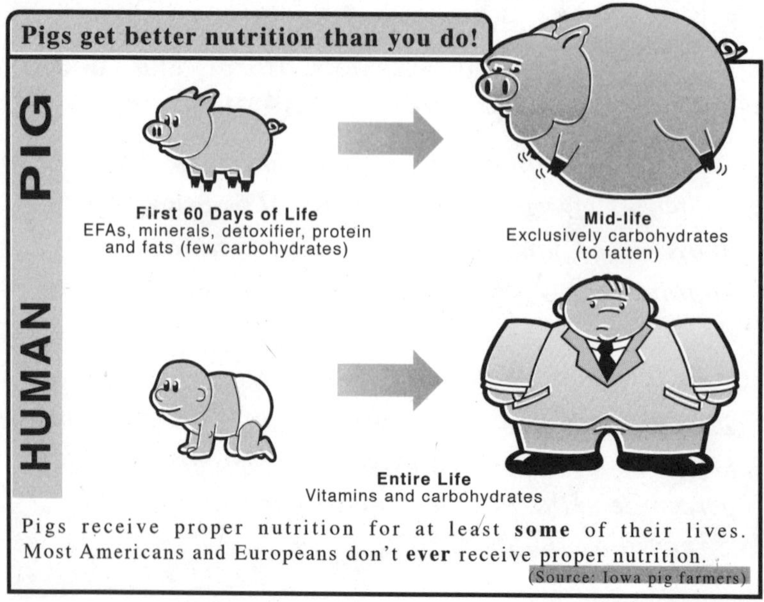

...You Still May Not Be!

in 2000

In 2000, these important findings were published. Did any nutritionist tell you about them?

A 60% carbohydrate / 25% fat* diet (high-carb / low fat) was clinically compared to a 40% carbohydrate / 45% fat diet (low carb / high fat). Here are the astonishing results:

- **"Elevated triglyceride levels [bad] persisted** throughout the day, induced by the **high carbohydrate diet**, *despite the decrease in fat* content of the meals."

- "...**high carbohydrate diets** are associated with **increases** in both **fasting and postprandial** [after eating] **triglyceride concentrations**."

- "...it seems apparent that **substituting carbohydrate for saturated fat leads to higher triglyceride and lower HDL**, associated with day-long increases of circulating triglyceride and remnant lipoprotein [RLP] cholesterol."

- **"All of these changes have been shown to be associated with enhanced atherogenesis [cardiovascular disease]."**

- "Given the atherogenic [heart damaging] potential of these changes in lipoprotein metabolism, **it seems appropriate to question the wisdom of recommending that all Americans should replace dietary saturated fat with carbohydrates.**"

Source: Stanford University School of Medicine, American Journal of Cardiology 2000; 85:45-48

***Life-Systems* Engineering analysis:** What we have been told to do, during the great 25-year carbohydrate eating *experiment*, causes the exact negative conditions we are trying so desperately to avoid.

Are you frustrated and "don't know who to believe" anymore? Isn't it time to learn the **science** of what really works? **It's called Radiant Health – and it's here today!**

*90%, or nearly all, polyunsaturated

We wish to thank, in particular, the following medical journals, publications, medical textbooks, universities, and institutions for making this work possible: (Listed in alphabetical order.)

Universities & Research Institutions: Harvard Medical School, Harvard School of Public Health, **Houston Academy of Medicine - Texas Medical Center (HAM-TMC) Library***, John Innes Institute, Massachusetts Institute of Technology, McGill University, Oxford University, Princeton University, Stanford University, Texas Southern University, Yale University School of Medicine, University of Alabama, University of Texas Medical School, University of Toronto, Efamol Research Institute, National Institutes of Health, Wysong Institute

***With nearly 3,000 current periodic subscriptions (more than 1,000 titles on-line), and more than 300,000 monographs, the HAM-TMC Library has one of the largest collections of medical literature in North America.**

Medically-Related Publications: *Albion Research Notes — A Compilation of Vital Research Updates On Human Nutrition, American Journal of Cancer, American Journal of Cardiology, American Journal of Clinical Nutrition, American Journal of Public Health, Basic Medical Biochemistry — A Clinical Approach, Body Fluids and Electrolytes, Bottom Line, Bowes & Church's Food Values, British Medical Journal, Cancer Research, Chemical Week, Condensed Chemical Dictionary, Consumer Reports On Health, Diabetes Interview, Dorland's Illustrated Medical Dictionary, Dr. Alexander Grant's Health Gazette, Drug Facts and Comparisons, Drug Topics, Energy Times, Enzymes, Essential Histology, Essentials of Biochemistry, FDA Consumer Health, International Journal of Sports Nutrition, Journal of the American Medical Association, Journal of Sports Medicine and Physical Fitness, Journal of Pharmacology, Lancet, Mayo Clinic Health Letter, Microbial Pathogenesis, Molecular Biology of the Cell, New England Journal of Medicine, Journal of Nutrition, Nutrition for Fitness & Sport, Science News, Official Journal of the American College of Sports Medicine, Pharmacist's Letter, Pharmacy Times, Photonics, Physician's Committee for Responsible Medicine, Physiology Coloring Book, Prevention, Prostaglandins and Control of Vascular Smooth Muscle Proliferation, Prostaglandins in the Cardiovascular System, Reuters Health Information Services, Roles of Amino Acid Chelates in Nutrition, Scientific American, Smart Fats, Stroke,* Stryer's *Biochemistry (4th Edition), Your Health, Textbook of Medical Physiology*

NOBEL PRIZE

TIME LINE OF SIGNIFICANT DISCOVERIES IN NUTRITION

EARLY 1900s: SPECIAL RECOGNITION NO PRIZES AWARDED
DR. JOHANNA BUDWIG FIRST TO RECOGNIZE IMPORTANCE OF EFAS; FOOD PROCESSORS LAUNCH CAMPAIGN TO DISCREDIT HER.

1904	IVAN PAVLOV – PHYSIOLOGY OF DIGESTION
1908	ILJA MECNIKOV – WORK ON IMMUNITY
1910	ALBRECHT KOSSEL – KNOWLEDGE OF CELLULAR CHEMISTRY, ESPECIALLY PROTEINS
1920	JULES BORDET – DISCOVERIES RELATING TO IMMUNITY
1923	SIR FREDERICK BANTING – DISCOVERY OF INSULIN
1931	OTTO WARBURG – NATURE AND MODE OF RESPIRATORY ENZYME
1937	ALBERT SZENT-GYORGYI – BIOLOGICAL COMBUSTION PROCESSES
1947	CARL & GERTY CORI – COURSE OF CATALYTIC CONVERSION OF GLYCOGEN BERNARDO HOUSSAY – METABOLISM OF SUGAR
1953	SIR HANS KREBBS – CITRIC ACID CYCLE [THE KREBBS CYCLE] FRITZ LIPMANN – DISCOVERY OF COENZYME A
1964	KONRAD BLOCH – MECHANISM AND REGULATION OF CHOLESTEROL AND FATTY ACID METABOLISM
1971	EARL SUTHERLAND – MECHANISMS AND ACTIONS OF HORMONES
1974	GEORGE PALADE – STRUCTURE AND FUNCTIONAL ORGANIZATION OF THE CELL
1982	JOHN VANE – PROSTAGLANDINS AND RELATED BIOLOGICALLY ACTIVE SUBSTANCES

Science Can Make Our Dreams Come True

"We need more research, not more physicians. ... There is so little truly effective medical technology available even in the very best of circumstances."

Dr. Handler would be delighted to know that the **dream of effortless better health has now been discovered.**

Dr. Phillip Handler, President – National Academy of Sciences (1971), W.O. Atwater Lecture, Third International Congress on Nutrition and Food Technology.

Unfortunately, We Were Right...

In *Beyond The Zone*, we predicted that the refined carbohydrate *experiment* would contribute to an epidemic in obesity. It did.

"Rarely do chronic conditions such as obesity spread with the speed and dispersion characteristic of a communicable disease epidemic. The greatest magnitude was in the following groups: 18-29-year-olds (7.1% to 12.1%) ..."

"The Spread of the Obesity Epidemic in the United States, 1991 - 1998," *Journal of the American Medical Association*, 1999; 282: 1519-1522.

Some Key Facts:

- **Obesity** costs **$230 billion per year** excluding treatment.
  (Dr. Robert Rubin, president, Lewin Group, American Obesity Association)
- **Sugar** consumption is **up** 28% since 1983.
  (Food Labeling and Nutrition News)
- **Soda** is the largest single source of **added sugar** in the U.S. diet – 33% of added sugar in the overall diet. Recent studies link frequent consumption of sugar-sweetened soft drinks to obesity.
  (New York Times, September 21, 1999)

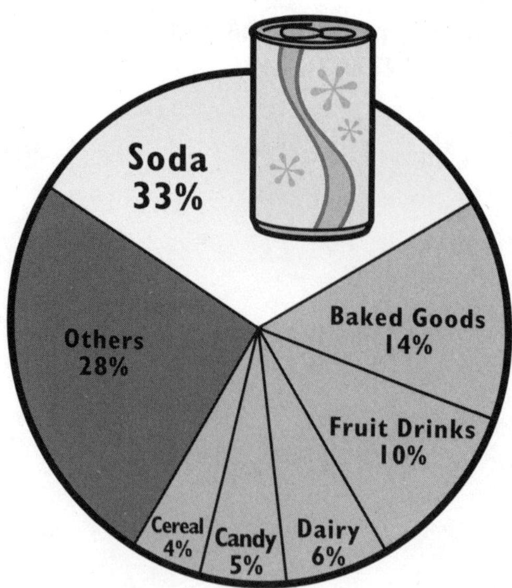

Contents

"It does not make any difference
how smart you are,
who made the guess,
or what his name is —
if it disagrees with real-life results,
it is wrong.
That is all there is to it."

Professor Richard Feynman
Nobel Prize-winner: physics

"Belief without understanding is stupidity. Mere generalized statements without ***sharp, specific conclusions*** *are meaningless."*

Professor Brian Peskin
Life-Systems Engineer

Chapter 1

Real Life Results

Real-Life Results Contradict Popular Theories

We told you this years ago...

Cholesterol Meaningless Compared to Triglycerides

"... 70% increased risk for cardiovascular disease [with high triglycerides] ... **independent** of total cholesterol."

Circulation 2000;101;2777-2782

Today, we are suffering from seemingly insoluble health problems: Chronic fatigue is the No.1 complaint of Americans, 60% of us are obese, diabetes has reached epidemic proportions, cancer now afflicts at least 40% of us and heart attacks and strokes will kill more than 42% of us. We Americans have a lot of material luxuries, but what is their value if we lose our health?

During the last 100 years, we have changed our food and diet on a grand scale. We have gone from a farm-fresh, all-natural food supply to a highly processed food supply. Natural, fresh food has been sacrificed to convenience and long shelf-life, leading us to a host of unforeseen problems.

The massive low-fat, high-*carbohydrate experiment* hasn't helped stop the terrible trend of chronic fatigue and ill-health. We have been bombarded with *theories* (guesses) along with reams of statistical studies. In fact, we will see how this experiment is actually causing the problem. The noble goal of achieving radiant health and being lean-for-life has continued to elude us – until now.

What went wrong? Years of detailed research in the new field of *Life-Systems* Engineering are paying off with answers that work.

Life-Systems Engineering starts with how the body actually works, according to established medical research.

Let's start with a brief review of some common theories compared with real-life experience.

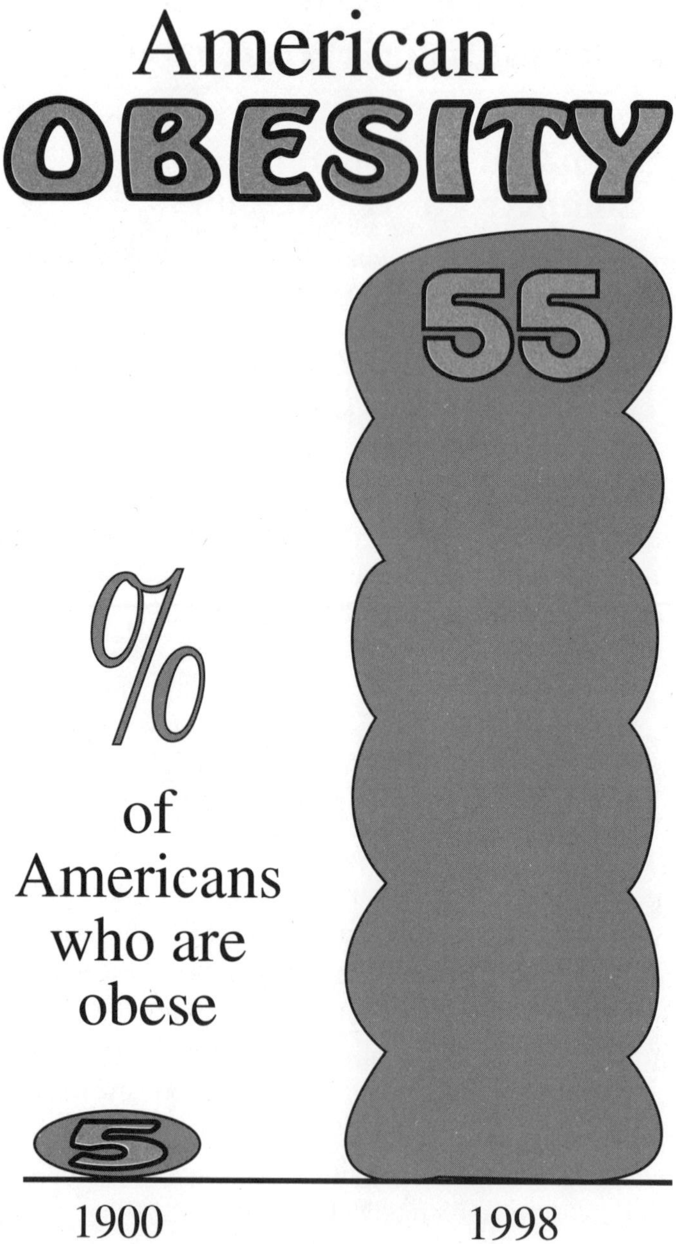

American OBESITY

55

%

of Americans who are obese

5

1900 1998

Source: National Heart, Lung, and Blood Institute

Theory:

A low-fat, high-carbohydrate diet keeps you lean and healthy. [FALSE]

Experience:

- More people than ever before are eating a low-fat, high-carbohydrate diet.
- In the last 10 years, obesity has become an epidemic, increasing by over 32%.
- Obesity afflicts *over half the world's population,* according to the World Health Organization.
- More than half of us are overweight, according to the National Institutes of Health.
- The *lowest* published obesity figures were from the American Medical Association, which stated that one in three women and one in five men are obese (now commonly defined as 25-30-percent above normal body weight).
- The average weight of young adults has increased more than 10 pounds in the last 7 years, according to the National Institutes of Health; *25% of children are obese!*

Comments:

The great low-fat, high-carbohydrate experiment, which was supposed to keep us lean and healthy, is only based on a theory (a guess). The real-life results are quite different.

To fatten cattle, ranchers feed them grain (carbohydrates).
In fact, to fatten any animal, you feed it carbohydrates.

Nobel Prize-winner James D. Watson and his co-authors, in their book, *Molecular Biology of The Cell*, tell us:
**"Carbohydrate:
General term for sugars and related compounds,...."**

Carbohydrate is another name for sugar

Learn more about preventing obesity. Read the chapter "Truth About Protein, Carbohydrates And Fats."

Sugar Consumption

[pounds per person, per year]

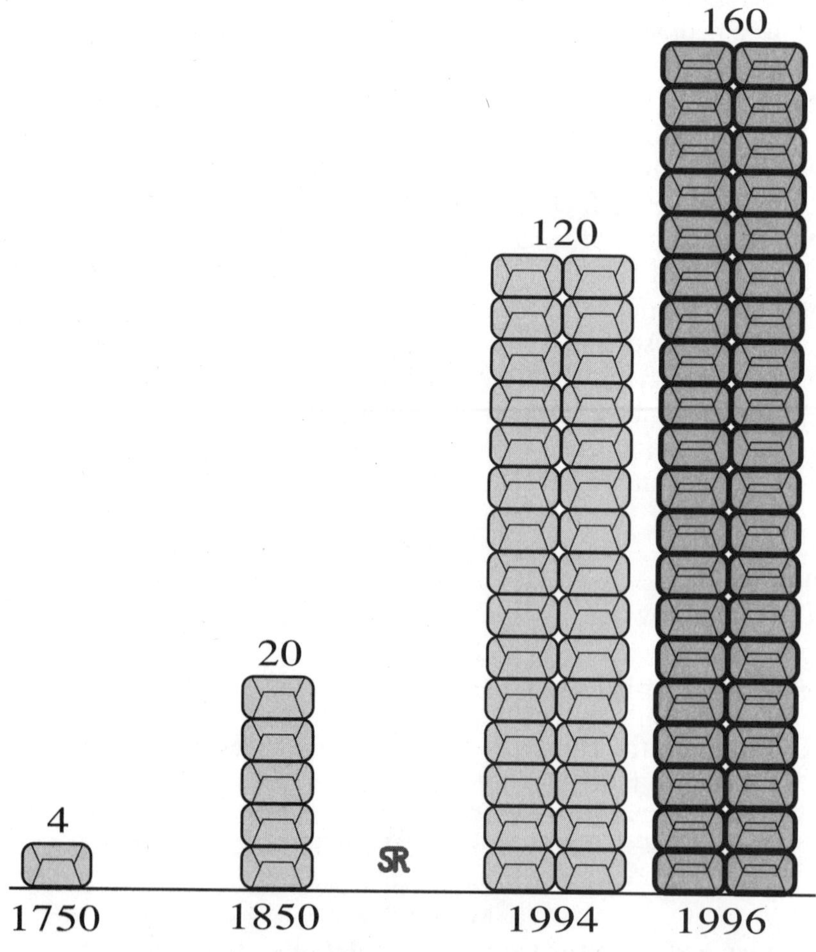

More than 21,648,000 metric tons of sugar was consumed in the United States in 1996

Source: Chemical Week, June 11, 1997, p. 32

Theory:

Too much sugar is harmful. [**TRUE**]

Experience:

- Sugar causes cavities.
- Excess sugar aggravates diabetes.
- Excess sugar may be linked to causing diabetes.
- Excess sugar may be linked to attention deficit.
- Excess sugar may be linked to obesity.

Comments:

How much sugar does the body require per day? No one has ever been diagnosed with a "sugar deficiency." The body doesn't require any sugar intake, although it does require protein and natural healthy oils.

Personal sugar consumption has soared during the last 100 years. In 1996, sugar consumption was more than 160 pounds per person.

According to *Nutrition For Fitness & Sport,* an 8-ounce glass of orange juice provides enough sugar energy to enable the average person to run about a mile. If you aren't immediately using this energy, it is quickly converted to bodyfat!

Surprise:
The body converts all carbohydrates to glucose. Glucose is sugar.

Learn more about sugar and cellulite. Read the chapter "Cellulite Takes A Hike."

Typical Lifetime Consumption

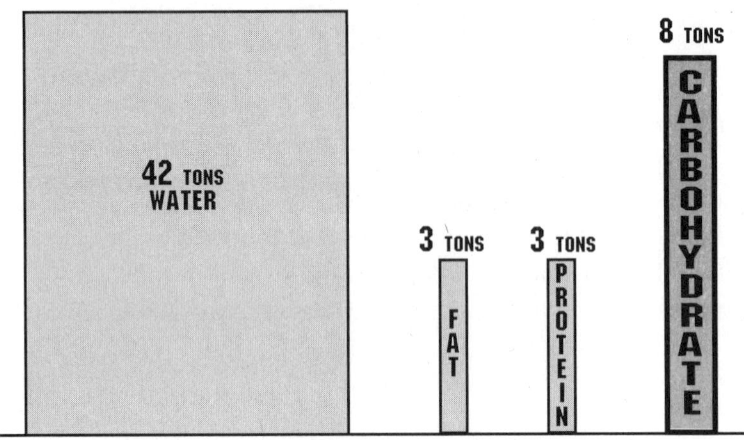

Body Content (pounds)

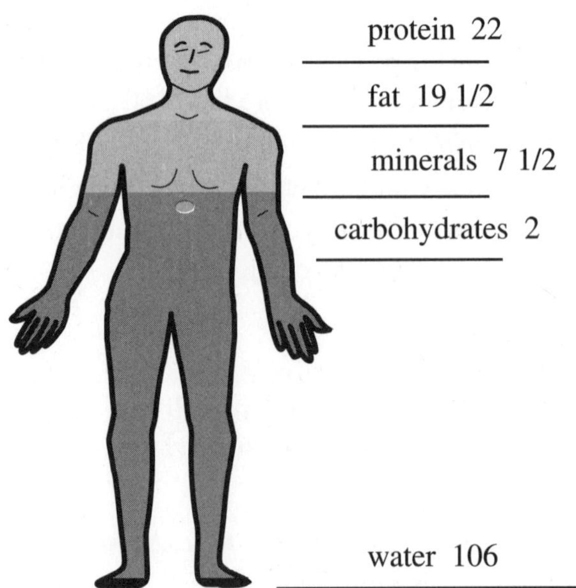

Excess carbohydrates go to fat.

Source: Jules Hirsch MD, Rockefeller University

Theory:

We need lots of carbohydrates. [FALSE]

Experience:

- Your body manufactures all the carbohydrates it needs, from proteins and the bodyfat you already have, according to the *Textbook of Medical Physiology.*
- The body stores only a small amount of carbohydrates.
- Excess carbohydrates are converted to fat.
- Carbohydrates contribute to cellulite.
- Excess carbohydrates reduce athletic performance.

Comments:

How much carbohydrate does the body require per day? According to *Nutrition For Fitness & Sport,* The National Research Council has not established an RDA for carbohydrates, because the body can operate on a completely carbohydrate-free diet. No one has ever been diagnosed with a "carbohydrate deficiency." The body fundamentally doesn't require any carbohydrate, but it does require protein and natural healthy oils.

The body converts all carbohydrates to sugar.

Learn more about carbohydrates. Read the chapter "Truth About Protein, Carbohydrates And Fats."

Dieter's Lament

Source: Beyond Pritikin

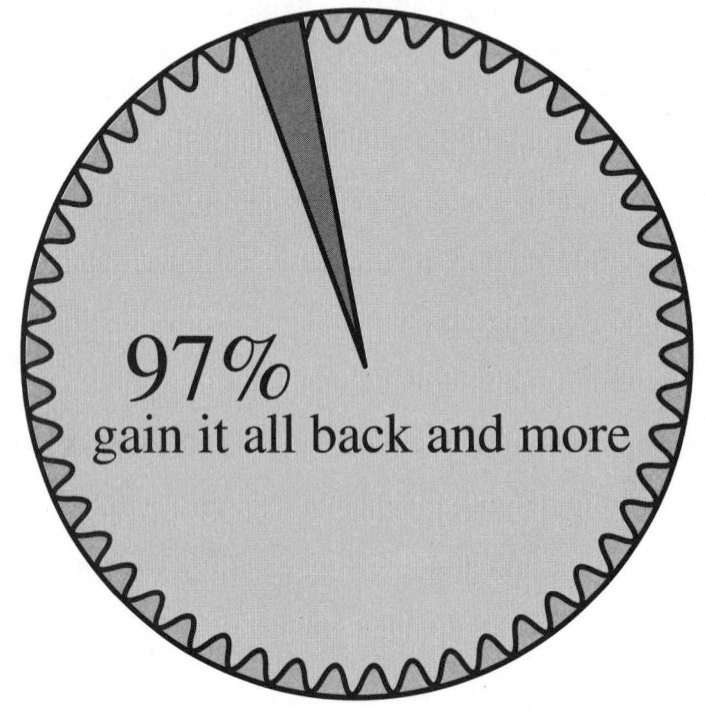

SR

Almost everyone on a diet gains back *more* than the weight lost within two years.

Theory:
A low-fat, reduced-calorie diet is the best way to lose weight. [FALSE]

Experience:

- Few people on low-fat diets lose weight permanently.
- More than 97% of the few people who actually lose weight this way put it all back on, plus more.
- Many people on low-fat, reduced-calorie diets gain weight.
- Many people on calorie-restricted diets have low energy and marginal health.

Comments:

Americans have shown incredible willpower in their efforts to lose weight, but willpower alone is not enough.

Until you are armed with the right information, it is impossible to take the right action.

The primary result of low-fat eating: your body craves high-sugar foods and makes you fatter — not leaner. Favorites include: chocolate, candy, and ice cream, all of which trigger release of serotonin in the brain. Serotonin gives you that tired feeling and makes you drowsy, according to Professor Wurtman at M.I.T.

The best efforts of eating a low-fat (carbohydrate-based) diet result in constant hunger and over-eating, which, in turn, reduces your energy level and continues a cycle of cravings all over again.

Learn about the nutritional discovery of the century.
Read the chapter
"Permanent Fat Loss – A Simple Solution."

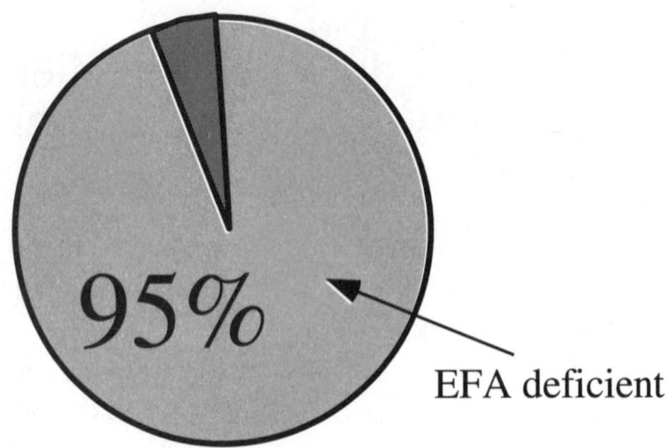

Most Americans Are Deficient In EFAs

Source: Fats That Heal, Fats That Kill

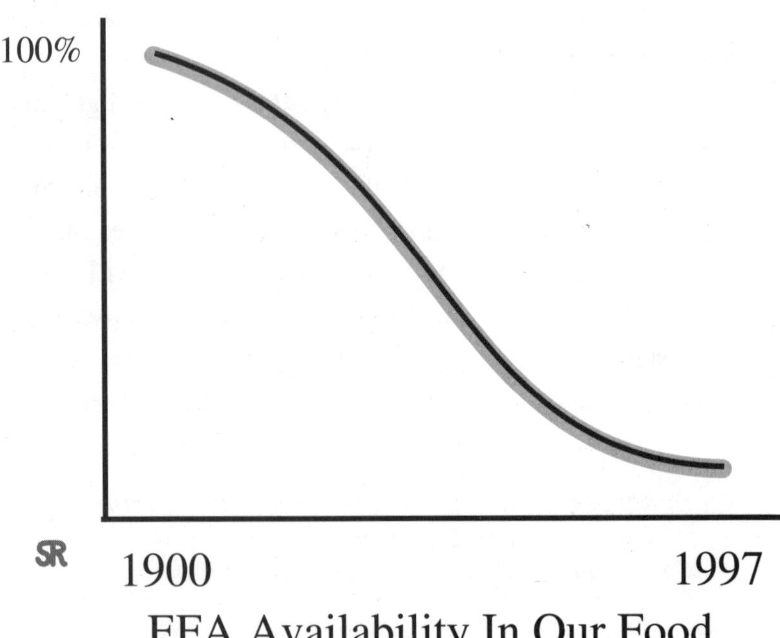

EFA Availability In Our Food

Theory:

We get all the healthy *essential* oils we need from our diet. [FALSE]

Experience:

- It is estimated that 95% of Americans are deficient in essential EFAs.
- EFAs are removed from processed foods.
- 6 months of consistent EFA supplements are usually required before the body develops an adequate reserve.

Comments:

While a huge increase in sugar consumption may be a major cause of the widespread obesity and health problems in the United States, another primary factor has been the reduced consumption of the healthy *essential* oils. All your cells are built on these components. Your body can't make them. They must come from the foods you eat. (According to the medical textbooks *Biochemistry and Disease* and *Basic Medical Biochemistry.*)

Without these basic building blocks your cells can't work the way they should. These EFAs play a central role in attaining peak performance and radiant health, including powering up your brain for peak performance.

Until the early 1900s, cultures around the world used simple means of extracting oils from seeds and nuts. In Europe, villages had at least one oil beater. The oil beater would gather flax and other seeds, crush the seeds, and collect their oil. Once or twice a week, the fresh oil would be delivered to the villagers.

Learn more about healthy essential oils. Read the chapter "Life-Systems Engineering Is Born."

Source: U.S. Senate Document #264, 74th Congress – 2nd Session, 1936

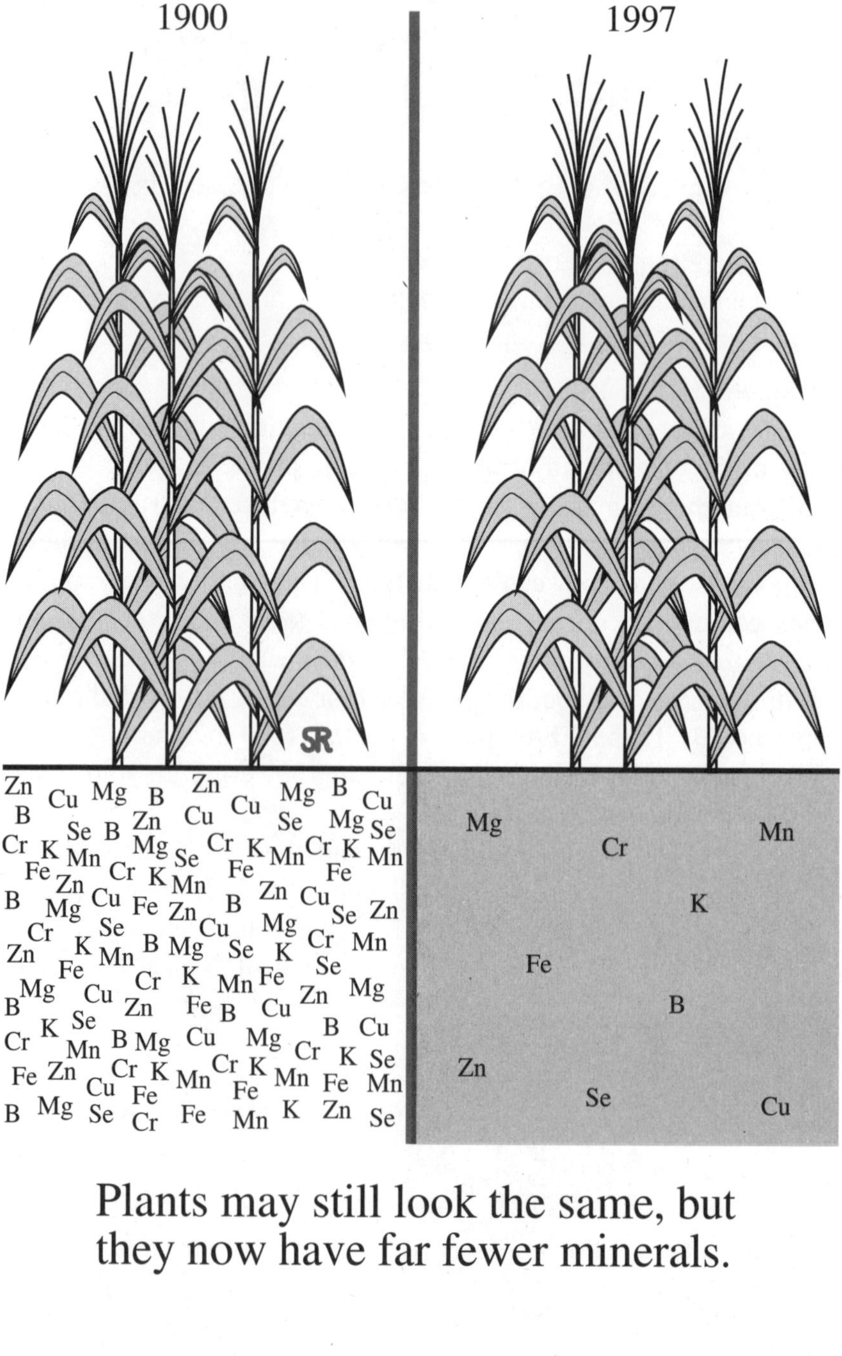

1900 | 1997

Plants may still look the same, but they now have far fewer minerals.

Theory:

We get all the minerals we need from our normal diet. [FALSE]

Experience:

- The U.S. government officially recognizes that Americans are deficient in essential minerals.
- Our soil is depleted of at least 9 essential minerals, so they are no longer in our food.
- Most mineral supplements are not bioavailable (the body can't use them effectively).
- Minerals significantly improve athletic performance, according to *Nutrition For Fitness & Sport.*
- Without proper minerals, vitamins can't be fully utilized.

Comments:

Because of overfarming the same land year-after-year, with synthetic fertilizers (chemicals), most soil is now deficient in minerals. Crops may grow with chemical fertilizers, but no longer give humans the full range of nutrients that Mother Nature intended.

Only minerals that are truly bioavailable support your peak performance and radiant health:

1. Minerals are building blocks for body tissue and other body structures.
2. Minerals enable enzymes and hormones which regulate the metabolism.
3. Minerals maximize the efficiency of healthy essential oils.
4. Vitamins don't work effectively without the proper minerals.

Most mineral supplements are not in the form the body can use.

Learn more about bioavailable minerals' role in peak performance and radiant health. Read the chapter "Something About Supplements."

How Much Bodyfat Do You Burn During The Day?

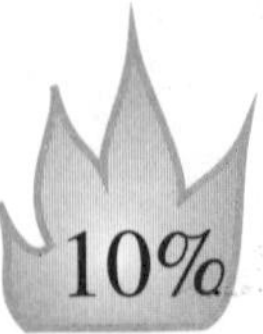

Nutritionally Deficient Foods

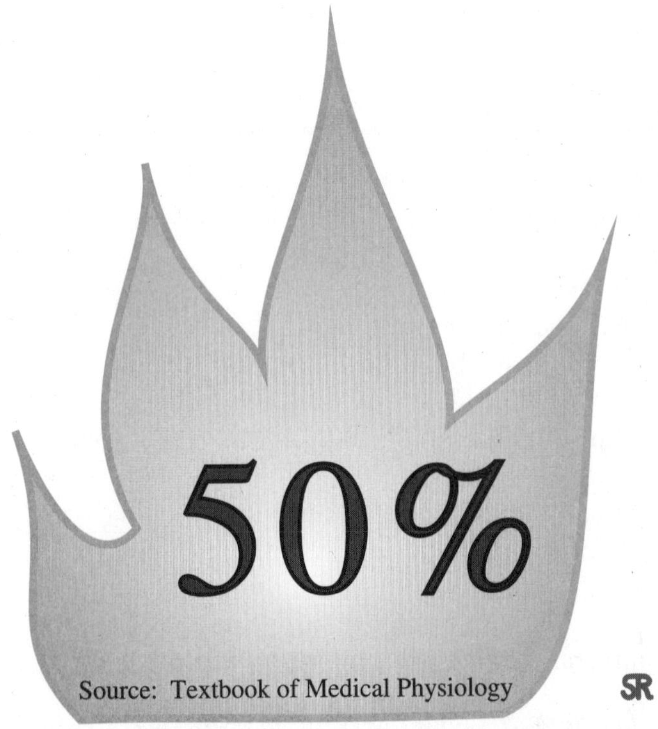

SR

Beyond The Zone

Theory:

Eating fat makes you fat. [FALSE]

More that you haven't been told...

Primitive Man, Meat-Eater *Not* Plant-Eater!

"[Based on scientific bone analysis] ... this research puts an end to the argument about whether the Neanderthals (primitive man) were primarily scavengers." **Their diet was predominantly *protein and fat*, NOT grains, plants, fruits, or vegetables like we have previously been told!**

John Noble Wilford, *New York Times* 2000

Experience:

- Eating the right kind of fats reduces bodyfat.
- Shortage of natural fats significantly reduces effectiveness of fat-soluble vitamins (A, D, E, K).
- Replacing fat with carbohydrate causes obesity.
- Eating enough of the right kind of fat is essential for
  - a. hormone production
  - b. prostaglandin production (heart and cardiovascular protectors)
  - c. peak brain performance
  - d. cellular immunity to disease.

Comments:

Remember a time when you were too busy to eat. You still had plenty of energy. You were effectively running on your own bodyfat. When you are Beyond the Zone and eat equal amounts of protein, natural fat, and carbohydrate, you will burn 3 times as much bodyfat as after a "high carbohydrate" meal. That's because protein and natural fats trigger your body's fat-burning hormone, glucagon, which tells the body to burn fat.

Life Beyond the Zone means peak performance and radiant health. Reducing your waistline comes naturally.

Learn more about essential healthy fats. Read the chapter "Truth About Protein, Carbohydrates, And Fats."

Carbohydrates
STOP you
from using the
best fuel available
–
the fat stored in
your own body.

Source: Textbook of Medical Physiology

Theory:

Carbohydrates are the best fuel for achieving peak energy levels. [FALSE]

Experience:

- Carbohydrates stop you from using the best fuel available – the fat stored in your own body.
- All excess carbohydrates are converted to bodyfat.
- Business professionals typically lose $1^1/_2$ hours of productivity after eating a high-carbohydrate lunch.
- How do you feel shortly after eating a plate of pasta? Energized or sluggish?

Comments:

Your body is designed to handle only a small amount of carbohydrates. Carbohydrates trigger insulin in your system. The Nobel Prize was awarded for the discovery of insulin and its functions — a fat-storage hormone. It quickly eliminates the sugar, because the body doesn't want it, and stores it as fat. That's why, after eating a plate of pasta or Chinese food, even though you may feel stuffed, you'll soon feel hungry again. The vicious eat, crave ..., eat, crave ... cycle never ends.

What impact would you expect from dumping more than 450 teaspoons of sugar per week into a system designed to run regularly on less than 1 teaspoon of sugar? We should expect a national health disaster with a multitude of symptoms ranging from increased cellulite to constant food cravings. Indeed, we find these symptoms everywhere.

Each pound of bodyfat could release 3,500 calories for peak performance potential.

The optimum fuel for peak performance is your own bodyfat.

Learn more about sugar metabolism. Read the chapter "Truth About Protein, Carbohydrates and Fats."

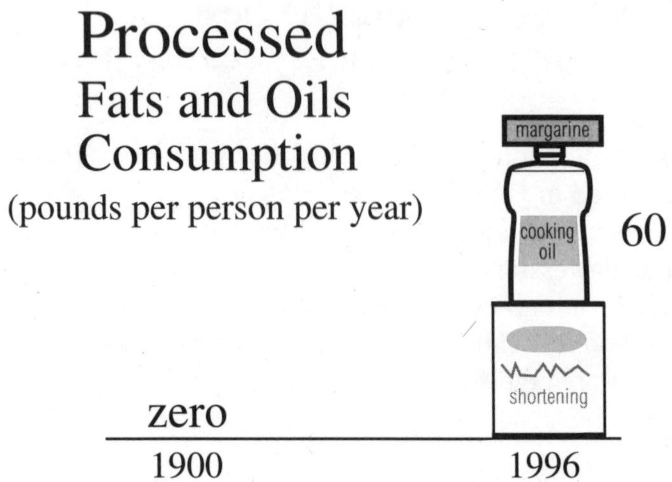

Source: Information Please Almanac, 1997

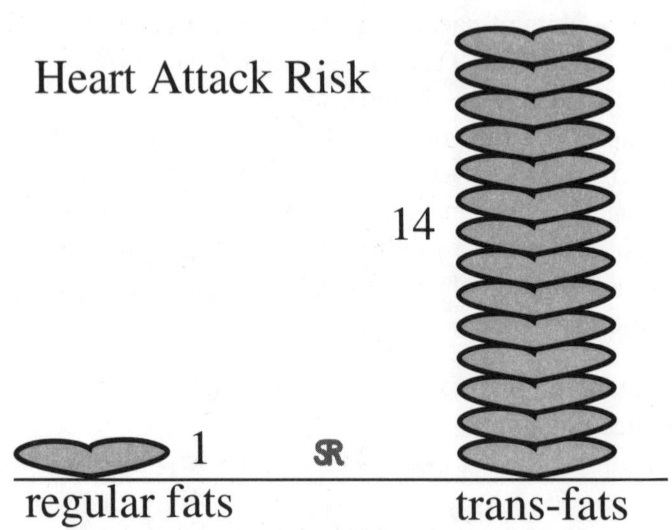

Source: Boston Globe, based on Harvard Study published in New England Journal of Medicine

Theory:
*Trans*fats are harmful. [TRUE]

Experience:

- A 14-year Harvard-directed study of more than 80,000 nurses showed *trans*fats (chemically distorted fats) are a much greater heart-risk factor than even saturated fats.
- According to *Cancer Research,* back in 1975, there was evidence that the *trans*fat link to cancer was greater than the animal fat link to cancer.
- *The Lancet* (a medical publication) stated, back in 1956, that "hydrogenation factories of our modern food industry may have turned out to contribute to the causation of a major disease." [referring to heart disease]
- Eating distorted cottonseed oil (containing *trans*fats) caused an increase in skin cancer from ultraviolet light. This was reported in the *American Journal of Cancer* back in 1939.

Comments:

According to Larry Tye, of the *Boston Globe*, referring, in December 1997, to a new study by Harvard and Boston University reserachers, "While the overall association between strokes and fat was surpirsing to scientists, they were even more intrigued – and upset – by the notion that **eating saturated fat can lower the risk of stroke**."

As can be seen, there is a long history of studies correlating *trans*fats with cancer and cardiovascular disease.

Learn more about transfats. Read the chapter "What You Don't Know Can Hurt You."

American Death Rate From Heart Attacks and Strokes

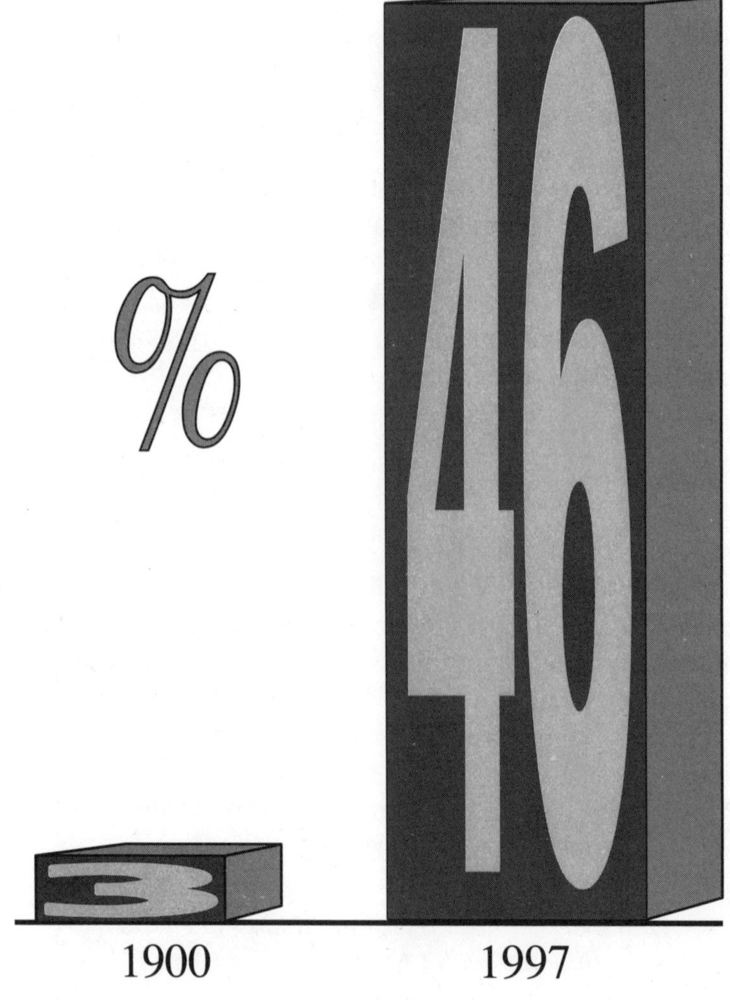

Sources: National Center for Health Statistics & World Health Organization

Theory:
Low-fat diets are "heart-healthy."[FALSE]

Experience:

- Despite the widespread adoption of low-fat diets, heart attacks remain America's number one killer.
- 46% of us died from cardiovascular-related disease in 1997, according to the World Health Organization.
- EFAs (typically missing from low-fat diets) can lower cholesterol, triglyceride levels, and blood-pressure.

Comments:

In 1900 only one in thirty (3%) of us died of heart-related disease. Today, more than two of every five Americans (46%) will die of heart-related problems. What could have caused this HUGE increase in heart-related problems? What's so different today? First, there has been a massive increase in sugar consumption. Second, there has been a dramatic drop in the consumption of EFAs, the healthy essential oils, that are vital to every cell in the body. The greatest jump in death rate from cardiovascular disease and cancer started after 1925 and is still increasing.

In the late 1930s, processed cooking oil began to be widely used by homemakers in America. A few years later, consumption of margarine increased, and processed oils replaced lard. "Cholesterol mania" began in the 1950s. Showing remarkable willpower and willingness to follow logical-sounding (but unproven) theories, Americans switched from eating butter and other natural fats and oils to eating highly refined unsaturated oils, margarine, and hydrogenated shortening.

Today, margarine far outsells butter. The average American now consumes 10 pounds of chemically processed shortening and 20 pounds of chemically processed margarine each year.

Deaths caused by heart disease decrease 44% with omega 3 oils. (New England Journal of Medicine)

Learn more about the healthy heart. Read the chapter "Is Cholesterol A Scapegoat?"

Arteries and Blood Vessels

Source: Prostaglandins in the Cardiovascular System

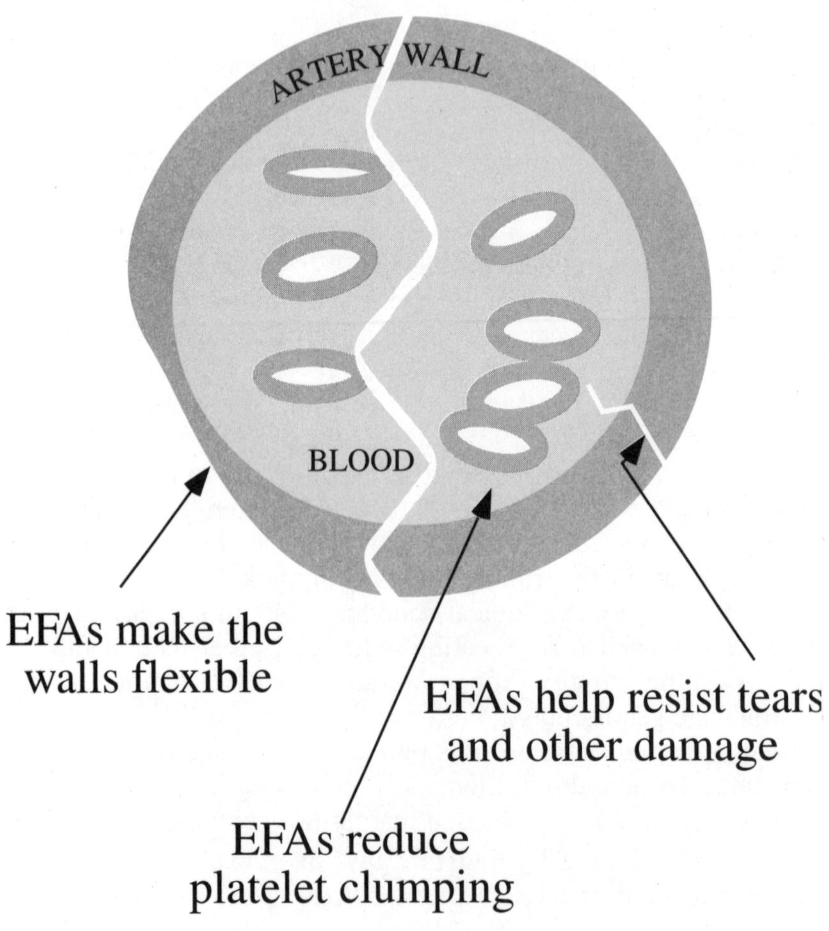

Theory:
EFAs reduce the risk of heart attack.[TRUE]

Experience:

- According to a study published in the *New England Journal of Medicine*, those eating at least 8 ounces of fish a week have a 40% lower risk of fatal heart attack.
- Eskimos in Greenland have a low incidence of coronary heart disease, diabetes, and cancer. They eat fatty meat and fish containing lots of EFAs.
- The Japanese have one of the higher life expectancies in the world. Their diet includes lots of Omega 3.
- In 1982, Professor John Vane was awarded a Nobel Prize for discovering prostaglandins – they prevent heart disease.

Comments:

Every cell in our body is made up largely of EFAs. *EFAs are the building blocks for prostaglandins* — Mother Nature's natural heart-protectors.

EFAs can support your heart's health in 4 ways:

1. Naturally "thin the blood" for ease of passage through the arteries (EFAs help reduce platelet clumping).
2. Help keep the arteries flexible.
3. Help keep the inner protective layer of veins and arteries strong and resistant to tears.
4. Naturally help reduce your desire for carbohydrates.

Carbohydrates are now considered to be a significant risk factor in cardiovascular disease, because they auto-oxidize in the blood.

Learn more about healthy circulation. Read the chapter "What You Don't Know Can Hurt You."

American Cancer Rate

Sources:
National Center for Health Statistics
and American Cancer Society

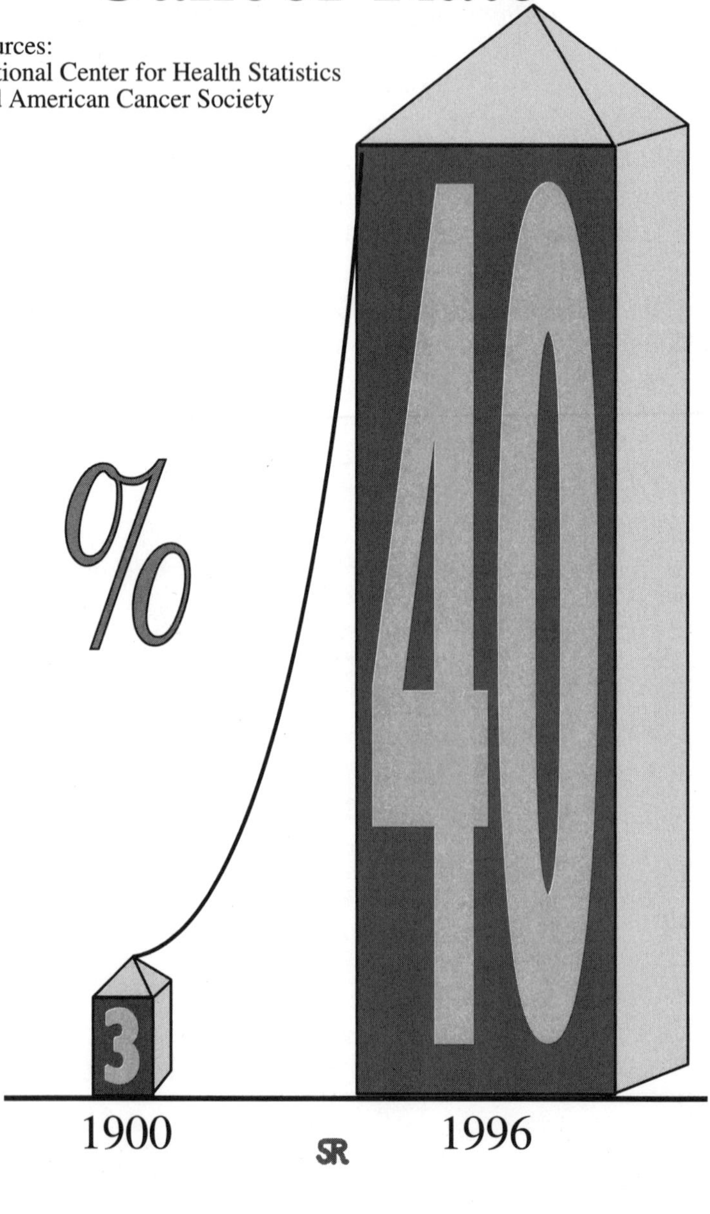

%

3

40

1900

SR

1996

Theory:

Low-fat, high-carbohydrate diets will reduce the incidence of cancer. [FALSE]

Experience:

- Low-fat, high-carbohydrate diets are at an all-time high.
- Cancer has steadily increased since the 1920s and is at an all-time high – 40% of Americans will contract it.
- Our increased consumption of processed carbohydrates has steadily increased since the 1920s and is at an all-time high.
- Healthy oils (EFAs), missing from a low-fat diet, make up your cell membrane — the first line of defense against disease.
- *Carbohydrates are known to "auto-oxidize" in the bloodstream,* leading directly to decreased immunity.
- Fiber from carbohydrates has been shown not to reduce the risk of colon cancer.
- Massive 1999 study of 89,000 nurses shows no link between fat intake and breast cancer.

Comments:

A recent report from Harvard University showed that *trans*fats (chemically processed oils) were closely linked to breast cancer. Natural fats and essential healthy oils are required for virtually all normal body functions. A shortage of these critical nutrients inhibits the immune system.

EFAs help prevent cancer in 4 ways:

1. Help strengthen cell membranes so they can resist infections.

2. Allow maximum oxygen transfer in your cells. Nobel Prize winner Professor Warberg showed that decreasing oxygen in the cells by only one-third caused spontaneous cancer.

3. Help protect us against skin cancer, whereas sunlight hitting EFA-deficient skin may cause cancer. With EFAs in your skin, you are much safer out in the sun.

4. Help the body manufacture natural vitamin D. Natural vitamin D has been shown to help decrease cancer, including breast-cancer.

Learn about cancer prevention. Read the chapter "What You Don't Know Can Hurt You."

Diabetes is TEN Times More Common In Only 41 Years

Source: Centers for Disease Control and Prevention

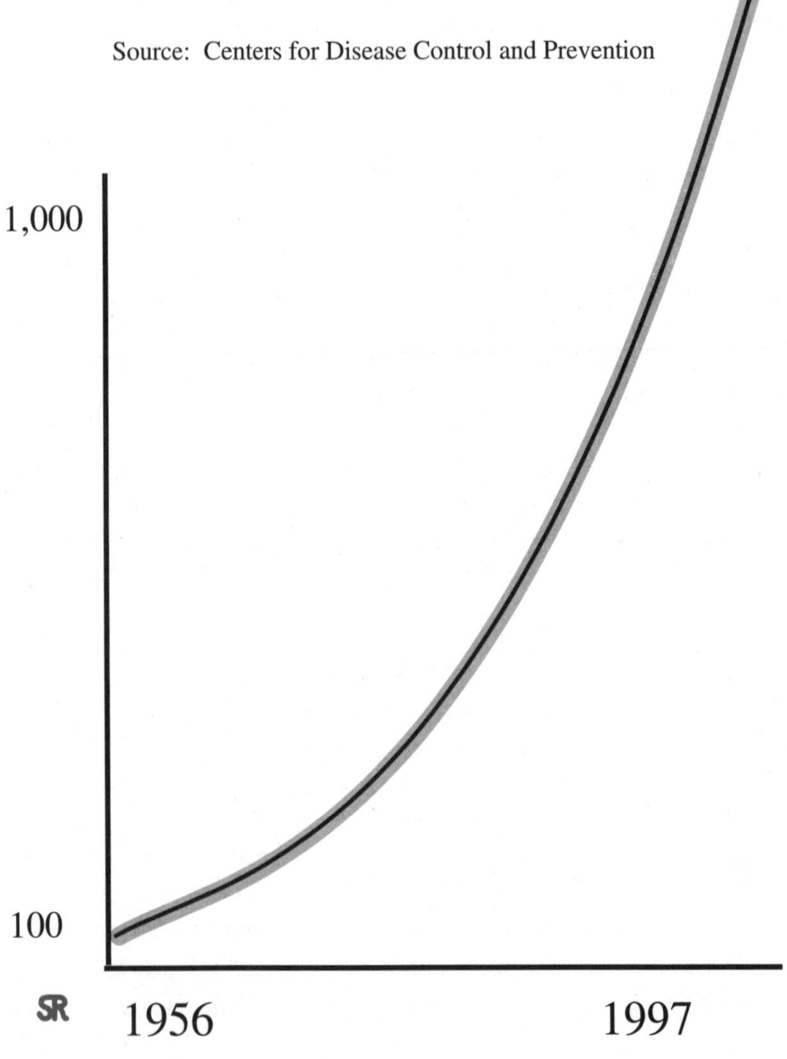

Theory:

Low-fat, high-carbohydrate diets reduce the incidence of diabetes. [FALSE]

Experience:

- There is a worldwide epidemic in diabetes. The Centers for Disease Control and Prevention and the World Health Organization estimate that 125 million people worldwide have developed diabetes, and the number is expected to double by 2025.
- Despite the widespread adoption of low-fat, high-carbohydrate diets, diabetes has increased ten-fold in just 41 years – a truly epidemic rate.
- Even children are developing diabetes, in epidemic proportions.
- "Complex" carbohydrates cause as much insulin release as "simple" carbohydrates – *Textbook of Medical Physiology*.

Comments:

There has been a dramatic increase in the incidence of diabetes. This correlates with the continuing rapid growth of obesity. This also directly correlates with the massive increase in sugar and carbohydrate consumption. The overload of sugar and carbohydrates puts the pancreas into a panic situation demanding excessive insulin for quick relief.

EFAs help prevent diabetes
and its complications in 4 ways:

1. Help the body regulate insulin.
2. Help restore diabetes-induced nerve damage (including impotence).
3. Help prevent obesity, *naturally*, by reducing hunger.
4. Help reduce stress on your pancreas.

There are NO known cases of diabetes being cured!

Learn more about preventing diabetes. Read the chapter "Truth About Protein, Carbohydrates And Fats."

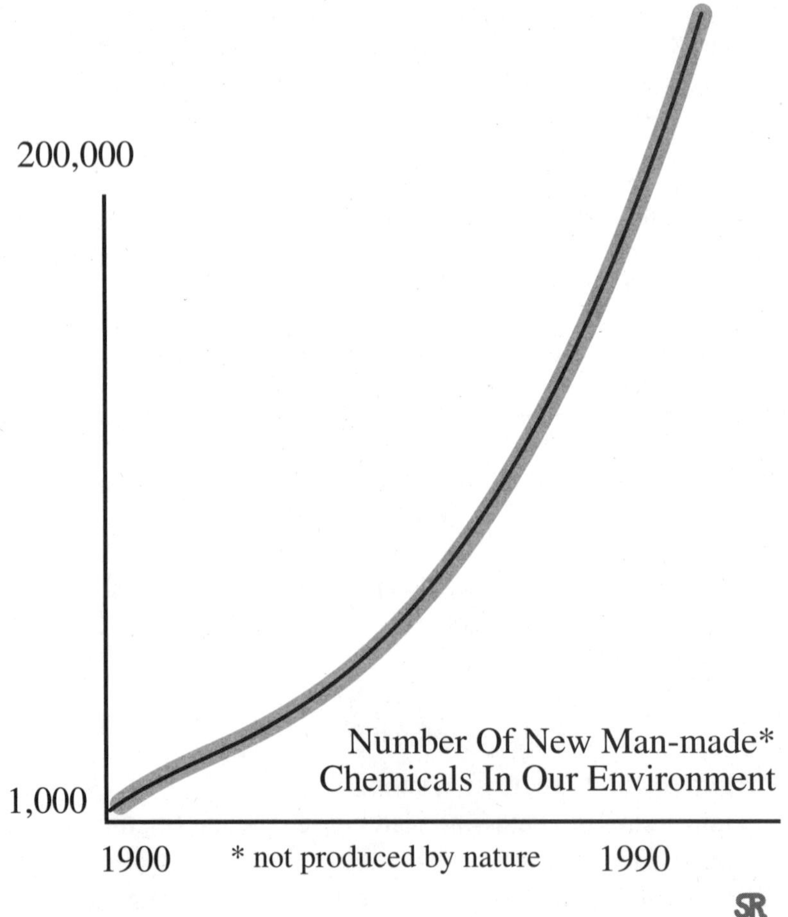

Over 600,000 Tons of Toxic Chemicals Are Pumped Into Our Environment Each Year

Source: Dr. Whitaker's Guide To Natural Healing, Julian Whitaker, MD, Prima Publishing, 1996, p.76

Theory:

Essiac-concept tonic is an exceptional detoxifier and is critically important when burning stored bodyfat. [**TRUE**]

Experience:

- Many toxic chemicals are found in our food, air, and water.
- The body stores toxins in bodyfat, according to Dr. Andrew Weil in *8 Weeks To Optimum Health.*
- When the fat is burned, what happens to the toxins? They are released into the body.
- Dr. Charles Brusch, President John F. Kennedy's personal physician, prescribed this tonic for President Kennedy and his family.

Comments:

Toxins disrupt proper body functions and place severe stress on numerous life-systems, resulting in ill-health and fatigue. As our body makes and stores fat, toxins in our system are stored in this fat. These toxins are released when bodyfat is used for energy production and cellular structure. Harmful effects of these toxins must be minimized for radiant health.

Essiac-concept tonic supports your peak performance and radiant health in 9 ways:

1. Gathers dissolved toxic waste material and helps discharge it harmlessly.
2. Helps cleanse the liver and colon.
3. Eliminates germs and inhibits growth of harmful bacteria.
4. Dramatically raises the oxygen level in tissues.
5. Natural "blood purifier."
6. Cleansing action helps keep arteries smooth and clean.
7. Natural diuretic — keeps you from retaining excess water.
8. Natural anti-inflammatory (reduces swollen tissue).
9. Helps generate new tissue.

The best nutrition in the world is no longer enough to provide peak performance and radiant health. A detoxifier is required.

Learn more about detoxification and radiant health. Read the chapter "Your Ultimate Detoxifier."

Healthy Eating Test

Do You Eat Healthy?

Many people **think** they eat well. Until now, we have misunderstood what really makes a healthful diet.

Take this simple test:

* Do you get food cravings?
* Do you frequently run low on energy?
* Do you need 8 hours [or more] of sleep?
* Do you have cellulite?
* Do you need three meals each day?
* Do you ever feel intensely hungry?
* Do you feel stressed out?

A "YES" answer to ANY of these questions shows *you are not eating healthy.*

Theory:

Authorities agree on what is defined as "eating healthy." [FALSE]

Experience:

- Highly respected medical textbooks provide a firm foundation of established medical research to help us clearly define "eating healthy."

  For example, read:
  Textbook of Medical Physiology
  Medical Biochemistry
  Molecular Biology of the Cell
  Biochemistry and Disease
- Outdated government recommendations disagree with current established medical research.
- Many "experts" have widely different meal "plans," based on *theories* – not facts.
- There is no government recommended EFA daily requirement, even though EFAs are an important part of every cell and the body can't make them.
- Americans have never been sicker, more overweight, or trying harder.

Comments:

Giving the body the nutrients that it is designed for is the first step to achieving peak performance and radiant health. Do you think that you are eating healthy? Then take the "Healthy Eating Test" on the opposite page.

If you failed the test, all is not lost.
It's time for a new perspective, based on
Nobel Prize-winning research.

Lots of vigorous exercise isn't required for good health.

Moderate exercise provides great benefit.

Source: Physical Activity, Fitness & Health – Harvard Alumni Study

Theory:

In order to protect your health and stay lean, you need a *lot of* intense, unpleasant, even painful, exercise. [**FALSE**]

Experience:

- Vigorous exercise offers virtually no additional mortality protection over moderate exercise, according to the extensive Harvard Alumni Study of 16,136 people.
- When you fill your EFA and mineral deficiencies, your endurance increases, so exercise becomes easier.

Comments:

Proper exercise may be a healthy pursuit, but few of us have time for lots of vigorous exercise. The good news is: studies have demonstrated that *moderate* exercise provides you with a good dose of health protection and decreased risk of heart disease.

Remember: all physical activity – even working around the house – is exercise. Simply increasing your activity level can improve your cardiovascular health.

Learn more about the role of exercise. Read the chapter "Exercise: Why Sweat It?"

New Ideas That Work – A Long History Of Delay

Discovery / Reaction	years before adoption
Discovery Pine needle "tea" cures scurvy ***Reaction*** Called witchcraft	50+
Discovery Dr. Semmelweis discovers washing hands prevents infection in 1848 ***Reaction*** He was fired	25
Discovery Dr. Fleming discovers penicillin ***Reaction*** Discovery ridiculed for 12 years (later he won the Nobel Prize for his discovery)	12
Discovery Dr. Budwig documents risks from *trans*-fats ***Reaction*** Margarine industry starts vicious personal attack in 1930s	70+
Discovery EFAs shown in 1982 to help prevent heart disease ***Reaction*** Still secret; low consumer awareness; growing support from medical community	?
Discovery Harvard recognizes trans-fats link to heart disease in 1997 ***Reaction*** Widespread media coverage – official dietary recommendations unchanged	?

Theory:

Once significant health benefits are known to society, they are quickly implemented. [**FALSE**]

Experience:

- Many important health discoveries were ignored or ridiculed.
- Recent exceptions have been high-cost, high-tech, high-profit equipment and pharmaceuticals.
- The U.S. government and nutritional "experts" still take many years to adopt the latest findings.

Comments:

We mistakenly assume good ideas that work are immediately recognized and implemented. Real-life experience is quite the opposite. Usually any new idea that challenges old ideas and theories is rejected. Given this long history of resistance to change, you can make your own estimate of how quickly the heart, diabetes, or cancer establishments will implement current findings.

New ideas that work often take a long time to be implemented.

Now, YOU don't have to wait 25 years.

> **"A new scientific truth does not triumph by convincing its opponents and making them see the light, but, rather, because its opponents die and a new generation grows up that is familiar with it."**
>
> Max Plank — Nobel Prize winner - physics

When you go Beyond The Zone, you get the benefits of peak performance and radiant health right now.

"One only sees what one looks for, one only looks for what one knows."

Goethe

Women...

Finally...the Truth Gets Reported!

Women **eating the lowest fat and most fiber** had almost **20% <u>less</u> calcium absorption (regardless of protein intake)!***

Dr. Wolf, Columbia University, said, "There is a need to assess public health recommendations for a low-fat, high-fiber diet."

***Life-Systems Engineering* analysis:** Now you know why calcium recommendations keep increasing year-after-year. If you still think you need extra calcium, this 20% variance in absorption means you may need two to three times more calcium intake to compensate. Women have been *mis*led about fiber and calcium requirements for 25 years. Ladies, have you seen this finding published in any popular publication?

Note: **There was no significant difference in calcium absorption based on eating more protein.** The idea that "protein leaches calcium from your bones" is scientific nonsense.

**American Journal of Clinical Nutrition* 2000; 71:466-471.

Chapter 2

Life-Systems Engineering Is Born

> *"It does not make any difference how smart you are, who made the guess, or what his name is – if it disagrees with real-life results, it is wrong. That's all there is to it."*
>
> Professor Richard Feynman – Nobel Prize-winner

Prior to commencing work on my thesis at the Massachusetts Institute of Technology (M.I.T.), I found an interesting article published in a respected journal. Because the article's conclusion shocked me, I brought it to Professor William Siebert for his analysis.

He looked at me as though I were an idiot and said, "You think just because something is published, it's true? Most of what is published is entirely wrong!" Those words never left me. Thank you, Dr. Siebert.

With everything I have read or researched since my M.I.T. days, I have utilized Professor Siebert's approach:

- Does the reasoning of the author make fundamental sense?
- Do the authors understand probability and statistics well enough to correctly interpret their own results?
- Who funded the study, and what results would they like to see?
- Are the study's initial criteria fair and unbiased?
- Are there inconsistencies in test results?
- Are all significant factors accounted for?
- Are there portions of the results that I may not be told about which would change my opinion of the conclusion?

The real meaning of the latest nutritional theory is: "This is our current *guess.*"

As you can see, there are many issues. Most nutritional "studies" and clinical "test results" that we hear about on television, or see in newspapers and popular books, leave many of these issues poorly answered or totally ignored. Some of those presenting the research prefer it that way.

A theory is only a formal guess about how something works. At least this guess should be highly accurate in predicting observed results, just as with physics equations.

If I were to tell a colleague that my new theory (equation) works 40% of the time, I would be laughed at. This is hardly the case in the nutritional field – where a 40% success rate might be considered outstanding. Fifty percent of disk surgeries give unsatisfactory results.* Researchers mustn't be prejudiced. Given all the wild nutritional claims that we are subjected to, it's really hard for us, as consumers, to know what to believe. Intelligence, logic, and analytical thinking are needed by consumers at all times.

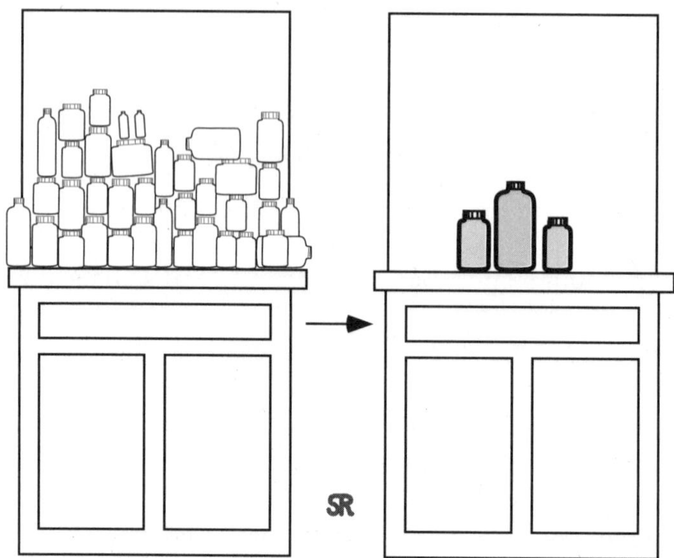

The Life-Systems Engineering transformation

* 200,000 spinal disk operations are performed every year. *Future — the Hoecht Magazine*, March 1998, page 44.

In an effort to "do the right thing," many of us have collected a variety of dietary supplements taking up counter space and promising a spectacular range of health benefits. Yet, we frequently don't look or feel significantly better whether we take them or not. The real solution to our nutrition needs isn't taking more and more "stuff." It lies in discovering just a few items that really work.

For hundreds of years everyone thought the earth was flat. It wasn't then and isn't now. For many years, doctors thought blood-letting with leeches cured disease. It isn't generally done anymore. In 1535, a French explorer, Jacques Cartier, learned from American Indians that pine-needle tea prevents and cures scurvy, a deficiency of vitamin C. French doctors called this "witchcraft" and refused to listen.

In 1750, it was known by the British Navy that citrus fruits prevented and cured scurvy. Yet, it took 50 more years before lime juice was given to sailors to prevent scurvy, thus introducing the word "limey" into the English language.

In 1848, Dr. Semmelweis, a physician at the Vienna Obstetrical Clinic, conclusively proved that sterilizing his hands prior to surgery prevented infection. Over 25 years elapsed before the practice was adopted. In fact, he was fired from the hospital for asking everyone to follow his sterilization procedure! How many patients needlessly died?

Sir Alexander Fleming's discovery of the antibiotic penicillin was ridiculed and ignored for 12 years before becoming commonly used. Later, Dr. Fleming was awarded a Nobel Prize for this discovery.[1]

There is a long history of important medical and nutritional discoveries taking too long to achieve recognition and widespread use.

The discoveries in this book are established facts. You don't need to wait 25-50 years to benefit!

Life expectancy in the U.S. has increased from an average of 47 years in 1900 to 73 years today – mainly because our infant mortality has declined. Improved baby survival is due to better hygiene and improved food distribution.

---

1 Racketeering In Medicine, James P. Carter, M.D., Hampton Roads Publishing Company, Inc., pages 17-21.

According to the Vital Statistics and Health and Medical Care historical tables, today's average adult lives only 11 years longer than adults did in 1900. This is a surprisingly small improvement considering the billions of dollars and millions of manhours spent on new drugs and technology. Modern nutrition, medicine, and technology haven't helped to lengthen adults' life-span significantly no matter how much we may think they have. In fact, the U.S. only ranks number six in worldwide life expectancy.

Since President Nixon's 1971 campaign on cancer some twenty billion dollars ($20,000,000,000) has been spent on cancer research. That's eight hundred million dollars ($800,000,000) each year for the last 25 years. Why are we still without a cure?

We have bright people and great technological machines to work with. In 1900 only one out of thirty people (three percent) died of cancer. Today, one out of five (20 percent) die of cancer, and one out of four (25 percent) will get cancer before they die.

A staggering 50 percent of us will die of heart-related diseases.[2]

Could it be that everyone is looking in the wrong places?

Given 90 years of technological and medical advancement, one would think we should be living well beyond the age of 120. There must be a significant reason why we don't.

Our team thinks that the many advances made in medicine and technology are more than offset by the destruction and removal of necessary nutrients from our food by the food processing industry. EFA (Essential Fatty Acid) removal and adulteration heads the list.

Can invalid conclusions about nutrition continue to be preached year-after-year? Can nearly everyone be wrong? The answer is a resounding Yes!

One of the reasons our health has not improved substantially over the years is that many of the newly published "solutions" don't work as well as advertised. The great physical chemist Linus Pauling raved about the power of vitamin C. Massive doses were supposed to prevent cancer and most other ailments. What did he die of? Cancer.

---

[2] *A 30-Minute Interview With Dr. Wysong*, Wysong Institute, 1994.

The "experts" are often *too quick* to offer the latest "truth" (guess), which later turns out to be incorrect!

Yet, even subjects widely considered to be "well known" offer occasional surprises. In March of 1996 scientists discovered that hemoglobin carries nitric oxide as well as oxygen. Nitric oxide causes blood vessels to expand and contract. This came as a complete surprise.

To quote Dr. Jonathan Stamler in a *New York Times* article dated March 20, 1996, "People thought they knew everything there was to know about hemoglobin. It is perhaps the most studied protein in all of biology, and its intricate workings have been examined for more than 60 years. That it has another function is a stunning revelation." One must now ask, how much does this new information influence previous blood-pressure theories which do not consider it? What other surprising discoveries regarding our life-systems are yet to come?

> "For years cancer specialists repeated their hypothesis as if it were a mantra: virtually all breast cancer has spread by the time it is detected. But now, seemingly overnight, that prevailing view has changed.
>
> ...It helps explain a puzzling fact about mammograms for women in their 40's: although X-ray screening tests can find cancers in these women's breasts, regular mammograms have little or no effect in decreasing their death rate from breast cancer.
>
> According to Dr. Hellman in his 1993 paper on breast cancer: **'This truly is dogma, rather than hypothesis generation and testing....Current practices seem more consistent with religious excesses than with the conditional nature of scientific hypotheses and learning.'**
>
> ...But in fact, mammography has not slashed breast cancer death rates. For women in their 40s there's a tiny benefit, if any. For women over 50, only a tiny proportion of those who have regular mammograms live longer as a result."[3]

[3] "Breast Cancer Is Now Being Viewed as Three Separate Diseases," *New York Times*, April 1, 1997, pages B9-10.

Health magazine published a highly slanted article promoting the high-carbohydrate, low-fat tradition, called "The New Diet Food," in September 1996. It blasted four authors' higher protein-based diets. Critic David Levitsky, a nutritionist at Cornell University, was quoted as saying, "High protein is a gimmick. It will cause a decrease in appetite – and it will sell books. But you can't stay on this diet forever, and *it's in direct opposition to everything we in nutrition have been doing for years.*" (emphasis added) Mr. Levitsky appeared to be trying to maintain status quo whether or not his supposition was right.

The nutritional field has a particularly abundant opportunity for misunderstandings and erroneous conclusions. Animal studies cannot be haphazardly generalized to humans. In many cases, the nutritional needs of animals and humans are quite different. For example, humans can't make vitamin C, while most animals do. Mice produce melatonin during the day. Humans produce it during the night. Wouldn't this lead you to believe melatonin's function may be different for the two species?

Years ago researchers incorrectly **assumed** that only specific oils would cause arterial buildup in rats. From this, they incorrectly classified certain oils as "good" or "bad" for humans. **All vegetable oils** are now known to cause arterial buildup in rats. Rats and mice do not always react the same as people!

One must also be aware that laboratory animals are subjected to unnatural conditions. These could alter the metabolism of the animal. The animal's physiological responses to the stresses encountered during experimentation are rarely considered. Once again, this alerts us to be cautious when relating animal testing to human response.

Furthermore, humans are not placed in a cage under controlled conditions. Researchers must rely heavily on what the subjects say they did. If you agreed not to eat pizza or jelly donuts for a month, would you admit to violating the agreement? Would you tell the researcher? Maybe you would, maybe you wouldn't.

Over and over, significant results have been misapplied or misunderstood by the nutritional researchers themselves. Low-fat, low-cholesterol, high-carbohydrate diets are *claimed* to be healthy; yet they produce strangely inconsistent and unexpected results.

In the meantime, how much damage has been done to unsuspecting followers? How much credibility has been lost?

Often, cause-effect relationships which the author claims to be true are flawed, or an inconsistent finding is simply ignored.

Many in the scientific community, as well as the population in general, blindly accept and parrot the idea that cholesterol from food clogs the arteries. Actually, as you'll discover, dietary cholesterol has virtually no connection with the cholesterol level in the blood.

We have seen powerful results with a nutritional product called Essiac-concept tonic. One of the benefits from its use is that arterial walls apparently become very slick, so that plaque doesn't build up. It appears to act like a non-stick coating. Even where there was previous plaque buildup, that buildup can actually decrease over time. Since this product can produce such results, do the dietary cholesterol numbers really mean what we have been told they mean? – absolutely not.

Many people in nutrition and related fields simply repeat, with no thought to the sensibility or logic of what they have seen or heard from another source. Others make "educated" **guesses** about cause-and-effect and promote them to anyone who will listen. Of course, they don't tell us that they are just guessing. We are often led to believe that those guesses are established facts. More often than not, the proof is faulty or absent altogether. Consumers accepting the claims of these two types of "authorities" can too readily suffer a lot of damage.

Our *Life-Systems* Engineering team understands that routine food processing destroys many active components in our food, especially EFAs. They are essential because they are required for life. Our body can't make them. Our bodies use EFAs to make cell membranes and other structures, including hormones. EFAs, when taken in the right amounts and ratios, optimize cell structure. They are fundamental to proper nutrition – truly a major part of the foundation of good health.

Our Life-Systems team considers nutrient-destroying food processing to be the *prime cause* of many ailments so prevalent today.

Much is already known about EFAs, but they have been one of the food processing industry's best-kept secrets. Our team has identified something **fundamental to basic nutrition** in this EFA-link, and its importance is just now starting to receive attention from mainstream media.

Basic essence deserves recognition as "the nutritional discovery of the century." **Basic essence is my term for a balanced combination of omega 3 and omega 6 EFAs your body needs but isn't getting.** It optimizes your body's systems from the individual cells on up.

Life-Systems Engineering also recognizes that our body's systems work automatically without our conscious intervention. We don't count our breaths each day, nor do we program our heartbeats. While it is possible to override the natural controls for a little while, such attempts at artificial manipulation don't provide satisfactory long-term solutions to problems with the body.

Years ago it was fashionable to attempt to control breathing patterns as described in some popular Yoga books. Many people got sick doing it. These changes in breathing caused a big change in their digestive process. When we do anything to override our automatic systems, we usually cause other unexpected changes, too.

Attempts to artificially alter the body's systems by trying to control a "short-circuited" automatic pilot are very common practice.

For example, our "hunger system" is designed to work automatically. It encourages us – when to eat, how much, and what to eat – without conscious intervention. A shortage of EFAs throws this "automatic pilot" out-of-whack.

Diet plans and eating programs typically fail because they interfere with the body's control system **instead of correcting a basic deficiency**. A long history of diet plan failures clearly demonstrates that the manipulation approach doesn't work. It also explains why there are so many nutritional products on the market, each trying to offer another "high-tech" solution to controlling appetite and "increasing the metabolic rate." None of these methods can work if there is a basic essence deficiency.

When the body does get the basic essence it needs, it works properly without any artificial manipulation.

Life-Systems Engineer Stephen Ruback maintains, "Because most people are deficient in biologically-active EFAs, any nutritional research which hasn't accounted for this fact yields highly questionable conclusions. The purported results of past research could be meaningless, or even dangerous to your health."

Could lack of these EFAs be the true cause for many of our diet-related health problems? If EFA deficiency were the cause of a certain problem, could other factors, like cholesterol or saturated fats, be mistakenly blamed?

Maybe it is the lack of EFAs – not cholesterol or fats in eggs, cheese, and steak – that causes the problems. After seeing our evidence, you too, may agree with such a conclusion.

Personal example: During a 2-month interval, I consumed many more fatty foods than I normally would have eaten (along with the Foundation of Radiant Health). I ate lots of steak, hamburgers, eggs, cheese, and butter. I cut back a little on my carbohydrate intake. Interesting results occurred: My LDL cholesterol – labeled "bad" – increased by 20%, yet my HDL cholesterol – labeled "good" – increased by 30% (the HDL/LDL ratio went positive)! But the best surprise was that my triglycerides (fluid blood fats) **decreased** by 25%. With such a diet, the commonly expected result would have been for both cholesterol components to have increased, along with triglycerides. The results for triglycerides were just the opposite!

Furthermore, **my around-the-middle "love handle" fat roll shrunk by half** during this time. During the past 20 years, neither intensive exercise, lots of nutritional supplements, nor stringent dieting made a dent in decreasing this "love handle" problem for me.

There was one more pleasant surprise: Instead of feeling exhausted from the high-fat meals, I had tremendous energy the whole time.

Clearly, these nutritional supplements are significant. This book will detail our far-reaching findings and conclusions. This book will help you to draw your own conclusions. Because prior nutritional theories didn't take into account EFA deficiency, you will be surprised at the powerful improvements eliminating this deficiency will bring you. Our conclusions are clearly and soundly presented – with the reasons why.

Albert Einstein succeeded because he *abandoned preconceived notions.* This is difficult to do!

My associates have provided deep insight into the meaning of this discovery about EFAs. Our team always tries to address results in a "systems" fashion. We say: "If one thing changes, everything changes." If I change my breathing, I automatically change my digestion, too; yet how many people are even aware of such a cause-effect relationship?

When evaluating anyone's proposed conclusions, including ours, keep the following in mind:

To know means to <u>know</u> <u>all</u>.
Not to know <u>all</u> is not to know.
Incomplete knowledge is dangerous.

Many nutritional researchers say calorie deprivation extends life. Does it make sense that we must always feel hungry or constantly starve ourselves to achieve or maintain appropriate body weight? Similar mistaken logic could say that reducing my breathing will make me live longer. The lungs would presumably work less (if I didn't suffer brain damage in the process)!

We are often misled by **not asking the right question** about the facts, **accepting the wrong answer**, or **not questioning** whether the conclusion even makes sense.

Life-Systems Engineering starts with what today's science overlooks.

Physiologists and biologists specialize in putting names on things. When we put a name on something, we *assume* we know about it and understand it. Nothing could be further from the truth. A name for something only makes it easier to talk about. How many diseases have been named, yet both the cause and cure remain unknown? The nutritional field has plenty of names, yet we still suffer from poor health.

Just because someone describes and classifies something with a name doesn't mean he understands it.

We are pleased to announce:

Finally, the *quantum breakthrough* in nutrition is here. Basic essence makes ancient history of today's torturous starvation-based diet plans. Now you can enjoy the foods you like, have more energy, achieve optimal overall health, and lose excess fat – all at the same time.

Read this book. *Then experience for yourself* why basic essence is being hailed as the **greatest nutritional discovery of the *century!***

Basic essence is a balanced combination of "parent" omega 3 + "parent" omega 6 healthy essential oils.

Life-Systems Engineering:
The new science of producing
desired results by working
cooperatively with the *natural*
processes of living systems.

Your Food: A Life-Systems Analysis

> *"I see what others see, then think of what others have not thought."*
>
> Albert Einstein – Nobel Prize-winner

As stated in the introduction, "To know means to know all. Not to know all means not to know." This standard is required of true experts. Many people simply repeat the latest nutritional theory with no understanding of whether it does or does not make sense from a *Life-Systems* perspective. This approach can even be harmful to our health.

An especially noteworthy definition appears in an out-of-print book, *On Love*, by A.R. Orange.[1]

> **"Ordinary scientist: one who possesses an assortment of information not verified by personal experience, and which is often disproved by another 'scientist'."**

This is common in the nutritional field, where the latest health food fad is often later shown to be of minimal benefit to most people.

In the book *Exploding the Gene Myth*, the section "A Word About Scientists," states, "I want to emphasize...that, contrary to popular belief, scientists are *not detached observers of nature* and the facts they discover are not simply inherent in the natural phenomena they observe. Scientists *construct facts by constantly making decisions about what they consider significant*, what experiments they should pursue and *how they will describe their observations*. These choices are not merely individual or idiosyncratic but *reflect the society in which the scientists live and work*."[2] (emphasis added)

---

1 *On Love*, A.R. Orange, The Janus Press, London, England, 1966, page 57.

2 *Exploding The Gene Myth*, Ruth Hubbard and Elijah Wald, Beacon Press, Boston, 1993, page 7.

I practice a martial art called Aikido. Its principles are based on the laws of physics – specifically centrifugal acceleration. Because I possess knowledge and understanding of these physical laws in a *personal* capacity, I appreciate these laws in a different way than most people or other scientists who lack this kind of intimate connection. Our team's understanding of the benefits from basic essence is more than theoretical. Knowledge without *personal* understanding is often incomplete.

Science is too often preoccupied with "how" rather than "why." To discover the truth or real relation of things is part of what distinguishes men from the animals. The cholesterol issue illustrates this perfectly. Almost nowhere in the literature is the question "why?" discussed – or even raised. What **causes** the initial "break" in the artery lining that triggers the body to send cholesterol to help in healing? Why do these tiny "cuts" keep happening, calling for more and more cholesterol to be deposited? Reams of studies are devoted to "how" plaque builds up, but they ignore "why" it starts in the first place.

Approximately 2,000 gallons of blood flow past any section of artery *each day.*[3] A tremendous amount of material is carried in this huge volume. Each of us would die within a few days (if not within a few hours) if *any* blood-component caused a serious problem in and of itself. Because this blood flow is so essential, any arterial obstruction would have to be specifically initiated by the body for some purpose.

Effective researchers must distinguish between what is more important and what is less important. Everything does not have the same level of influence on a result.

Many nutritional studies have been incomplete because they have not considered the whole system – as we do in *Life-Systems* Engineering. There are specialists in the biological functioning of salt, specialists in metabolism of fats, specialists in protein metabolism and so on. Because these "experts" have little understanding of other biological areas outside of their main area of expertise, their results are often based on ***incomplete knowledge***.

3 *The Physiology Coloring Book* (a medical school text), Wynn Kapit, Robert I. Macey, and Esamail Meisami, HarperCollins Publishers, New York, 1987, page 36.

Imagine a group of scientists disassembling and studying a mechanical watch for the first time. A metallurgist would analyze the different metals required for all the parts with great precision. Another expert would examine the crystal in great detail. Likewise with the case and all the other parts. Yet, no one would necessarily have the slightest idea that the sole purpose of all of these parts working together as a *system* was to tell time.

Years ago, the human appendix had no known function, so it was routinely cut out. Some physicians decided they knew more than Mother Nature and assumed she would design a part with no function – simply because they didn't understand it!

We still don't fully understand the appendix, but lots of experience shows us very clearly: if Mother Nature designed it, there is a purpose for it. The function continues, whether or not we understand it.

Imagine the absurdity of having an experienced company design and build a race car, then allowing a driver, unfamiliar with the car, to take off a critical part because he thought it wasn't needed or didn't like how it looked.

Much has been known about the metabolism of fats, proteins and carbohydrates for many years. *In the late 1800s, laboratory results clearly suggested that eating fat didn't contribute to adding excess bodyfat.* Indeed, **carbohydrates were well known to be a significant cause of adding excess bodyfat.** Even more research confirmed this in the 1940s. It's interesting to trace how this fact became distorted by the food processing industry.

When we look at the body in a Life-Systems fashion, we find that many biological substances follow a certain path. If the path has a beginning, it must have an ending. Before we go any further, it is important for you to clearly see how the words "good" and "bad" are often misused and are usually misleading. You'll see clear examples where the labels "good" and "bad" have been inappropriately applied. There is no better example than cholesterol.

"Good" and "bad" labels are frequently someone's biased opinion.
Be cautious in your conclusions whenever you see these terms used.

The following quotation illustrates the rationale for designating cholesterol transported by HDL (high density lipoproteins) as "good" and cholesterol transported by LDL (low density lipoproteins) as "bad." (emphasis added)

Here's the "reasoning":

> "**Presumably**, the cholesterol in the LDL, coming from the liver to the tissues, is more likely to be deposited at the sites of the arterial wall lesions, and cholesterol in the HDL, traveling to the liver, is less likely to contribute to the lesion." [4]

Note the key word "presumably." It means probably or likely– in other words, a guess! No mention is made of what causes the lesions in the first place. The cholesterol is performing *a natural healing function*. We are "shooting the messenger" instead of reading the message!

The terms "high," "low," and "lite," often mean very little. One may ask, "How high is up?" An inch off the ground, the height of a tall building, or the moon's orbit?

Each of these definitions might be used. Relevance and significance are the keys to understanding. Don't be fooled by labels such as "lite" or "low-fat." **These terms seldom mean what we incorrectly assume**. This is very important.

Typically, a low-fat or "lite" version has only about 20 percent less fat than the regular version. When the product is still more than half fat, the "low" fat designation isn't as significant as it may appear.[5]

Many people try to lose weight by restricting calories and fat. For most of us this is not a realistic option – we don't have the long-term willpower or adequate incentives. A million-dollar movie actress may have the financial motivation to starve herself on an 800-calorie "juice diet," but I don't. Do you? Don't worry about it, though – the starvation method is wrong.

Let's look at what happens when we restrict calories.

First, your food craving goes into overdrive. We burn food for energy in the same fashion as a motor burns gasoline. Excessively cut back on how much gas you give the engine, and it won't run well.

---

4 *The Physiology Coloring Book*, page 129.

5 A regular 80% fat hot dog is "litened" to 20% less fat, leaving 64% total fat remaining (80% of 80%). While the fat is less, it's hardly "lite" in fat.

Likewise with calories – if your body signals for food, you need to eat. How many people do you know who are slim, yet excessively tired and fatigued, or sick too much of the time, because they starve themselves?

Appetite is a real desire, so by fighting with our appetite we invite failure!

Basic essence is the only nutritional supplement that will naturally satisfy the appetite – it is a very special and critically needed food. When it is added to your diet, your appetite shrinks and food cravings disappear because your body *finally* gets what it truly needs.

In fact, there is no other food where so little gives the body so much.

Second, when calories are restricted too much, your body goes into a kind of "hibernation." Your resting metabolic rate decreases. Your body senses you are starving, so it begins to function at a low level of existence, instead of at an optimum level. A new, lower "set point" is reached.

I was told this story time and again by body-building experts. Does it make sense? Yes, from a *Life-Systems* perspective, it does. This explains why so many of us reach weight "plateaus" where we can't seem to lose more excess fat no matter how little we eat. Your body is very good at adapting to conditions you place on it. Fortunately, you no longer need to starve yourself!

Life-Systems Engineering Principle:

One must always be aware that the human machine, whether functioning regularly or irregularly, is always in mechanical equilibrium. Consequently, any change in one direction is bound to bring about a change in another direction. **It is absolutely essential to foresee this new change.**

With the proper blend of EFAs you won't have to worry about calorie restriction, because *your body automatically desires the right amount of food.* In fact, when your body gets the EFAs it

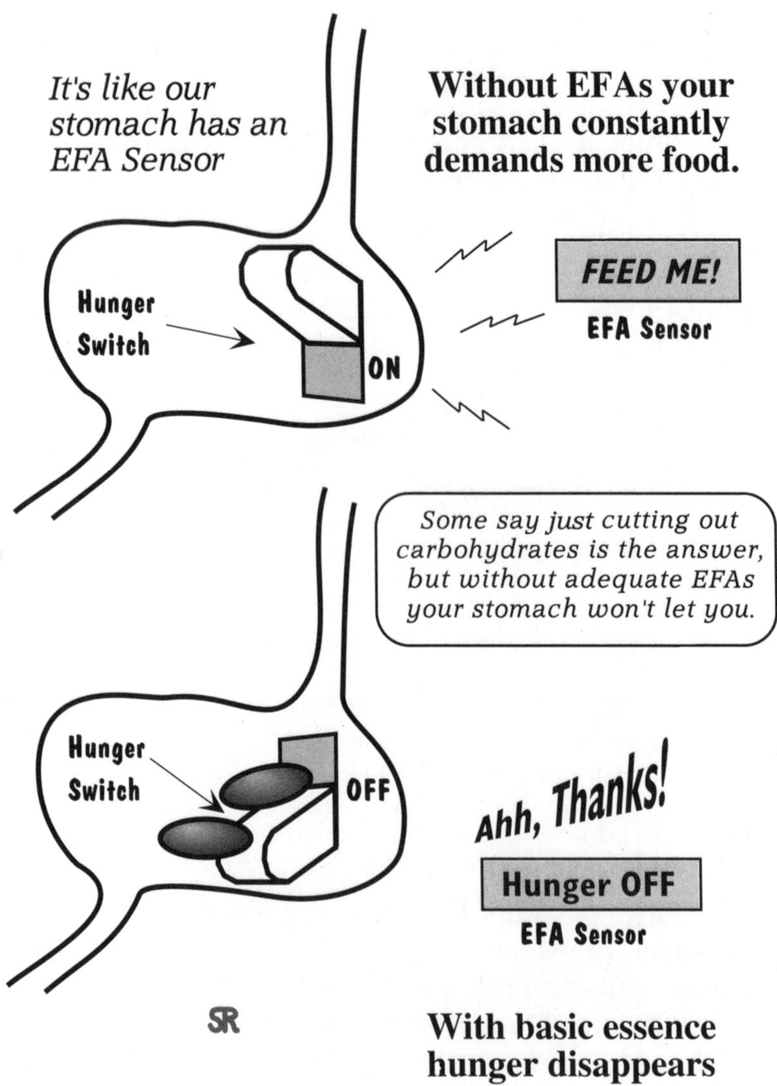

needs, total calorie requirements actually decrease by as much as 30-50 percent. The only reason we are eating so many calories is because food processing removes or destroys essential nutrients. We no longer receive sufficient amounts of these vital ingredients in our food. Therefore, we are always hungry.

Your calorie requirements can decrease by 30-50%!

Most people don't know this, but your stomach acts as though it has an EFA sensor. Because we don't obtain enough life-supporting EFAs in our diet, the "EFA-switch" is always on. No matter how much food we consume, we don't satisfy this critical need. *Eating more of these same EFA-deficient processed foods fails to fill the need.* So the cycle continues: Eat, Crave, Eat, Crave ... **we never seem to get enough food**. This deficiency keeps us constantly hungry. Once your EFA sensor is satisfied, you simply aren't hungry all the time.

A big bag of potato chips or popcorn goes well with the Sunday football game – and that's OK. Once you start taking basic essence, you can still eat the potato chips and popcorn. However, when EFA levels are satisfied, you no longer desire to eat the whole bag. A few handfuls will be satisfying, and then you can easily stop. In fact, you will probably want to stop before you feel stuffed.

Many express amazement at how effectively an all-natural substance can reduce excess hunger and help decrease calorie intake. Because *basic essence isn't a drug – it's a real food* – few understand how powerful it is, until they try it.

If you've never been able to eat just one piece of pie or a few spoonfuls of a hot fudge sundae without wanting to eat the whole thing, you'll be amazed at the power of unprocessed EFAs.

In today's "drugs for everything" culture, we often forget the beginning of drug and pharmaceutical development: all drugs originally came from plants! The plants came first, and the drugs were then synthesized from what chemists decided were the plant's most active ingredients.

Even today, the principle ingredients for many pharmaceuticals come from plants.[6]

6 *NOVA* (PBS), "The Hidden Power of Plants," 1987.

The Solution To Modern Health Problems...

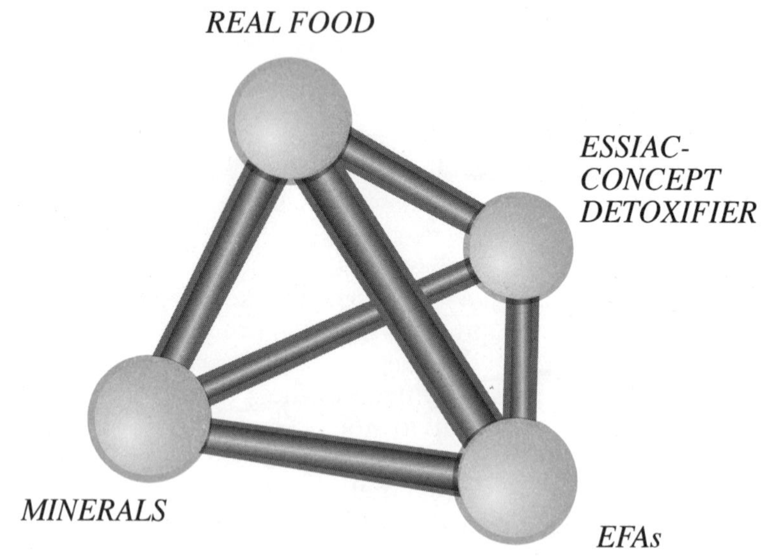

Radiant Health

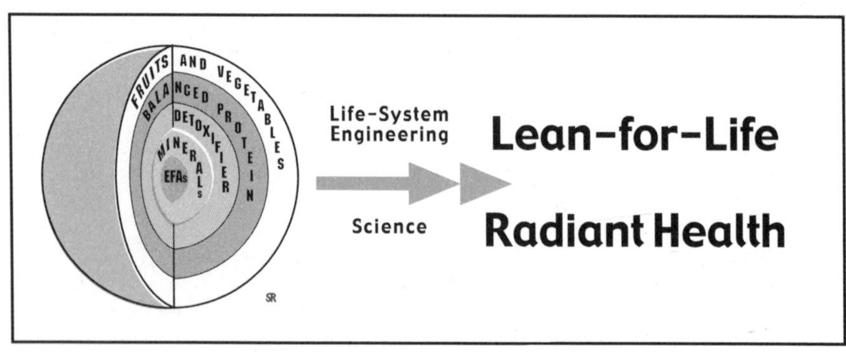

Chapter 4
Permanent Fat Loss - A Simple Solution!

> *"The facts are relative, but the laws are absolute."*
>
> Albert Einstein – Nobel Prize-winner

For more than 20 years, like most Americans, I wrestled with my weight. As a teenager, I was underweight. When I hit my thirties, I became overweight.

My lifestyle as a business traveler – eating fast-food and indulging in fine restaurants – took its toll. I won the "fat middle" award that couldn't be given back. Exposing my condition in a swimming suit was embarrassing. I began to understand the agony most women go through when bathing suit season comes each summer.

I started training with a professional body-builder. Over a 2-year period I lost 25 pounds and gained a good amount of muscle, yet I still held on to the "love handles." This demonstrated that adding muscle and even losing weight doesn't automatically decrease bodyfat. I followed a "politically correct" high-carbohydrate, low-fat diet during this period. Later, after I stopped the intense body-building, I continued a similar diet.

My job was demanding. Food was one of the few pleasures I didn't want to deny myself. I would eat little fat or sweets 5-days-a-week, then I would indulge on the weekends. This system took enormous willpower during the work week. After years of effort, I couldn't understand why my excess waistline still wouldn't come off. It didn't appear "genetic" because my parents' waistlines were slender.

Then, one day, I started awakening to new possibilities. While watching an old movie, I noticed that all the actors appeared to be in good shape. Although I knew Hollywood feeds us selected images, I started to wonder if something was different back then compared with now. Could the answer to the obesity epidemic be hidden in these old movies, I wondered. What was different back then?

Soon after watching some of the old movies, I visited a dog kennel, hoping to find a German Shepherd puppy. I had owned two previous German Shepherds over the years, and they had both developed hip disorders in later life. (This has long been considered a genetic weakness of German Shepherd breeding.)

I wanted to minimize the potential problem. So, I asked the kennel owner what could be done. What he said shocked me. His kennel virtually never found this disorder in their dogs – at any age. I didn't believe him at first. Having heard that the disorder was a genetic problem, I asked how his results could be so good. His reply was very clear: "We feed them proper food – the type of food an animal in the wild would eat. The hip disorder has to be food-related, because it takes 5-10 years to develop."

This explanation sparked an explosion of new ideas, with a whole new train of thought. I started thinking about degenerative conditions that take many years for their effects to be seen.

The breeder then showed me what was in typical commercial dog food. One of the components is ground chicken feathers. "Only a starving dog would ever voluntarily eat these, and no responsible breeder would knowingly feed this to his dogs – regardless of how much advertising hype was used to describe them as good," he said.

From that moment, nutritional topics started taking on a different focus for me.

The solution to my waistline problem had to be powerful enough to fix the cause of the obesity. After months of thinking about this, it occurred to me that food processing could be the answer. If this was true, it also would answer many unanswered questions. It could explain why all the common approaches – like lots of vigorous exercise and low-fat, low-cholesterol diets – don't really work.

For the first time, I started thinking about what was really going on. It was time to throw out all the popular theories and actually look at the problem. As a *Life-Systems* Engineer, I knew that any valid theory has to be based on real facts. The deeper I looked into it, the more I realized we are surrounded with nutritional misinformation:

- **The low-fat, high-carbohydrate plan doesn't work.**

  Too many people I know (including myself) remained overweight on it.

- **The low-cholesterol concept doesn't add up, either:**

  Research clearly shows that blood cholesterol doesn't rise when high-cholesterol food is eaten.

  Several physiology books clearly state that there is no known cholesterol-sensing mechanism in the body.

  The body doesn't seem to adjust or control blood cholesterol levels directly.

One author said there should be a cholesterol sensor in the blood, and the absence of one was a genetic oversight. This is an excellent example of nutritional researchers being so sure of their theories that they'll state them as truth – second-guessing Mother Nature – even when it means ignoring the facts. If there is no cholesterol sensor in the bloodstream, (yet, there are sensors for many important substances that require regulation) then, like it or not, we must recognize that *a cholesterol sensor is not required.*

I started researching the literature and discovered that most recommendations we have been "fed" are based on limited studies with small groups of people. These special results have been generalized and applied to everyone – a matter of convenience overrunning logic.

I began to realize that we must be careful not to make generalizations based on elite groups, such as professional athletes. Although some specialized nutritional programs may work for them, these individuals are by no means representative of the general population.

Elite or specialized groups are not representative of the general population.

While listening to the radio, I once heard a guest say that the degree of flexibility between men and women is the same, because world-class male gymnasts can do the splits as easily as world-class women gymnasts. Yet, it is generally conceded that the average man has much less flexibility than the average woman.

The one nutritional concept that seems to have virtually universal agreement is that many nutritional researchers feel the others are wrong. Credibility in the nutritional field has reached an all-time low, and no wonder, given the low success rates.

Our team's personal experience illustrates the need for a completely different theory.

Our team's conclusions have none of the inconsistencies of the popular theories. You will be able to draw your own conclusions as to both their correctness and effectiveness.

Let's look at some popular misconceptions which have supported researchers' invalid conclusions:

- **My gut's better than your gut**

You may hear the argument that man's gut is closer to the length of a vegetarian's gut than to a carnivore's. (Here we go comparing man with animals again.) The average human's gut is proportionately many times longer than that of a strict carnivore (meat eater). Humans have a weaker acid concentration in the stomach (10 times weaker than a carnivore's). Carnivores need a shorter, more powerful gut to quickly digest raw meat, bone and feathers. Humans can't digest bone and feathers – that may be why we have no desire to eat them. Nor do we normally eat raw meat – so we wouldn't need a shorter or more acidic gut.

However, people like to eat fish. Fish gives us necessary protein plus a few parent omega 3 EFAs and is easier for us to digest than red meat. Did primitive man rely heavily on fish? If he did, this could readily explain the difference in digestive systems between man and carnivores.

Most of us aren't fortunate enough to obtain really fresh fish. Store-bought fish smells unpleasant. *A "fishy" smell is a sign that the EFAs are going bad.* Fresh fish has no smell and tastes buttery – not at all like most store-bought fish. If you don't particularly like fish, it may be because you have never had truly fresh fish.

The fact that certain cultures like raw fish (sashimi and sushi are routinely served in Japan and many other countries) is direct verification that we may have had raw fish as our protein basis thousands of years ago.

Furthermore, we must account for the fact that man likes to eat meat, fish and fowl. Most of us do enjoy it frequently. Even if we stop eating meat for a while, our desire for it remains.

Unlike most animals, man is capable of eating many types of food. Animal protein plays a significant role in the human diet. We have teeth suited for eating meat as well as teeth for eating plants. We are called omnivores – because *we are designed to eat both plants and animals!*

- **Ancient history argument**

We sometimes hear the claim that 5,000 to 10,000 years ago man ate such and such .... This cannot be substantiated, because no complete or reliable records are available. Yet, several very important differences become clear.

1. There were no man-made food preservatives, chemicals, or additives like we have today.
2. Farming was done without the use of synthetic fertilizers or man-made pesticides.
3. Commercial food processing didn't exist.
4. Minerals were still plentiful in the soil.

Those people of long ago apparently received the full nutritional value from the food they ate. When these factors are accounted for, it is obvious that such comparisons aren't "apples to apples."

- **"We're all different"**

Other theories suggest that differences between blood types (A, B, AB, or O) are the reason food is metabolized differently. This goes back to the "We're all different" school of thought. Are we really all that different? I have one heart; so does everyone I know. We can each live with only small variances in most important parameters. Sodium in the blood can range between 135 and 145 milli-equivalents per liter. So the sodium range varies just 4%. This is a rather narrow range. If it could vary by as much as 50%, then perhaps there would be some real differences – at least in physiological terms. If your sodium level was too "different" from the 4% range, you would surely die. Blood plasma calcium levels are rigidly regulated to stay within a 3% range.

Blood glucose (sugar) levels are tightly controlled, too, at approximately 70 milligrams per deciliter – about 1 teaspoon per gallon of blood.* The body tolerates only very small variances.

* *Basic Medical Biochemistry*, page 483.

If you consistently have too high a glucose level above this teaspoon per gallon, you'd be diabetic. Until this century, when we have learned to influence glucose levels with insulin, this disease nearly always led to severe complications and death.

- **Pick a favorite food and build a case for it**

The typical diet of the Mediterranean region is often praised because these people apparently have fewer heart problems, are said to be less overweight, and are supposedly healthier. Use of olive oil is usually claimed to be a key factor contributing to this superior state of health.

Let's look at olive oil a little closer.

* This is one of the few oils that, generally, undergoes very little processing.

* There is much less food processing in the Mediterranean region than in the U.S.

* People who use olive oil tend to use little of other oils.

* Olive oil itself isn't particularly special in its nutritional factors, compared to other unprocessed oils. In fact, it has few EFAs. So, we have to ask whether the observed difference in regional health is because of how good the olive oil is or how bad it isn't. Note this subtle, yet critical, difference.

There is a big difference between how good something is and how bad something isn't.

When we look closely at all the evidence, better health and a lot less obesity in the Mediterranean area may well be attributed to their lack of nutrient-destroying food processing. While there could be still other possibilities, this is one of the strongest. Several other contributing factors include: positive effects from drinking moderate amounts of wine, consumption of more fresh seafood, lower carbohydrate intake, higher garlic consumption and a more relaxed lifestyle, compared with Americans.

- **Recent history sheds some insight**

Various books describing the mid-1800s highlight frequent eating feasts, yet the people weren't overweight. Some people will suggest that our ancestors performed much more physical exercise than the average person today. This may be true, although to less an extent than often claimed. The lower classes toiled, but there were also many people in the wealthy class, and you can be certain these people didn't do much physical work, nor were they generally obese.

- **The great glucose lie**

Many people claim that glucose (classified as both a simple sugar and a carbohydrate) is the body's preferred energy source. **That is only true if their definition of "preferred" is quick conversion to bodyfat!** Lipids (fat) make up 15% (proteins make up 15%).* "**Fatty acids — [not carbohydrates] are the major fuels of the body.**"** *(See page 6.)* A *Life-Systems* study of how the body works leads us to suggest that fats are preferred by the body. Here's why: Per unit weight, fats occupy less volume and produce more energy than carbohydrates or proteins. One gram of fat produces two-and-a-half times as much energy as one gram of carbohydrate. That translates to a more efficient energy source, and nature loves efficiency! The average American has enough fat reserves to last for weeks without eating any food. We have a maximum of only about 24 hours of glucose reserves. But, the body converts fat to glucose as needed, so we don't require more.

Eating large amounts of carbohydrates or sugar causes an excess of glucose in the blood. This stops fat burning and upsets the natural body rhythm. With high blood glucose levels, there is no reason for the body to convert stored fat into more glucose. The excess fat stays on our bodies.

Nature loves efficiency. A major physics concept, called the "Principle of Least Action," suggests the body wants to use the highest caloric fuel it can get.

---

* *Essentials of Biochemistry,* pages 145, 203.

** *Basic Medical Biochemistry*, pages 29, 272, 357.

- **What about countries which use rice as a mainstay?**

It is true that certain countries use rice as a staple food and that the majority of the people in those countries aren't overweight. China, Cambodia, Laos and Vietnam are examples. The rest of the story is that many people living in these countries barely survive and live on the brink of starvation. A starving person living in a sub-standard economy may subsist with a small bowl of rice a day. It's cheap. No one has excess bodyfat when they are starving. In this case, carbohydrates can be considered beneficial.

In the U.S., the majority of us face a different kind of "starvation." Even after stuffing yourself with 3,000 carbohydrate-loaded calories during the day, you'll still get a "starving feeling" in the late evening!

- **Ignoring the digestive process**

Some theories suggest that every bit of fat we eat goes directly to bodyfat. With a little more information, you'll quickly be able to see through this fallacy.

"Fat turns to fat" is a gem of incorrectness with no basis, except that it may sound true. But it is not true! Eating fat does not usually add bodyfat. There is a connection between carbohydrate, fat and protein which must be clearly understood.

A 1996 study appeared in the *American Journal of Clinical Nutrition*. Researchers tested over 300 people and concluded that the association between dietary fat and abdominal fat increase was insignificant! Their results showed dietary fat independently plays a very minor role in an increase of overall bodyfat and does not specifically influence fat accumulation in the intra-abdominal region.[1] In other words, eating fat does not put fat on our gut.

Physiological fact:
All food, including fat, is broken down to basic components in the digestive system. These components are recombined by the body as needed.

1 *The American Journal of Clinical Nutrition*, Department of Human Studies and Nutritional Sciences, University of Alabama at Birmingham, 1996, vol. 64, pages 667-84.

Animals don't count calories of protein, carbohydrate and fat. How often are they overweight? Never, in the wild. Domesticated animals can become overweight, though, if we intervene and feed them processed foods! Even horse feed now comes fortified with EFAs to counteract the negative effects of food processing.

Animal nutritionists appear to understand the digestive process better than their human nutritionist counterparts.

Throughout the wild animal kingdom, the largest variance of weight among adult individuals of the same sex within a species is only about 50%. Wild animals have an advantage: Their food doesn't undergo nutrient-destroying food processing.

Today's men and women weigh 85 - 400 pounds and more. Something isn't right. The variance is too high. The upper-end is way too heavy, and too many of us are quickly heading there.

- **Playing with the numbers**

"Games" are often played with numbers and "clinical studies." Various mathematical results can even be used to denote different types of "averages." Most common are the mean, median and mode. Each has a quite different meaning and interpretation. The different types of averages are useful in different situations. In most nutritional reports the type of average isn't identified. We are easily misled.

The bottom line: no matter how "average" is defined, too many people are far heavier than is desirable or biologically safe. "Safe" is defined as not overtaxing the body systems.

The subject of statistics and clinical studies is so important that an entire chapter is devoted to them. Don't worry, though. We've made the information as fun to read as it is startling.

- **A bit of engineering**

Our skeletal structure is designed to function properly within reasonable limits. It's an engineering fact that the skeletal structure simply can't grow enough to handle excessive increases in weight. Just a minimal weight increase beyond "normal" causes skeletal stress. Excess weight cannot be considered safe under any

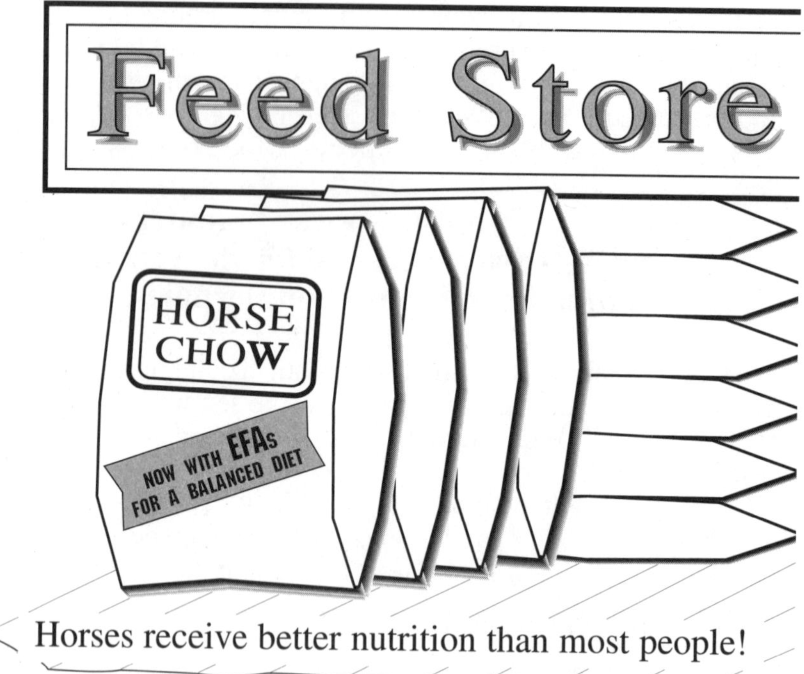

circumstances – no matter how loudly or frequently a special group may claim it is all right to be obese. Animals aren't overweight – and neither should we be.

- **We are diseased but don't know it**

Prior to 1920 there was virtually no cardiovascular disease. Nowadays, this disease is right at the top of the killers. Why? It can't be that people didn't live long enough to be affected, because the age of the average adult has remained almost constant. Could this disease be related to nutrient-destroying food processing?

As reported in Scientific American,[2] according to a 1995 report by the Institute of Medicine, 59-percent of the adult population now meets the current definition of clinical obesity (overweight by 20-percent.[3]) This is astonishing! Researchers at Harvard University

2 *Scientific American*, August 1996, pages 88-94.

3 If you weigh 150 pounds and are 20% overweight, you *should* weigh only 125 pounds.

estimated $45 billion (in 1990) was spent in the obesity-related diseases. Another $33 billion was spen loss products. With more than half of the adult populatio obese, the traditional methods of weight control clearl worked.

Although this article goes on to state, "obesity isn't curab we beg to differ. Remember,

virtually all research is conducted on test subjects who are EFA-*deficient!*

According to Bikram Choudhury, frequently called the best yogi of the 20th century and the world's foremost yoga teacher,

> The United States has 5% of the world's population. *That 5% has more back problems than the rest of the world combined.* Every day doctors write half a million prescriptions for mental disorders, but many of these people are not mentally sick. Their physical body is damaged, so they cannot fully use their brain and mind. The spine is ruined, and the nervous system doesn't work anymore.

With our bodies so out-of-whack it's no wonder our systems don't work as well as they could. Could there be a fundamental lack of nutritional components in our diets – which we have overlooked?

A *deficiency* of basic essence (EFAs) produces a *disease state.*

Obesity is a *symptom* of EFA deficiency – just as the disease scurvy is a *symptom* of severe vitamin C deficiency.

- **Myth: Adding more muscle automatically replaces fat.**

Most exercise trainers tell us the metabolic rate of muscle at rest is higher than the metabolic rate of fat at rest. Muscles obviously use more energy (calories) when active. More muscle won't automatically decrease bodyfat, because, with bigger muscles, you will eat more.

Adding *more muscle increases appetite*. That's why bodybuilders must eat all the time!

• **Forced intervention is not the answer**

Does it make sense that we should have to go hungry or go on forced calorie restriction to maintain a reasonable weight? The body automatically regulates everything else, doesn't it?

Do we wake each morning to calculate how many heartbeats we require, then give the command to our heart? Do we consciously regulate our blood pressure? Certainly not! Do we calculate how many breaths will be required during the day, then give the lungs their command? There is unlimited air for us to breathe, yet we don't die from too many breaths or too much oxygen extracted from the air.

Do you know anyone who has become sick from drinking too much water? Our bodies automatically excrete the excess. Then, what leads us to believe that eating should require calculating?

Our bodies don't need our conscious control: The functions are automatically performed. Likewise, when we function correctly, true hunger is an automatic and proper response to the need for nutritious food.

Doesn't it make logical sense that we automatically know what to eat?

* Food cravings drive us nuts – this verifies that we have a built-in mechanism (hunger) which tries to tell us when and what to eat (taste).

* We are gaining too much weight, feeling constantly hungry and tiring too easily. Clearly, the mechanism isn't working properly.

There has been a major advertising campaign reinforcing the myth that we require three glasses of milk a day to be healthy. Does this make sense? No.

Drinking processed cow's milk makes no sense from a *Life-Systems* Engineering perspective. Yet, we are told to drink it three time a day. We are the only animal that routinely drinks another animal's milk. Milk is naturally designed to provide the correct nourishment to an infant – of the milk bearer's species only. Should we be feeding processed cow's milk to our children? No.

Strangely enough, our taste mechanism isn't working right. We are surrounded by a flood of diet plans and eating programs. These artificial plans rarely work, because they try to control a function that shouldn't be artificially controlled. Eating doesn't need to be controlled if we consume the nutritious fuel we were designed for. How do we know this? By personal experience. Taking EFAs – in the proper form – fixes the system.

Unfortunately, most of us are malfunctioning, so the built-in mechanism can't work correctly – lack of EFAs causes something like a "short circuit." The body has a very efficient automatic mechanism for controlling body weight, like it has for every life-system.

We use gasoline instead of diesel fuel in our (gasoline-designed) automobile engine because gas engines can make use of more of its energy. It's interesting to note that the actual energy content of both gasoline and diesel fuel is similar. If anything, diesel fuel has more inherent energy. Yet, a gasoline engine won't run on diesel fuel. It was designed to run on gasoline. When choosing fuel (food) for our bodies, we must always be sure to consider our specific machine requirements – providing it with the appropriate fuel.

We need optimum functioning to maintain GREAT HEALTH. Just because our body can tolerate certain foods doesn't mean it will thrive on them.

It is only logical to start from the basis that our Creator didn't make a mistake regarding food. People did. It's called food processing.

Why haven't others picked up on this line of reasoning? Surely, someone spending a career in the nutrition field would have thought about this.

One answer may be that most nutritional studies are funded by special interest groups. Perhaps certain groups have no interest in widespread dissemination of this information. Certainly, the results are clear enough. However, **foods that nutritionists advise us to eat frequently yield only marginal weight-control, and often, even harmful results follow from their suggestions.**

I first became involved in the nutrition field as a process engineering consultant. I was introduced to a remarkable herbal formula called Essiac-concept tonic[4] which has the property of minimizing the negative effects of many food additives, chemicals and toxins in our air and water. We added a remarkable herb called "Cat's Claw" to the brewing process. User results have been extraordinary.

Basic essence – a blend of both essential "parent" EFAs (omega 3 and omega 6) – proved just as amazing. Taking a small daily amount significantly decreased my appetite, took away food cravings and eliminated constant hunger.

My wife has been a body-builder and a runner for years, and she also does aerobics twice a week. None of these efforts ever made a dent in her cellulite. She started taking basic essence, and the cellulite on the back of her legs decreased by 50 percent in just 90 days and virtually disappeared within nine months. Whether you are a body-builder, marathon runner, or couch potato, basic essence will work for you!

None of that vigorous exercise eliminated the cellulite – but basic essence did!

I was amazed that just a little of this EFA blend could accomplish so much. This product isn't a drug – it's a real food. I wanted to know why and how it worked. There is little about EFAs in the general literature. The literature only said that our bodies can't make EFAs. All cell membranes and most hormones use EFAs as "building blocks" in the same way that amino acids are building blocks for protein synthesis (muscles).

It was several years before the results of new research were published explaining why the results I saw had to be the way they were.

Assuming a person received the minimum requirements of vitamins and minerals, I suspected most excess bodyfat (and many other health issues, too) could be traced directly to EFA-deficiency.

At last, I had a predictive theory which consistently agreed with observations.

4 Essiac is a registered trademark of the Resperin Corporation.

No calories had to be counted nor compromises made in a person's lifestyle.

AND

A powerful side benefit:
You can eat whatever you wish (although your desires will probably change).

Finally, I could ACCURATELY trace the reasons behind the results. Most studies are performed backwards. The researcher has a specific result he wishes to prove. I work in the opposite direction – simply to find out *why* a certain result occurs.

No special interest groups were involved in this analysis. It is based on observed results and pure reason. "EFA deficiency causes obesity" accurately describes observable results, as any valid scientific theory *must* do.

Virtually all of us are deficient in EFAs. The modern diet *doesn't* include them.

The few EFAs that we do get are altered or heat-destroyed during food processing. **An adulterated EFA is no longer an EFA**. This fact is known, yet rarely publicized.

EFAs are extensively used throughout the body – without them we'd die. Yet, surprisingly few researchers have analyzed how scarce unadulterated EFAs are in today's diet – **after nutrients have been destroyed by food processing**.

Our bodies, being the incredible machines they are, try to hobble along with what's available. As in the race car analogy, our undernourished bodies are like a race car forced to run on diesel oil instead of high grade gasoline. The race car wouldn't run at all; our bodies do – though inefficiently. That's why most of us are so run-down, tired, stressed-out, sick and overweight.

Most human test subjects are deficient in EFAs which are so basic to proper physiological functioning.

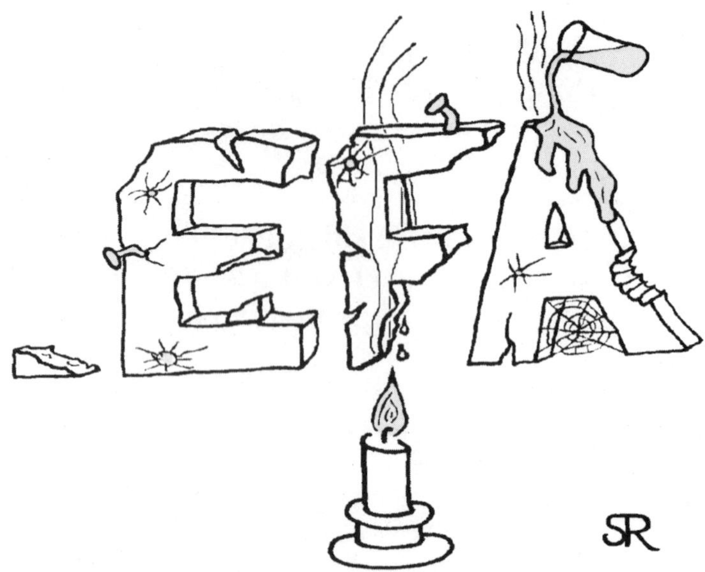

An Adulterated EFA is NOT an EFA.

What is the value of the conclusions from all the tests and studies that don't account for EFA deficiency? <u>Often</u> <u>very</u> <u>little</u>!

Little controlled testing has been done to determine the range of effects from a deficiency of EFAs (few big companies are interested in funding this type of study).

Yet, the role EFAs perform in the body is so basic, powerful and essential, that the effects of any deficiency must be profound and system-wide. The speed and power of their positive improvements in bodily functioning demonstrate they make a substantial difference.

Readers may be shocked at how they have been manipulated by certain industries to consume harmful, EFA-deficient foods while being misled into thinking these foods are healthy.

We must understand the nutritional picture from a life-systems viewpoint.

Here's an example. I once read an article that stated some researchers have "conclusive proof " that eating fat causes an increase in breast cancer. This is an interesting contrast with results from a recent extensive review of dietary studies published in the *New England Journal of Medicine*, involving more than 300,000 women. That study concluded that a low-fat diet (less than 20-percent calories from fat) did not reduce breast cancer risk – contrary to many reports issued over the last five years.[5] A Harvard University directed 14-year study of 89,000 women published in 1999 found "**... no increased risk of breast cancer with increased intake of animal fat, ...**" They conclude "... reductions in total fat intake during midlife are unlikely to prevent breast cancer and should receive less emphasis."*

The air we breathe and water we drink contain all sorts of toxic chemicals, and their amounts increase every year. Animals (including humans) store toxins in their fat cells. When we eat meat, we also take in those concentrated toxins. **Even "fat-free" foods contain toxic substances.** (Especially processed foods – only organically raised and pesticide-free foods are the exceptions.) Today's foods contain many times the amount of harmful chemicals compared to past years!

For example, here are some of the chemicals you can get from eating a typical "commercial" apple. The effect on the body is often as bad as the chemical names are hard to pronounce.

Chemically-grown apples can contain:
...fructose, complex carbohydrates, and are a fair source of Vitamin C. They may also contain: 2,4-Xylenolor 2,4-Dimenthylophenol, 6-Benzyl-aminopurine, Amitrole, AzinphosMethyl, Benomyl, Bentazon, Captan, Carbaryl, Chinomethionat, Clofentezine, Copper Sulphate, Cypermethrin, Deltamethrin, Diazinon, Dichlone, Dicofol, Dimethoate, Diphenylamine, Diquat, Dodine, Endosulfan, Etherfon, Ethion, Ethoxyquin, Fenbutatin Oxide, Fenitrothion, Fenvalerate, Ferbam, Fluazifop-Butyl, Fluazifop-P-Butyl, Folpet, Formetanate Hydrochloride, Gibberellic Acid, Glyphosate (present as isopropylamine salt), Lime Sulphur or Calcium Polysulphide, Linuron, M-Cresol, Malathion, Manoozeb, Metaidehyde, Methidathion, Methomyl, Methoxychlor, Metriram, Metribuzin, Mineral Oil, Naphthaleneacetimide, Napropamide, 0-Phenylphenol, Oxamyl, Oxy-demeton-Methyl, Parrafin Base

5 "Breast Cancer: The Fighting Forties," Michelle Stacey, *Town and Country* magazine, September 1996. (source: *New England Journal of Medicine*)

* *Journal of the American Medical Association*, 1999;281: 914-920.

Our bodies tend to concentrate toxins in the fatty tissues. The female breast contains a very high proportion of fat cells. Therefore, we should expect toxins taken in from air, water and food to build up in a woman's breast tissue. That could easily account for the highly publicized increase in women's breast cancer. Did fat cause the cancer, or did the concentrated toxins in the fat do it?

When we eat various food products containing fats, our bodies have to deal with all of the additives and preservatives from food processing. Keep in mind that these chemicals are man-made. **They have only existed within the last 100 years or less.** Our bodies haven't learned how to adequately deal with them.

There is no mechanism for effective elimination of such high concentrations of these toxins, so the body gets them out of the way temporarily by shoving them into excess bodyfat. Unfortunately, "temporarily" easily becomes a lifetime – especially when we continue to ingest more of these toxins each day. The fact that toxins are quickly stashed into bodyfat has been known for years.

Our body today doesn't even get a chance to recuperate, because we are constantly ingesting, drinking and breathing in more toxins.

Cause-effect relationships are often claimed erroneously by researchers. For example, we often hear that excess blood cholesterol causes problems in arteries. Is the problem really caused by the cholesterol, or is there an underlying cause beyond the cholesterol? Is the cholesterol just a symptom of the true cause? If the arterial wall was smooth and slick, then nothing could attach to it. What if there was a natural product that assists in making the arterial walls smooth and resistant to scarring? If it couldn't stick to the arterial walls, then "excess" cholesterol wouldn't matter. There is a product that appears to do that. It's an Essiac-concept tonic, which is fully described in Chapter 14.

We eat when we are hungry. We also eat when we aren't hungry! With the arrival of the supermarket, convenience stores and endless snack foods, we use any social occasion as an excuse to eat. Even food preparation has become almost effortless. At the same time, most of today's controlled or planned eating control programs (diets) leave people hungry too much of the time.

Does an eating plan of four to six small meals a day make sense? Few of us even have time for eating this frequently. I tried it myself during my "bodybuilding days." After careful study, I concluded it wasn't beneficial to fat loss or increased energy.

Interestingly, just the opposite effects occurred – I became tired after eating.

Also, it's not very efficient from a *Life-Systems* viewpoint. Nor is it consistent with how other mammals eat in the wild. Our domesticated cats and dogs may eat three meals a day because we train them to eat this often. They wouldn't eat this way in the wild.

No common mammal except humans spends such a preponderance of time eating. As we shall discover, the fewer times we eat each day, the better.

Some "eating programs" tell you to eat even when you aren't hungry. Would you go to sleep in the middle of the day even if you weren't tired?

While on my "low-fat (EFA-deficient) plan," I was always hungry. I'll bet you're hungry much of the time, also. Once you attain an adequate intake of unadulterated EFAs, you won't be hungry, because you now enable your body to function properly.

Could these frequent-eating plans be another example of manipulating conditions in an attempt to make an incorrect theory work? The evidence suggests the answer is YES.

• The genetic excuse

Could genetic problems be causing this rise in obesity? No. This explanation doesn't stand up to any examination of the facts.

First, the overweight problem has grown faster during the last twenty years than during the previous twenty. The number of overweight children 6-17 years old has doubled in just two decades.

Second, we don't want excess weight, so there is no conscious effort to gain excessive weight. There are no human breeding programs encouraging this effect, to our knowledge. Nor is it a mutation – *mutations can't reproduce this rapidly*.

Third, in *Exploding the Gene Myth*, the author says,

> Molecular biologists, as well as the press, use verbs like "control," "program," or "determine" when speaking about what genes or DNA do. These are all inappropriate because

> they assign far too active a role to DNA. The fact is that DNA doesn't do anything; it is a remarkably inert molecule. It just sits in our cells and waits for other molecules to interact with it.[6]

This book, written by Ruth Hubbard – Professor of Biology Emerita at Harvard University – explains in detail what you need to know about genes and DNA. A gene does not determine a noticeable trait by itself. It does so only in combination with other genes and the environment. Biologists sometimes use misleading terminology when describing genetics. **A gene cannot act by itself.** Relatively few diseases or disabilities are genetic. Genes and DNA are not what most people think they are!

In a 1996 Reuters Health Information Services article, Dr. Robert V. Considine, of Jefferson Medical College in Philadelphia, noted that obese subjects have high levels of the hormone leptin. Supposedly, this hormone signals the level of bodyfat to the brain. Mouse experiments showed that a genetic mutation at the leptin-receptor gene could cause obesity to develop in mice. They thought they had found the "fat gene." Nevertheless, as we will see time and time again, humans aren't always like other animals. The leptin receptor has since been shown to be the same in both fat and thin people – so it is not the key to human obesity.

There is no known genetic cause of obesity. Therefore, medical intervention shouldn't be required.

None of this, however, will stop research funded by drug companies. There are billions of dollars to be made by having tens of millions of people drugged for a lifetime trying to keep fat off. The numerous harmful side-effects of such medication – although quite significant – will be downplayed.

From a *Life-Systems* Engineering viewpoint we don't want to try and trick Mother Nature.

---

6 *Exploding The Gene Myth*, page 11.

The results would be disastrous.

The answers are in front of us –if we have the sense to see them.

An August 1996 article in the *Seattle Times* described University of Washington scientists causing mutations of the RII enzyme in mice, (involved in fat storage and regulation) hoping to artificially regulate bodyfat levels. They claim the mice stay thin even when consuming foods with a calorie content from fat as high as 50-percent.

The fact that you don't gain weight from eating fat was known in 1920. Don't today's researchers read prior work? The high fat content of the DIET, not the mutation, was the cause of not gaining weight. Did anyone try giving the same 50-percent fat diet to the mice who didn't have their enzymes altered and record the results? It wasn't mentioned.

What has changed the most during the last few years? The biggest change has been the type of foods we eat and where we eat them (restaurants). Many children eat at fast-food restaurants more often than at home. Is there a correlation here with the phenomenal increase in ADD (attention deficit disorder), hypertension and other obvious malfunctions? The mystery disappears when we focus on the increase of nutrient-destroying food processing which has become routine in everything we eat.

The stomach acts as if it has a sensor for EFA levels. When we don't get sufficient quantities of basic essence, we remain hungry – no matter how much we eat. With consumption of just a small amount of basic essence, food cravings and "edginess" disappear.

**For the first time,
taste and hunger work together!**

Even bubbly *cellulite takes a hike*

Finally we do have a chance at winning the "battle of the bulge."

Any "eating plan" which doesn't naturally eliminate cravings and constant hunger, or which requires "control" through willpower or calculation, is wrong.

Such plans cannot work for long – and they don't!

The information presented in this book has a physiological (biological) basis. The basic essence connection does everything described. It has to, because of the nature of our biosystem.

The only variables are: how much basic essence you need (based on body weight) and how long it will take for you to see the effects (based on your current internal condition). No willpower or wishful thinking is required.

Your appetite can decrease significantly. Caloric consumption goes down because your body finally gets the unadulterated EFAs it has been craving. Thus, you no longer seek vast overloads of food while your body hopes that it will finally get some EFAs in the next bite.

> ***Incorrectly,* we are taught to *attempt* to control our body through dieting instead of learning how to *allow* our body to work for us, *effortlessly – with EFAs.***

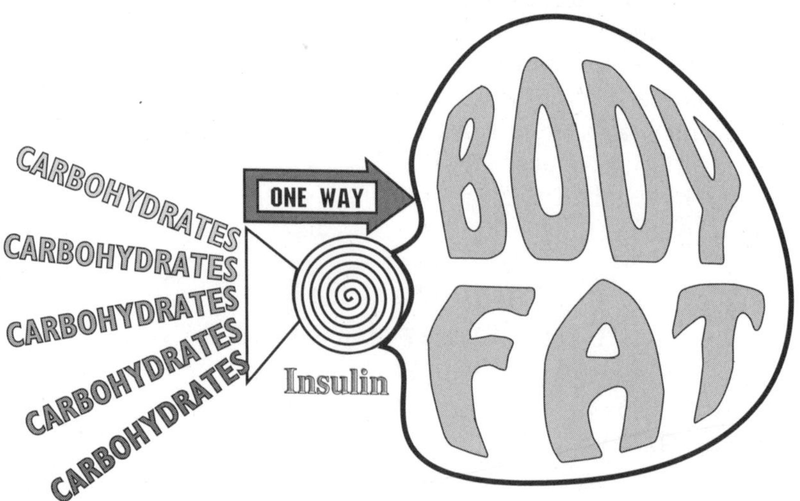

Bodyfat can't be burned when the body is busy converting carbohydrates into more bodyfat.

Truth About Protein, Carbohydrates and Fats

"The universe is a mechanism run by rules."

Sir Isaac Newton

In the delightful foreword of *Martinis and Whipped Cream*,[1] Milton Kemp, M.D., tells us:

> Physicians have known the truth about carbohydrates in weight control for decades. **Eating excessively of carbohydrates is the prime cause of excess poundage**. (emphasis added)
>
> Suppose you ate nothing but apple pie all day long, for breakfast, lunch, and dinner, and another piece thrown in for good measure. Would these be filling meals? Not in the least. You would still be hungry even though you ate approximately 1,600 calories. Apple pie is almost 100 percent carbohydrate. You might also gain weight....
>
> On the other hand, just for comparison, if you had four meals consisting of two strips of bacon and two eggs each, you would be eating less than 1,000 calories and thus, probably would lose weight because this type of meal is 100 percent free of carbohydrate. Furthermore, you'd have that "full feeling" for a longer period of time.

Isn't this interesting, especially since it was written back in 1966? Dr. Kemp is pointing out that the non-carbohydrate meal has 37% less calories, yet is more filling, and you could lose weight too! Dr. Kemp continues:

> I am not suggesting you cut down your carbohydrate intake to zero. The body needs a certain amount of carbohydrate to properly assimilate and metabolize the protein and fats. If you gave it none, it might borrow from its own carbohydrate storeroom for a while, but then troubles would arise. The exact amount of carbohydrate that is needed for any given individual is presently unknown. The author suggests that you take about 250 calories a day.

1 *Martinis and Whipped Cream*, Sidney Petrie, Parker Publishing, West Nyack, NY, 1966 (out of print).

I find two things particularly noteworthy. First, it was well known at least by 1965 that excess carbohydrates are converted to extra bodyfat, although many people still think "fat goes to fat." Second, Dr. Kemp admitted that he didn't know how much carbohydrate the body needs. How often has an "expert" admitted he didn't know something? Today, virtually everyone feels compelled to supply an answer – whether true or not – it doesn't seem to matter.

One reason that the body has to quickly convert carbohydrates (sugar and starch) to fat is because toxic by-products are formed during the cell's use and breakdown of glucose (sugar). If these by-products can't be used by the body fast enough, they are converted directly to fat and cholesterol to protect us from self-poisoning and eventual death.[2]

Your body wasn't designed by Mother Nature to use glucose (sugar) as its "preferred" fuel, even though we have been led to believe this myth. Quick conversion to bodyfat and cholesterol is the body's way of eliminating excess glucose's toxic by-products. If this didn't happen, the affected cells would die of excess internal waste. So, even natural unprocessed carbohydrates can cause problems if we eat too much of them – and *"too much" is much less than we have been led to believe*.

The human body was not designed to accommodate today's processed carbohydrate (sugar) feeding frenzy.

The preface of *Martinis and Whipped Cream* also states: "The carbohydrate calorie is more fattening than any other kind of calorie. This is the scientific fact that is now revolutionizing the eating habits of millions. Only the villain carbohydrates need be watched."

This was written in 1966. What happened? Has Dr. Kemp's warning been heeded? No, instead, nutrient-destroying food processing is even more widespread. More and more of the nutritious EFAs have been removed or deactivated in foods. At the same time, more and more processed carbohydrates have been put on the market. Processed carbohydrates (sugar) are cheap and have a long, stable shelf-life. Carbohydrate consumption has continued

2 *Fats That Heal, Fats That Kill*, page 35.

to grow by leaps and bounds. EFA-deficiency causes constant hunger, which drives us to eat almost anything – nutritious or not!

Way back in the 1950s, Dr. Pennington wrote, "Contrary to the claims of the low-calorie school of thought, low-calorie diets have failed."[3]

Gayelord Hauser's Treasury of Secrets goes on to state, "The metabolism of the foods we eat – the proteins, fats, and carbohydrates – is no longer a mystery. What Banning found out the hard way (in the 1800's), scientists can vouch for today: **It is the large group of carbohydrates, especially the denatured, over-refined ones, that are the real troublemakers; they are the real enemies of the millions of men and women who gain weight easily and who are hard to reduce.**" (emphasis added)[4]

Here was the exact cause and the partial solution – published more than 45 years ago! The missing link was that they didn't know a deficiency of EFAs drives carbohydrate cravings. They did know, full well, about the evils that processed carbohydrates (sugar) do.

With a shortage of metabolically-active EFAs, our body increases our hunger.
It doesn't know what else to do.

This wouldn't be quite as bad if the carbohydrates we stuff ourselves with weren't so stripped and devoid of nutrients and fiber. We end up with a vicious cycle: Eat, Crave; Eat, Crave ... We never seem to get enough food.

There is a lot of truth to the old joke about eating Chinese food and being hungry an hour later: Chinese food is mostly carbohydrates and water. Unfortunately, that is true of most of our typical diets now.

In 1966, although the scientific community had been informed of insulin's function, few scientists could adequately explain why carbohydrates are quickly converted to bodyfat whereas the fat in our food is not converted to bodyfat. Two decades earlier, in 1944, Dr. Blake F. Donaldson had proved under comprehensive scientific conditions that this is the case (although he could not explain why), and the medical community took note. This research was conducted at New York City Hospital.

3 *Gayelord Hauser's Treasury of Secret*s, Gayelord Hauser, Farrar, Straus and Company, 1951, page 384 (out of print).

4 *Gayelord Hauser's Treasury of Secrets*, page 383.

By using radioisotope tagging, Dr. Donaldson could accurately follow a substance's path as it traveled through the body. Dr. Donaldson found that carbohydrates quickly produce bodyfat.

Today, we also know that rapid fat buildup is tied to insulin production – which, in turn, is triggered by eating carbohydrates (sugar). Newly diagnosed diabetics typically gain weight when they start taking insulin. The more carbohydrates consumed, the more insulin is required, and this translates directly to excess bodyfat. Ask any newly diagnosed diabetic how much weight they gained during their first ninety days after they started taking insulin.

On page 314 of *Dr. Bernstein's Diabetes Solution,* published by Little, Brown and Company, Richard Bernstein, M.D., states,

> The evidence is now overwhelming that **elevated blood sugar is the major cause** of the high serum lipid [blood fat] level among diabetics and, more significantly, **the major factor in the high rates of various heart and vascular diseases** associated with diabetes. Many diabetics were put on low-fat diets for so many years, and these problems didn't stop. It is only logical to look elsewhere, to elevated blood sugar and hyperinsulinemia, for the cause of what kills and disables so many of us. My personal experience is very simple. **When we reduce dietary carbohydrate, blood sugars improve dramatically**. I abandoned the high-carbohydrate, low-fat diet that I had been following since 1947. [emphasis added]

Congratulations to Dr. Bernstein! He finally looked "elsewhere" for the cause of the problem, instead of continuing to beat the same dead horse.

From a *Life-Systems* Engineering analysis, the next logical step is to see if the same result happens with non-diabetics. Does a widely recommended low-fat diet lead to decreased cardiovascular problems? The answer is NO, it does not.

Research done in the 1980s, by Dr. Sheldon Reiser of the United States Department of Agriculture, conclusively showed that sugar (carbohydrates) was a major culprit in raising both cholesterol levels and triglyceride levels in the blood. Later studies showed that insulin released because of the sugar produces a number of negative effects.

It is well-known among diabetics and their doctors that diabetics have increased internal scarring at their insulin injection sites. It's not because of the needle, **it's because of the insulin itself**. Rarely is this mentioned in the general literature. Eating any carbohydrate causes the release of insulin, so this is another strong indication that excessive carbohydrates, especially processed carbohydrates, could be a prime factor in causing cardiovascular problems.

The average American consumed one hundred-sixty (160) pounds of sugar in 1996! Compare this with four (4) pounds consumed in 1750. We eat even more today. Where do the excess carbohydrates go? – to a fat stomach, fat thighs, and fat hips!

It's amazing that the low-fat, high-carbohydrate diet would be recommended once this became known. How could the nutritional community ignore this research?

As a former bodybuilder, I was always told to eat carbohydrates, including spaghetti, bagels, whole wheat bread, and juice. Each of these foods undergoes lots of processing.

I was surprised that over an intense 3-year period, I never lost the annoying love handles around my waist. It didn't matter how well I adhered to my personal trainer's low-fat, high-carbohydrate diet. I trained like an animal, and I got plenty of rest. I recall a few of the bodybuilders on the low-fat, high-carbohydrate diet looked impressive, but most others didn't have razor-sharp abs or an ideal waistline, either.

> **"[In type II diabetics], the carbohydrate diet led to impaired glycemic and insulin responses as well as to hypertriglyceridema."***
>
> ***Life-Systems* Engineering analysis: These are the conditions that anyone, especially diabetics, will want to avoid - not aggravate!**

You can perform a simple test yourself: Eat a big bowl of spaghetti with just some tomato sauce – no meat – or eat four slices of bread, or two plain bagels. If you can do this, you'll feel like you have an anchor in your stomach, and you'll be hungry just a few hours later.

* *American Journal of Clinical Nutrition*, "Fats and Oil Consumption in Health and Disease", October 1997; 66: 4 (S)

Now try this: At another meal time, eat a big piece of cheese, several eggs fried in real butter, or a broiled rib-eye steak (minus the baked potato, which is carbohydrate). You won't have the anchor-in-the-stomach feeling you get from eating the carbohydrates. Neither will you be hungry again in just a few hours. Nor will you feel like taking a nap. Most people are absolutely shocked by the difference.

Rarely does anyone perform a test eating protein and (natural) fats and oils without carbohydrates. When we honestly perform this personal test, we quickly find that carbohydrates – not the natural fats or proteins – are the villains!

Most of us think crackers are good for us because they have little fat. They are almost pure carbohydrate (sugar). Most of us have assumed that the fat in food gives us a heavy feeling in the stomach or a tired feeling overall, but the facts don't support this view. If you don't believe this, then perform the meal comparison above, for yourself.

Are we "hooked on carbohydrates"?... Television, magazines and billboards bombard us with commercials for soft drinks, breads, cereals, crackers, chips, cookies and other processed carbohydrate (sugar) products. Why? Well, for one thing, these are high-profit items. By contrast, there are comparatively few meat or roast turkey commercials; these have lower profit margins. In a typical supermarket, just try to find bread that is made without sugar and that also includes the more nutritious whole wheat berry (the whole grain). You often won't. We are physiologically conditioned – through EFA removal by the processed food industry – to become addicted to processed carbohydrates. Then, for added impact, we are psychologically influenced – brainwashed by massive advertising campaigns – to accept our new fate.

Basic essence – the missing ingredient ... I call the combination of life-sustaining essential healthy oils,[5] or EFAs, "basic essence" to emphasize their importance and necessity. EFAs occur in two forms: **omega 3** and **omega 6**. Technically, they are called "parent" alpha-linolenic acid and "parent" linoleic acid. **We need both because our bodies can't make either of them, so *they must come from our food.*** Once they are eaten, our body makes use of them through many complex biochemical reactions. These are the

5 Essential healthy oils are known as "essential fatty acids," or EFAs. They are essential because our body can't make them. They must come from the food we eat.

"parent" (source) molecules which *the body uses to make many other important molecules, such as hormones, and the controllers in the cells – prostaglandins.*

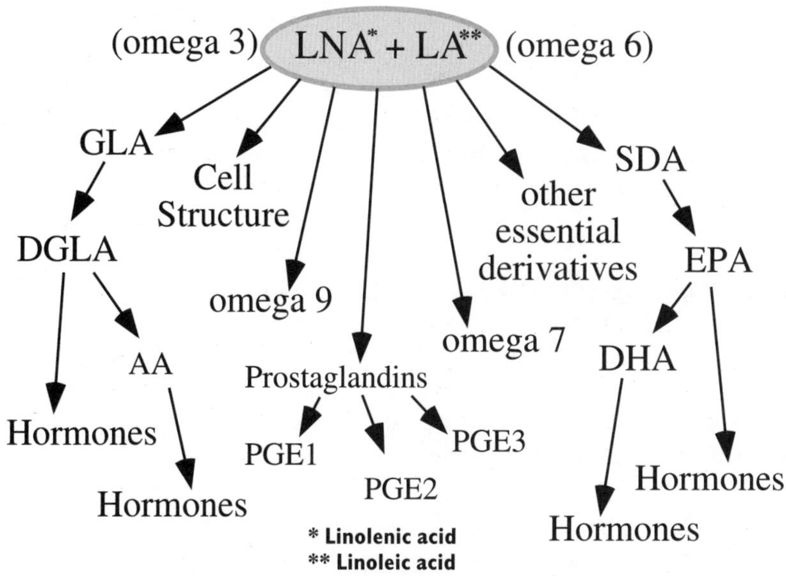

Basic essence contains the critical parent components for many body functions and structures.

Why do we associate eating healthy fats and oils with becoming fat? Here's one reason: carbohydrates are usually combined with the fats we eat, so we rarely eat fat without carbohydrates. When we eat these meals, the effects of fats and carbohydrates are intermixed. French fries are fried in oil (fat), but potato is mainly carbohydrate. If a large order of greasy french fries gives you gas and bloats you, blame the potato, not the grease, because carbohydrates (unlike fats and oils) routinely cause trouble.

Your favorite hamburger or hot dog or barbeque sandwich is usually served on a roll or bun loaded with (processed) carbohydrates. A tuna sandwich is served on bread. Steak or roast beef is served with potatoes. Turkey is served with dressing and mashed potatoes. And so on it goes ....

We combine carbohydrates with fats and oils and then blame the fat or oil for feeling bloated, tired, and gaining weight.
The carbohydrates are the real culprit.

In doing the meal comparison, unless you eat a piece of cheese without bread, you won't be doing a fair test. And this is what has happened time and time again. Have a breakfast of bacon, cheese, eggs fried in butter (no bread), and you will feel satisfied, not bloated or tired. I ate this breakfast myself and ran a full mile just twenty minutes later. My wife thought I was crazy and was very concerned that I'd be sick to my stomach running this soon after a meal, especially with such a high-fat breakfast.

I didn't get sick to my stomach. Instead of becoming quickly exhausted because I don't run frequently, I outran her! Now that she's taking the basic essence, too, she can keep up with me.

Performing your own eating experiments will show you how radically different you will feel – depending on whether you eat carbohydrate, protein, or fat. For most of us, consuming carbohydrate has a much different effect than eating protein or fat.

Basic essence has the effect of automatically reducing your desire for carbohydrates (sugar), especially the unhealthiest ones: processed carbohydrates.

Since the early 1980s the American public has become bloated with excess bodyfat and consumed by the desire to lose it. You already know that most nutritionists and the government recommend a low-fat and high-carbohydrate diet as the method of choice.

Dr. Louis Aronne of Cornell University Medical School knows that you can't cut out carbohydrates. He is a well-known obesity specialist and has monitored high protein diets. In his *Bottom Line/Health* article he states, "Sooner or later people find themselves unable to resist bread, pasta, bagels and other carbohydrate foods. Once they resume eating a 'normal' diet, the weight comes back."[6]

6 "High Protein Diets, Why They are Dangerous," Louis Aronne, M.D., Associate Professor of Medicine, Cornell University Medical School, *Bottom Line/Health*, January 1998, page 7.

If you recall, to determine a cause-effect relationship, you must change only one thing at a time. I ate few processed carbohydrates and took basic essence concurrently, so which was significant? Not eating carbohydrates or taking basic essence? The results show that, **if you have a basic essence deficiency, you can't cut back enough on the carbohydrates**. Your appestat won't let you! So the answer is that both are significant. Without basic essence, you will desire an endless supply of processed carbohydrates, just like Dr. Aronne stated.

A nutrition scientist must be primarily concerned with one thing: Is the outcome consistently predicted by the theory? That is, *are the results consistent with the evidence?* The *results* speak for themselves. Americans are eating less natural fats and oils and more processed carbohydrates. This should be great – just what the doctors ordered: low fat and higher carbohydrate! But what has happened since this trend began? **Our nation has become even fatter.** What went wrong? For one thing, more of those carbohydrates are highly processed.

Prepared foods offer us convenience and more leisure time. Nutritionally-lacking processed carbohydrates (sugar) fill the supermarket shelves. We are starving ourselves into obesity! We all know that eating sweets and drinking beer make us fat. Both are carbohydrates.

Cattle ranchers know how to fatten cattle:
Feed them lots of grain (carbohydrates).
Cattle ranchers don't feed fat to cattle to fatten them for market. It would make sense to see if this pattern holds for people, too.

The top two commercial markets for corn are:

1. high-fructose corn syrup for sweetening drinks and processed foods
2. animal feed to fatten up hogs, cattle, chickens and other animals for market.

Most of the sugar in soft drinks comes from corn.

According to the *Mayo Clinic Health Letter,*[7] dieticians recommend we obtain our calories from: " Six to eleven servings of bread, cereal, rice or pasta, two (2) to 3 servings of fruit, two (2) to 3 servings of milk, yogurt or cheese, two to four servings of meat, poultry, fish, dry beans [a carbohydrate], eggs or nuts, and three to five servings of vegetables a day." The newsletter goes on to say that the recommended number of servings sounds like a lot of food, but the serving sizes are smaller than one would assume. This adds up to 11-20 servings of carbohydrates, four to six servings of proteins, and few EFAs. Even the U.S. government today suggests that a "typical 2,000 calorie/day diet contain as much as 1,200 calories from carbohydrates (equivalent to as much as 60 teaspoons of sugar). As you will see, that's too much!

Eating this much carbohydrate will keep you fat, exhausted, and headed toward diabetes. Once the Foundation of Radiant Health is implemented in your diet, your body won't desire these vast amounts of carbohydrate – the cravings disappear.

Some people may say that they know thin men and women who eat lots of processed carbohydrates all the time, do little exercise, yet stay thin. Let's make this really clear.

This *"eating like a horse" and not gaining weight is often the main symptom of the onset of diabetes*, because the person is not metabolizing much of the food.

The glucose (sugar) stays in the blood too long. I've seen this happen in the past, but never knew why. Now, I know exactly why it happens. **If you are in this category, speak with your physician about getting a glycohemoglobin test** to check for this condition, soon. You may be a walking diabetic time bomb! You may even stay thin, *possibly for years, until diabetes hits.* That's a problem you don't want to have!

The portion of the adult population that is considered overweight in the 1990s ranges from 33 percent to more than 59 percent, depending on which study you read. That's right. Between 3 and 6 out of every ten adults are overweight. Between 1960 and 1980 it was estimated that only 25 percent (1 out of 4) of the adult

7 "Food Servings," *Mayo Clinic Health Letter*, April 1997, page 7.

population was overweight. So **we have jumped as much as 34 percentage points in obesity in less than twenty years**.

These overweight statistics are even more shocking when another bit of information is added. In 1982, fewer excess pounds were required for a person to be considered obese. Back then, if you should have weighed 100 pounds, twenty extra pounds was considered obese. Now, if you are supposed to weigh 100 pounds, an extra thirty pounds is allowed before being labeled obese. Our standards are more lenient today. The women's fashion industry takes this into consideration. *They adjust the sizes every few years, so that a "size 8," for example, keeps getting bigger.*

And what about children? Judging by the number of obese children today, their problem is at least equal to, if not worse than, that of adults. For the period between 1960 and 1980, the National Institutes of Health reported that the average weight of younger Americans increased by 10 pounds while the consumption of saturated fat and cholesterol remained about the same.

We may ask the question: How does a more sedentary lifestyle – including more television, more computer-related activity and less physical activity – relate to this increase in weight? Could that explain our population's weight increase?

Think of children as health "markers" for the population the same way that canaries are markers for miners: they are often the first ones to succumb when something goes wrong. Inactivity, alone, does not make children overweight. The natural process of growing requires tremendous amounts of energy. A growing child doesn't have to perform vigorous exercise to avoid becoming overweight. Yet, our children are increasingly overweight. There has to be an additional cause – something Nature didn't anticipate.

A *Life-Systems* Engineering analysis concludes that EFA deficiency is the culprit, and EFA supplements are the only natural way to stop the carbohydrate feeding frenzy.

With such poor results from eating programs, it's no wonder that people are disillusioned and many of the experts are losing their credibility.

The National Research Council's Committee on Diet and Health recommends that we eat a diet of 30 percent fat, 55 percent carbohydrate, and 15 percent protein measured by calories, (not weight).[8]

Consumer Reports magazine polled a panel of sixty nutrition experts. "The answer" to what we should eat was that fat should constitute as little as 20 percent of overall calories and that we should get more than half of our calories from carbohydrates. This group advocated eating significantly less fat by calories than the National Research Council recommended!

When questioned about protein requirements, the National Research Council's panel said not to worry about protein. They reported that most Americans get enough protein. The polled panel had a different answer. They said to maintain moderate protein levels.

We are not told what they meant by "moderate." Does it appear that there is some confusion and uncertainty here? It looks that way.

Have you ever noticed women who are mostly skin and bone but who still have hips or thighs that are disproportionally large compared with their skinny arms? This happens all too frequently with most common eating plans largely because these plans are out of balance with what the body was designed to run on.

Even if you were born with a pear-shaped body type, an EFA-deficiency will likely exaggerate this kind of physical imbalance.

Important Difference:
Fat loss isn't the same as weight loss.

There are all sorts of calculations available and tables to provide numbers suggesting the ideal amount of bodyfat for your height and weight. Don't waste your time. *Simply looking, front and back, in the mirror will give you all the information you need.* If your belly is flat, if you have little excess around the middle, if your rear end isn't huge, and women, if the backs of your legs don't have cellulite, what more evidence do you need to tell you that you look fine?

---

8 *Enter The Zone*, Barry Sears, Ph.D., HarperCollins Publishers, Inc., New York, 1995, pages 10-11.

Just look once a week, first thing in the morning before you eat. This is all the feedback you need. (Note that when you sit, there will naturally be a small fold in the stomach. You are bending your body, so this is like bending the binding on a book. There has to be some excess there to allow your body to straighten out.) What counts is when you are standing (with your stomach pulled slightly in – not pushed out.)

Let's individually explore the three classes of foods:

- carbohydrate
- fats and oils
- protein

Carbohydrate

Aside from fresh whole fruits and vegetables, virtually all carbohydrate sources are heavily processed before reaching the consumer. Processing changes the raw foods to make them easier to market and transport and more suitable for long shelf-life. Unfortunately, this means that the majority of the original nutrients are destroyed, biologically altered, or removed in the finished product. This is the main reason why it is pointless to make comparisons with what man may have eaten a long time ago. There was no nutrient-destroying food processing back then.

An unprocessed whole grain, such as the whole wheat berry, contains natural healthy oils. Once the grain is processed, the oil and other nutrients are removed, destroyed, or altered. Wheat germ (which contains the EFAs) needs to be refrigerated. Otherwise, it becomes rancid (the oils go bad). The white bleached flour used in most baked goods doesn't require refrigeration because the wheat germ, and its EFAs, have been removed.

Even if the EFAs were still in the flour, heat can destroy them.

Food processing is driven by the need for non-refrigerated products with long shelf-life and high profit margins. Nutritional quality is way down on the list of priorities.

The majority of processed food is mostly processed carbohydrates with processed and hydrogenated oil added.

The processed carbohydrate industry has done a marvelous job of promoting its products – often to the detriment of other segments of the food industry. Processed carbohydrates offer us convenience in the form of packaged drinks, ready-to-eat breads, cookies, crackers, chips, popcorn, cereals, cakes, pies, bagels, pasta, and rice, to name a few examples.

Although there is little fat in a processed carbohydrate food, such as spaghetti, there is also very little nutrition. Processing takes out most beneficial nutrients, such as *essential* (required for life) natural oils. Essential nutrients are stripped away and often sold as separate products.

Organic processed carbohydrates may be a little healthier than their common non-organic counterparts. At least organic carbohydrates don't have the chemical residue from pesticides or synthetic fertilizers, but even they have few nutrients or essential oil-containing components. Have you been lulled into thinking that, as long as you eat "enriched" flour, you are getting all the nutrition that Mother Nature put into wheat? Well, did you ever stop to consider why the flour needs to be "enriched" in the first place?

How Much Sugar Do We Eat?

In 1996, in the U.S. alone, we consumed 23 million tons (46 billion pounds) of pure sugar.[9]

The average American sugar consumption was about 160 pounds per person in 1996!

Here's a table showing the amount of artificial sweeteners along with natural sweeteners. The amount of natural sweeteners (sugars) was 21,648,000 metric tons.[10]

A hundred years ago, and in the 1930s and 1940s, during depression and war time, sugar was a luxury. Nowadays, Americans are hard-pressed to find anything made without sugar. Few of us know what home-made bread should taste like. Modern society has paid a high nutritional price – in both nutrition and taste – for foods altered by processing. We have become the starving obese!

9 This does **not** include carbohydrates such as grains that the body converts to sugar.
10 A metric ton is about 10% more than a U.S. ton (2,240 pounds vs. 2,000 pounds).

U.S. SWEET TOOTH

1996 Consumption

	(IN THOUSANDS OF M.T.)	(IN MILLIONS OF DOLLARS)
NONNUTRITIVE		
Aspartame	9.2	$749
Saccharin	1.8	13
Acesulfame	5.7	502
Total	16.7	1,264
NATURAL SWEETENERS		
Refined sugar	8,600	4,541
High fructose corn syrup	10,285	4,799
Glucose	2,635	722
Sorbitol	41	67
Xylitol	9	66
Mannitol	10	39
Crystalline fructose	68	20
Total	21,648	10,254

Source: SRI International (Menlo Park, CA).

32 CHEMICAL WEEK, JUNE 11, 1997

Are Only Sweets and Grains Considered Carbohydrates?

No, not at all. Although many people recognize desserts, bread, pasta and cereals as carbohydrates, *most fruits and many vegetables, especially beans, rice and potatoes, are also primarily carbohydrate.*

A carbohydrate is a molecular structure made of sugars linked together. There are two classes of carbohydrates: simple and complex. One of the main differences between them is the time it takes for the body to break them into their more basic components – the simple sugars – and finally to glucose.

Complex carbohydrates, such as starch, take longer to break down, slowing the transport of sugar into the bloodstream after the food is eaten. But the elevated glucose level stays for a longer period of time than it does with a simple sugar. The end result is that the body receives the same total amount of sugar overall, but spread over a longer time.

In terms of calories, nutrients, and sugar content, it makes little difference whether you eat simple carbohydrates, such as white rice, or more complex carbohydrates, such as brown rice. There is no advantage from eating the vast amount of complex carbohydrates that the standard bodybuilding diet and other eating programs are famous for. Actually, as we will see, this may be much worse from a *Life-Systems* analysis – your glucose stays elevated far longer.

Surprise! Salt is required for cellular sugar (glucose) transfer.
Many Americans are actually salt-deficient!*

* *Essentials of Biochemistry,* page 241.

To legitimize the high-carbohydrate preferences of these plans, the promoters tell us that glucose is the preferred energy source of the body. This is only partly true.

Our brain feeds on glucose, and the brain uses about two-thirds of the circulating glucose in the bloodstream. Other organs don't need much glucose. **The body can convert glycogen (a substance readily stored by the body) into glucose whenever needed. It can also convert our fat reserves to glucose as needed.*** Furthermore, as the *Textbook of Medical Physiology* clearly states on page 973, "During much of the day, muscle tissue depends not on glucose for its energy but on fatty acids. The principle reason for this is that the normal resting muscle membrane is only slightly permeable to glucose except when the muscle fiber is stimulated by insulin...." During moderate or heavy exercise, glucose is used, but not during the majority of the day. Few of us are told this medical fact.

An average 180-pound male carries about 15 percent bodyfat (about 27 pounds). Twenty percent (5-7 pounds) is used structurally throughout the body, so he is left with about 20 pounds of excess bodyfat called *adipose* tissue. An average 130-pound woman should have about 22 percent bodyfat (about 29 pounds).[11] Each pound of fat is capable of liberating 3,500 calories of energy, so the average adult has over 70,000 (3,500 x 20) calories available for conversion to energy. We burn about 300 calories per hour walking or about 600 calories per hour running. So, with about 70,000 calories stored up, we have enough fat stores to walk 230 hours or run 115 hours! At 8 hours per day, we would have a full-time job walking non-stop for a month in order to burn off that much fat.

Most of us have over a month of bodyfat reserves — enough energy to walk from Miami to Houston *without eating.*

The bottom line:

We don't require many carbohydrates at all.*

---

11 *Protein Power*, page 151.

* Your body makes glucose with glycerol (from bodyfat) combined with amino acids (from protein). *Basic Medical Biochemistry,* pages 28-29, 394, 428.

Remember, researchers knew many years ago that any carbohydrates not immediately used by the body are stored as fat.[12]

What happens when excess carbohydrates are eaten after the liver's and muscles' reserves are already full? They go *directly to fat.* Insulin, which is triggered by carbohydrates, not fats, stimulates conversion of glucose to fat, which is then stored in the existing fat cells. Carbohydrates are not primarily used for energy. *They just get added to the existing fat.* Wouldn't it be nice if our body just magically vaporized excess carbohydrates and excess calories? As most of us know all too well, it doesn't. The main function of carbohydrates is making fat.

The closest thing to magically vaporizing excess calories is EFAs. EFAs help to burn excess calories as fuel.

We have a special type of bodyfat called "brown adipose tissue" (BAT). Scientists have known about BAT for at least twenty years, but BAT has received little attention. A *Life-Systems* Engineering approach leads us to surmise that the body may have an automatic safeguard against obesity – when it isn't short-circuited.

Our team of *Life-Systems* Engineers believe this BAT could be one of the body's *automatic regulators* against becoming overweight. Its function is simply to turn excess calories into heat – instead of excess bodyfat. BAT is made from EFAs. When the body has enough EFAs for its life-supporting functions, it can then funnel more calories into the BAT. So with EFAs, we gain increased resistance to becoming overweight, and any excess fat we already have will burn more readily, too.

At the same time, your desire for processed carbohydrates significantly decreases, so the fat-depositing mechanism slows down.

---

12 Glucose, stored as glycogen, can be stored in two areas: the liver and the muscles. The brain can only use the glycogen stored in the liver; the glycogen in the muscles can only be used by the muscle where it is stored. The liver doesn't store much glycogen—enough for 10-12 hours of normal daily activities. This is the equivalent of about three candy bars or a small plate of spaghetti. There is only a small reserve of about 1,200 calories in all the muscles. It only takes a few minutes of intense muscle activity for its glycogen to get completely used up! So we use very few carbohydrates to keep these little reserves full. As soon as these reserves are full, extra carbohydrates are converted to bodyfat.

This is a powerful attack:

- Reduce desire for carbohydrates;
- Increase burning of stored excess bodyfat.

Even though the "fat-free" carbohydrate has achieved legendary status, ***it is your worst enemy*** **– while *EFAs* (basic essence) *are your best friend.***

Whenever excess carbohydrates are consumed, the body doesn't want them and pours out insulin. Virtually *no insulin is generated from eating fats or proteins.* From a *Life-Systems* Engineering analysis, this is a major impact that must be kept in mind.

The body normally uses insulin to tightly control blood glucose (sugar) levels – approximately 70-90 milligrams per deciliter – **less than one teaspoon of sugar for your entire bloodstream.**[13]

Let's look at how much glucose (sugar) eating a bagel produces. The package says about 40 grams of carbohydrate. We must subtract the insoluble (indigestible and not usable by humans) fiber content, so we have approximately 30 grams of carbohydrate that gets converted into liquid glucose. Five grams equals approximately one teaspoon. So from one bagel we get about six teaspoons of glucose. If we eat two bagels we get 12 teaspoons worth – many meals pack a lot more carbohydrates.

This overloads our system with about **10 times the carbohydrates the body normally allows in the bloodstream**.

In engineering terms, we call this an *order of magnitude effect.* In other words, this carbohydrate overload is very significant.

---

13 A "ballpark" calculation shows that normal blood glucose concentration is about one gram per liter — just one part per thousand (a gram is approximately one-fifth of a teaspoon and a liter is a little more than a quart). Adults have about five liters of blood, so we have five grams of glucose in our bloodstream. One teaspoon has about one-hundred-twenty drops, so a typical adult has about one hundred twenty (120) drops of glucose in their bloodstream.

Approximate glucose (sugar) equivalents in just one average serving:

	Glucose (teaspoons of sugar)		Glucose (teaspoons of sugar)
Beer	3	Pecan pie slice	9
Fruit juice	5	Pizza slice (one)	4
Glazed donut	3	Soda	3
Honey bun	5	White bread (2 thin slices)	5

Total allowed in bloodstream <1

Few of us stop after only 1 portion. Before the discovery of the Foundation of Radiant Health, I routinely craved and ate an entire large pizza (10 slices) amounting to an incredible 40 times the blood's resting glucose level! How many portions do you usually eat? Doesn't it make sense, when we keep overloading and stressing our system like this, that sooner or later, something will fail? For safety (prevention of *glycosuria*), hospital patients **receive no more than 7 tsp. sugar (carbohydrate) per hour** during intravenous feeding.* The average American frequently eats more than 20 tsp. sugar (carbohydrate) per meal several times a day!**

There are four major types of carbohydrate in the human diet: *fructose*, found in fruits; *sucrose*, found in sugar cane; *lactose*, found in milk; and *starches*, which are large polysaccharides (sugars linked together) present in almost all non-animal foods and particularly in grains.[14] Our processed food diet contains large amounts of cellulose, which is a carbohydrate. However, humans have no enzyme to digest cellulose (purified sawdust). Cellulose is the same stuff (sawdust) that termites eat. Therefore, cellulose provides us no nutrients and can't be considered a food for humans. Its only function in our diets is to control the absorption of water from our food and to help form stools for easy elimination of solid waste – particularly useful with a diet high in processed carbohydrates.

Do you think a diet of fruit is better? It is estimated that 50% of adults *can't digest the fructose from more than* 2 pieces of fruit!***

14 Other carbohydrates include: amylose, glycogen, pectins, and dextrins. Meat has very small quantities of carbohydrates.

* *Body Fluids And Electrolytes*, pages 71-72.

** *Beyond The Zone*, pages 316-320.

*** *Basic Medical Biochemistry*, page 404.

Carbohydrates are broken down and absorbed by the body as the simple sugar (or monosaccharide), glucose. All sugars are absorbed by the liver, where they are converted into glucose. Milk sugar is called galactose, and fruit sugar is called fructose. **Both are converted quickly into glucose**, just like common table sugar.[15] It happens very quickly. Glucose is the only sugar which can be released directly into the bloodstream. Foods containing glucose hit you quickly, because their sugar doesn't require any time for conversion. A can of soda or sweetened juice drink's sugar effects are immediate.

Nothing makes you feel more bloated than consuming carbohydrates, plus, you'll be hungry again in just a few hours.

If your blood glucose levels run higher than average (above 90 milligrams/dl.) and remain elevated long-term, the number of potential physical problems is enormous. Ask any person who has diabetes, or your physician. Excess blood sugar levels make you tired and increase the likelihood of numerous diseases.[16] High blood sugar levels promote the growth of unfavorable bacteria. A person suffering from diabetes with high blood glucose levels doesn't heal from injuries. There is no good reason to maintain elevated glucose levels. However, there are many good reasons to maintain normal (low) glucose levels.

Diabetics will be glad to know that EFAs help with neuropathy (loss of feeling due to nerve damage) even reversing it in many cases.[17] More than 50% (half) of all diabetics develop severe nerve loss (including impotence) and more than 95% of all diabetics have some degree of nerve damage. EFAs support production of Prostaglandin E4, shown to be highly significant in the neurophysiological improvement of diabetic neuropathy. If EFAs can do this, don't you want to have Prostaglandin's E4 benefits, too? Peak performance and radiant health demand it! Prostaglandins assist in the second-by-second regulation of all tissues, including the components of blood microcirculation and blood platelets.

---

15 Most table sugar is produced from beets — not sugar cane!

16 Two common diabetes-related disorders are gangrene and retinal (vision) problems. Gangrene can develop in wounds that don't heal quickly and can lead to amputation. Problems can develop involving the retina (at the back of the eye) and often lead to blindness.

17 "The use of gamma-linolenic acid in diabetic neuropathy," D.F. Horrobin, Efamol Research Institute, Kentville, Nova Scotia, Canada.

If you are short on EFAs, you are short on the resulting prostaglandins, too. Without them you get a more rigid blood cell and increased blood viscosity (high-viscosity fluids don't flow easily). These conditions, in turn, contribute to higher blood pressure. Both conditions are common in diabetics.

Glucose (sugar) auto-oxidizes in the bloodstream. *Life-Systems* Engineers wondered what was causing the "cut" in the artery in the first place, that causes plaque (buildup). Carbohydrates, because they are auto-oxidizers, raise havoc with all the substances in your blood. It has been a well-known fact among scientists for years that *oxidized* cholesterol and *other substances* in the blood are some of the causes of these arterial "cuts," and the subsequent healing becomes arterial blockage.

High glucose levels from carbohydrates are a prime cause of arterial damage, and ultimately arterial blockage. That's where the scientific evidence points. Think about the 10-fold increase in diabetes. Processed carbohydrates are at its root.

An article on page 1 of the May 1997 *Diabetes Interview* states:

> Glucose in the bloodstream auto-oxidizes. It produces free-radicals all by itself. Diabetes is now defined as a condition that speeds up the aging process. Preventing free-radical formation is what the anti-oxidant theory is all about. Outside of the immune system's specialized use of free-radicals, we don't need extra ones floating around, doing damage. We know oxidation damages blood vessels, and causes cardiovascular problems....

Also in the same issue, Keith Campbell, RPh, said,

> "Diabetes is now defined as a condition that speeds up the aging process. The disease is defined this way because these oxidized compounds damage blood vessels and cause complications, like cardiovascular problems, that are associated with old age."

If this sounds like a direct cause of blocked and inflamed arterial walls, you may then ask how can anybody in their right mind advocate eating an overload of processed carbohydrates?

No one could. Many people in the nutritional fields aren't in their right mind. They are misled – and the scary part is that so many of us, despite the best of intentions, including many of our physicians, have been misled, too.

Can the ability to produce insulin be compromised by eating excessive amounts of processed carbohydrates over many years? Certainly, by destroying your pancreas. That's how many adults acquire diabetes. *Your body doesn't need much carbohydrate, no matter whether the carbohydrates are simple or complex.* Insulin's job is to remove the resulting excess glucose from the bloodstream as fast as possible, which simply means these excess carbohydrates get stored in your body as fat.

It is now known that **insulin also tells the body not to burn any stored fat**. So there is a compound effect from excess carbohydrates: carbohydrates get converted to new fat, and the old fat doesn't get metabolized (burned).

You will notice a sugar-low typically within just a few minutes after eating a large serving of carbohydrates. If you eat a big plate of spaghetti or a couple of bagels, within just a few hours (or even minutes) you'll get mental fatigue and feel tired and sluggish. Many successful businessmen know this. That's why they don't eat high-carbohydrate lunches.

This sluggish feeling comes from the excess glucose (sugar) in the bloodstream. Ask a diabetic how he or she feels when their blood sugar level is above 200. They feel tired and don't have any energy.

Especially interesting information:

- ∞ Half of us say we have nothing in the cupboard but two boxes of cereal.
- ∞ Consumption of toaster pastries has tripled in the past decade. Kellogg's now sells more Pop-Tarts than Frosted Flakes, the top-selling cereal in the nation.
- ∞ Bagel sales will top 3 billion for 1995, double what they were just 2 years ago![18]

Marketing of processed carbohydrates has paid off. We have been turned into a nation of "carb-o-vores" by the processed food industry.

You may hear about "good" and "bad" parts of certain *Life-Systems*. For example: "good cholesterol" and "bad cholesterol." This is a poor choice of labels, because there are no good or bad parts in any life-system – just balancing forces.

---

18 "Outlook," *U.S. News & World Report*, November 10, 1997, page 14. Source: NPD Group: *Are You Normal?*, Bernice Kanner, St. Martin's Press, 1995.

A *good* and *bad* distinction concerning Life-Systems is misleading. Both parts of a biological process are required. One part cannot be separated from the other.

The "Indian National Rail Study" compared Northern Indians, who ate lots of meat and clarified butter (ghee), with Southern Indians, who were vegetarians and ate no meat. The Southern Indians did eat plenty of margarine and processed oils though.

While the Southern Indians ate only one-tenth the natural fat, they had 15 times more heart disease than their Northern neighbors.[19]

Higher cholesterol from foods like meat and butter, in and of themselves, *don't cause arteriosclerosis*.

Here's another example: The National Health Examination Follow-up Survey followed 4,700 people and reported in 1990, "in the instance of total blood cholesterol, we found no evidence in any age-sex group of a risk associated with elevated levels."[20]

With this many people, there were many incidences of extremely high blood cholesterol values. Yet, as we see time-and-time again, when the results of any blood cholesterol study are impartially analyzed, *cholesterol is not a cause for concern for the normal person*. On the same page, this study goes on to say that diabetes is the most important risk factor leading to death by cardiovascular dysfunction!

Also consider that the body has no blood sensor for cholesterol. This suggests that your body doesn't care what the circulating blood cholesterol level is. Your blood system does have many sensors for other critical nutrients. A *Life-Systems* Engineering analysis must ask: Is it possible that high-density transported and low-density transported cholesterol designations ("good" HDL and "bad" LDL) were invented simply to keep the cholesterol-lowering drug manufacturers in business? LDL is critical in bringing life-sustaining basic essence into the cell!

19 *American Journal of Clinical Nutrition, 20:471, 1967.*

20 *Diabetes Solution*, Richard Bernstein, M.D., Little, Brown & Company, New York, NY, 1997, page 314.

Glucagon, a hormone, releases stored glycogen and stored bodyfat for conversion into glucose. Unlike insulin, though, *glucagon's action is stimulated by protein.* When more protein and fats and less carbohydrates are eaten, excess fat stored in your body is more readily burned for fuel. *Basic Medical Biochemistry* (pages 23 and 394) clearly states that **bodyfat is made from glucose!**

There is a Life-System at work, and it involves significant differences between the roles of carbohydrates and proteins. It is much easier to lose bodyfat by eating protein than by eating carbohydrates, because the protein-influenced glucagon causes stored bodyfat to be converted to glucose. Then the glucose is used or burned. The *Textbook of Medical Physiology* has a section called "Formation of Carbohydrates From Proteins and Fats – Gluconeogenesis." With the glycerol portion of fat, the majority of amino acids (from proteins) can be easily converted into carbohydrates.[21] The great part is that, with basic essence, this lost bodyfat doesn't come right back!

Methods that attempt to alter our *Life-Systems* can be harmful. So beware. Keep in mind that EFAs allow your body to function as it was meant to. We lose our system balance when we artificially override natural, perfectly engineered, Life-System mechanisms.

The function of insulin, which is produced by the pancreas, is to get rid of excessive carbohydrates. When we take our system too far out of balance with carbohydrate overload, *the flood of insulin can bring the blood glucose level too low.*

Here's an illustration of what happens. If you walk into your house in the winter when the house is 40 degrees, you might set the thermostat for 72 degrees. The air temperature probably hits 74 to 76 degrees before shutting off. This overshoot is a common mechanical system occurrence.

To counteract this type of overshoot in a biological system, Nature provides a feedback mechanism: glucagon to balance insulin. The problem is that this feedback system is being forced to deal with higher glucose (sugar) levels than it was designed for!

Biosensors measure the residual glucose level in the blood and feed back that information to the insulin controller. This feedback

---

21 *Textbook of Medical Physiology*, Arthur C. Guyton, M.D., and John E. Hall, Ph.D., published by W.B. Saunders Company, ninth edition, 1996 Page 863.

system reacts to overloads of sugar the only way it can – with an overload of insulin. Here's where the concept of a "sugar-low" comes from.

That's how the feedback system works in the whole body. Another part of the feedback system works at the cellular level. The cell-by-cell counterparts of insulin and glucagon are system-balancing eicosanoids. Eicosanoids (prostaglandins) are your body's hormone controllers, only they work without entering the bloodstream. They act quickly and at extremely low concentrations. This makes them difficult to measure.

What are the building blocks of eicosanoids? You probably guessed it ... basic essence.

Research now shows that, if we don't have sufficient protein in the bloodstream compared to carbohydrate levels, glucagon is inhibited.[22] Remember, glucagon releases stored glycogen for conversion into glucose: If glucagon is inhibited, fat-burning is interrupted.

Another problem with too much insulin is that cellular oxygen transfer is cut way down.

When we eat too many carbohydrates, we get a quintuple whammy:
1) Low oxygen transfer (sluggishness)
2) Exhaustion from the excess insulin
3) Excessive hunger (cravings)
4) Bodyfat doesn't get burned
5) More fat is stored in the body.

Excessive carbohydrate consumption resulting in high glucose (sugar) levels gives the same result – all the time. We aren't meant to eat lots more carbohydrates than protein. What about unprocessed carbohydrates? There aren't very many of them today. Only a few fresh fruits and vegetables are in this category. Some common fruits and vegetables along with their carbohydrate levels

22 When glucagon is inhibited, glucose can't be converted from the fat reserves. Insulin takes priority over glucagon. With excess carbohydrates, the fat gets put on and can't easily be taken off.

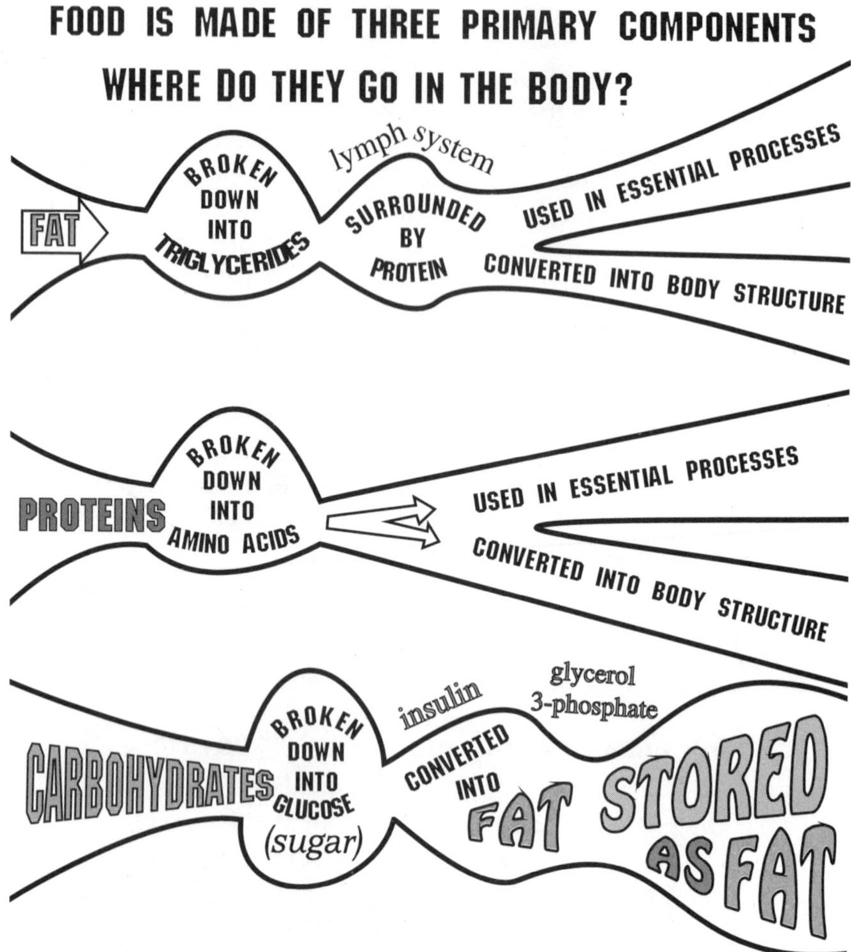

are listed at the end of this book. Processed carbohydrates have most nutrients removed. The unprocessed carbohydrates are better for you, but even unprocessed carbohydrates, eaten in excess, will upset the balance of your system.

Now, because of the basic essence discovery, there's an easy, no-effort solution to the problems caused by these detrimental carbohydrates. When you eat enough of the basic essence combination of EFAs, you will no longer desire many carbohydrates. Your body will finally get the nutrients it has been needing. Your taste for them will actually change – naturally.

Without basic essence, our diet is very different from what our bodies are designed to eat. Because of EFA-destroying food processing, it has been virtually impossible to overcome the desire to eat too much. Now you can see why traditional diets or eating programs are doomed to fail. They do not take into account food processing and the basic essence-connection. Plus, they typically promote overdosing on carbohydrates.

What about the people who can eat carbohydrates "all day long" and not get fat? We already discussed how this can be a symptom of diabetes.

Let's explore this group in more detail. Many thin women are in this category. Upon further analysis, many of them suffer from low energy and look sickly, too (especially without their makeup). They don't radiate healthiness. Some of these women, by consciously overriding their automatic *Life-Systems*' hunger mechanism, are starving themselves. Does this make sense? No. Any woman starving herself won't gain weight. Yet ...

The starvation (caloric restriction) method of weight control does not support radiant health and requires tenacious willpower.

This diet of drastically reducing calories while eating mostly carbohydrates has a big downside – these *starving people are not healthy*. Review the "Healthy Eating" test in Chapter 1, on page 30. A "YES" answer to *any* of those questions indicates you aren't eating healthy (as defined by what the body needs), nor are you in possession of radiant health. If we are honest with ourselves, many of these women (and men) will rate "poor" to "very poor" in overall health as evidenced by how they feel and look. The good news is that *achieving peak performance and radiant health is easy, once you know the secret.*

I have visited aerobics sessions many times over the years. A surprisingly frequent observation was that thin women typically had lots of cellulite and had no energy after just 15-20 minutes of exercise. I saw many of them leaving the session early due to their exhaustion.

Some athletes – for example, marathon runners – may be able to get by with consuming excessive carbohydrates and not get fat because they exercise so much. Vigorous exercise stimulates increased growth hormone production. Growth hormone has a tendency to burn excess fat. I lifted weights diligently for three years twice a week under professional guidance. Yet, exercise alone wasn't enough to get rid of my excess middle.

A specific and non-typical group, such as marathon runners, may be taken as the norm for all of us. Just because they more easily tolerate excessive carbohydrates doesn't automatically mean the rest of us can. We must be careful when we make generalizations based on specialized elite groups, like athletes. Exercise is only one part of a complex *Life-Systems* equation.

Generalizing results from specific groups is a classic method of distorted logic using incomplete knowledge. There is a significant difference between thriving and just surviving. To lose excess bodyfat in a healthy way, your body has to be operating very efficiently. I wasted years of effort trying to lose excess bodyfat on the high-carbohydrate, low-fat diets – barely surviving – and you may have, too.

Using the "small groups" technique described in the STAT-SMART chapter, a "researcher" can "prove" many things. Could it be that someone in the processed carbohydrate industry wanted to show that carbohydrates are healthful, and then found an elite athletic group to "prove" it so? They certainly wouldn't mind a scientist saying carbohydrates are great, would they? Virtually everyone already ***assumed*** *that dietary fat went directly to bodyfat,* so this convenient idea would have been instantly accepted by the public as "the answer" to our excess weight problems. Unfortunately, it doesn't work for the average person, as demonstrated by the results – high failure rates and unprecedented levels of obesity.

Because a non-typical group did not quickly become fat on carbohydrates, the food-processing industry may have decided that lots of carbohydrates were great for everyone!

We are even told by some nutritionists to eat a snack every two to three hours (eating four to six small meals a day) whether we are hungry or not. This is supposedly an attempt to keep glucose levels constant. But keeping the levels constantly high is not the answer. Something is drastically wrong here. Does this advice make sense? Should you drink an extra gallon of water even if you're not thirsty? No. Should you go to bed if you aren't tired? No. This frequent-eating approach doesn't make sense in terms of a systems understanding of our bodies.

A *Life-Systems* analysis concludes that frequent carbohydrate overload will destroy your pancreas.

When you consume even a few carbohydrates, like in a can of soda, your blood insulin concentration is increased 10-fold within a few minutes! Loads of insulin are dumped into your bloodstream. After about 10 minutes, the rate of insulin release slows down towards normal. Then, it springs back a second time, raising its concentration above the level of the first jolt.

This is illustrated with the graph on the next page.

*Insulin levels will reach 10 to 25 times above norma*l to get rid of the excess glucose (sugar), and continue to stay elevated *even 2 to 3 hours after the time carbohydrates are eaten.*[23]

Imagine eating carbohydrate-loaded meals 4-6 times a day. You haven't given the insulin enough time to get the last meal's glucose (sugar) out of the bloodstream yet. Now you force the cycle to begin again – only this time, the body doesn't have enough stored insulin because the pancreas was never equipped for you to eat so many (processed) carbohydrates so often. So, your resting blood sugar level stays even higher.

The third meal forces your poor pancreas to perform again, but by now it produces even less insulin, because your pancreas needs several hours to manufacture new insulin.

By the fourth meal, your pancreas is exhausted and cannot respond much at all. Now consider doing this day-after-day.

Bodybuilders are taught to never train the same body part two days in a row.

23 *Textbook of Medical Physiology*, page 977.

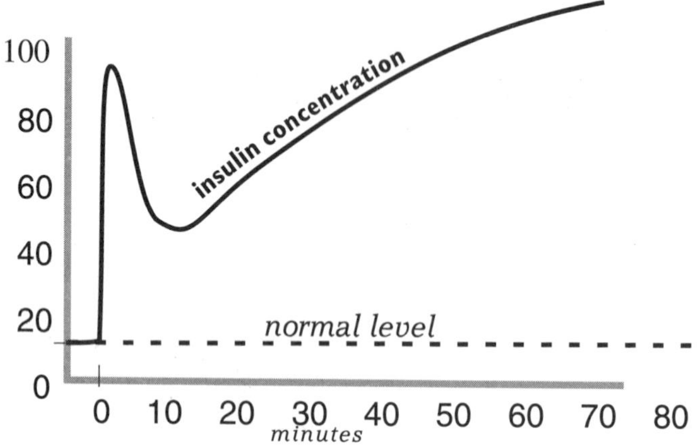

The sugar from 1/2 can of soda or a slice of bread generates more than 10 times the normal insulin level.

In the kidneys, peripheral nerves, and lenses (eyes) sugar (carbohydrate) consumption raises levels of intracellular *sorbitol* which can't escape. This causes increased osmotic pressure and cellular damage. Diabetics beware!*

Rest is required between workouts. Yet, we don't show the same consideration to our poor pancreas!

The medical textbook *Scientific Foundation of Biochemistry in Clinical Practice* states that only 1% of your pancreas can make insulin. The rest (99%) of the pancreas is involved in various digestive processes.

The pancreas isn't a muscle, like the heart, which works continuously. It isn't like the lungs, which also are designed to work continuously. **The pancreas is designed to secrete insulin once or twice a day in response to carbohydrates, with several hours between secretions.**

It doesn't make *Life-Systems* Engineering sense to eat so many carbohydrate meals. Eating this many times a day is a virtual guarantee for gaining fat, developing diabetes, and suffering a premature, often agonizing death.

* *Essentials of Biochemistry*, page 182.

For every 10 pounds overweight you become, your risk of contracting diabetes doubles during any 10-year period.[24] Is it any wonder that:

According to the National Institutes of Health, about 700,000 new diabetics will be diagnosed this year. That doesn't include people who become diabetic but don't know it yet.

That's more than two new diabetes cases each and every minute – 24 hours a day!

The body has very complex automatic systems to regulate numerous functions. We don't need to count the number of breaths we take during the day. Breathing is regulated automatically. Just try to alter your breathing pattern intentionally. It can't be accomplished for any length of time without tremendous difficulty. And even if you could alter your breathing, you'd have to be able to alter other related functions to maintain system balance. Remember, if you change one thing, you change many things.

Your body has many different components which act together in complex, balanced and integrated systems. When your body is hungry, it tells you to eat. There is a reason. Appetite suppressants are detrimental partly because they artificially interfere with a highly-regulated, automatic system. Many of my clients told me they had to force themselves to eat when taking prescribed appetite suppressants. This is a terrible condition. Once basic essence intake is adequate, you should never again have a need to consider hunger-suppressing drugs.

Most people can fast for a couple of days drinking only water. Numerous religious sects practice ritual fasts which last from 1 day to as long as 6 weeks. Your body will convert a modest amount of stored fat to glucose. When, in addition to fasting, you supplement the water with a small amount of basic essence, you'll see how little carbohydrate is required – you'll still have plenty of energy.

Because so few people fully understand the link between nutrition and basic essence, a multitude of incorrect theories and solutions that can't work, no matter how good they may sound, have been promoted.

24 *Bottom Line*, December 15, 1997. Source: David Williamson, Ph.D., Division of Diabetes Translation, Centers For Disease Control and Prevention (study based on 14,000 people).

The theorists haven't told you about basic essence and the nutritional connection because they simply don't know.

With adequate basic essence, cravings will ease and eventually cease, and you can eat virtually whatever you desire. You won't want two bagels anymore. Just one bagel (or even just a half) will do nicely. Within weeks, just half a bagel or less will be enough. Your body wants basic essence, so that it can work as it was meant to. With adequate basic essence, you will soon feel the improvement in your physical state. If you eat too many carbohydrates, you will feel stuffed and wonder why you ate what you did. *After receiving this new type of feedback from your body a few times, you'll gladly change your habits, because it takes no real effort.*

I used to eat a whole large pepperoni pizza in one sitting every week. In addition, I also "needed" a weekly hot fudge sundae (with extra fudge). Now if I have either of these, I just eat a small portion, and I enjoy eating it more – even in smaller amounts. I honestly don't want to gorge myself; and I don't like the feeling if I do. The difference is that basic essence makes this happen automatically. Other than taking the basic essence regularly, there is no special effort or action on my part.

No one can obtain the needed level of EFAs just from their food anymore because food processing distorts, destroys, or removes them.

Once you have established adequate basic essence intake, your body's systems begin to work together harmoniously. Fat is properly metabolized, and overeating becomes a non-issue. You'll enjoy the taste of food even better than before, but the cravings and compulsions will disappear. This is great for those of us who know what it's like to spend the better part of our day thinking about what to eat yet trying to stay slim.

We are too busy and stressed to make "proper eating" another job, and now we don't have to.

Here's a simple way to test how little carbohydrate you really need. While taking basic essence, eat as much protein and natural fats and oils as you care to and minimize your carbohydrates.

Be careful: hidden carbohydrates are everywhere. For example, milk has lots of carbohydrates, so be sure you count a glass of milk as carbohydrate when analyzing your results. Milk doesn't contain much protein. (Cream has virtually no carbohydrates – it is almost all fat.) Beans are almost all carbohydrate, as is most fruit. These all add up, so most of us eat many more carbohydrates than we realize. [At the end of this book is a short list of foods which have a high carbohydrate content.] The list is enclosed for reference purposes only, because you'll be able to eat whatever you desire. Further proof that your body doesn't need processed carbohydrates is that your desire for them decreases dramatically once the EFA deficiency is eliminated.

Here's the kind of menu I tried. I felt great. Try it for yourself:

Reduced carbohydrate menu:

* Breakfast – two-three eggs fried in butter, a big piece of cheddar cheese, two-three strips of bacon, and half a bagel. (Yes, I did eat this large amount.)

* Lunch – none was required – I took some basic essence and wasn't hungry at all.

* Dinner – half a can tuna fish, one tomato, some relish, two pieces minimally processed bread with mayonnaise.

If an adult's [25] weight is close to what it should be, typically, take two capsules (1,000 - 1,200 mg. each) or a half teaspoon of basic essence about twenty (20) to thirty (30) minutes before mealtime – whether you eat or not – two times per day. Five 1,000 mg size capsules equal about a teaspoon – you don't need a lot. Your body can only assimilate a little at a time, so taking more at once doesn't offer a benefit. If you take it 20 minutes or so before a meal, you'll desire less food at the meal. Remember, basic essence is real food.

With basic essence, many people find they can easily and comfortably skip some meals.

25 If you are larger, take proportionately more. You have more cells that need basic essence.

This shows how effectively basic essence satisfies the appetite.

If you only eat once a day (as some people say they do) take one-half the daily portion in the morning, and the remainder later in the day. Because basic essence is food, you can take it whenever you wish.

Most people see noticeable results within a few weeks.

It may take as long as 90-180 days, depending on your state of health and level of deficiency. If you are very deficient, it will take a bit longer to see obvious effects.

If you are like most people, you'll love the way you feel.

You won't feel bloated or experience those distressing sugar lows.

You'll finally be able to follow your body's natural response.

If you feel tired or sluggish after eating a meal, then your carbohydrate intake is probably out of balance. If so, review the high-carbohydrate list. Many people aren't aware that many varieties of beans are mostly carbohydrate. *One serving of beans provides almost all the carbohydrates you need for the entire day.*

After dining, you should never feel exhausted, bloated, or tired. If you do, something is WRONG! No one should feel like taking a nap after eating.

You should feel content after dining, yet remain easily capable of performing vigorous work. If you can't, it is a measure of your present dysfunctional biological system. Compare how you feel now, and again seven days later, and again thirty days after you start taking basic essence.

Many people have reported the following improvements:

- **More energy.** Cellular oxygen transfer is greatly increased. This isn't a caffeine high or a stimulant effect. This is a very subtle, yet noticeable, sustained improvement.
- **No cravings.** People quickly lost their cravings. It is delightful not to be controlled by food anymore. Hunger takes on its appropriate function, telling when you need to eat.
- **Increased overall well being**. Many feel better than ever before. Most people don't know what feeling well means anymore. Now you can.
- **Better hormone balance.** Because basic essence is fundamental to the manufacture of hormones and prostaglandins, many women have found their monthly cycles much less troublesome.
- **Attention Deficit Disorders** (ADDs) are helped, too. Scientific research confirms this. Purdue University conducted a study which was published in the *American Journal of Clinical Nutrition.* About 40 percent of children with ADD had deficiencies of EFAs as measured in their blood.[26]
- **Increased calm.** Stresses from everyday life are minimized. You will be much more at peace regardless of daily pressures.

Within approximately three to six months of adding basic essence to your diet, you probably won't want many carbohydrates anymore, because your body's signals will grow to tell you to eat less of them. You don't need willpower, either, though you may need to consciously monitor and gradually adjust your eating habits.

The high-carbohydrate proponents say that high fiber is important to optimal nutrition – especially colon efficiency. This is false!* Fiber is just indigestible carbohydrate. Many bodily wastes attach to fiber so they can be eliminated. The mistake that many of these proponents make is misleading us into thinking that, to get enough fiber, we need a lot of processed carbohydrates, such as high-fiber cereal.

26 *Energy Times*, "Attention Please," Rafael Avila, December 1996, pages 52 - 58.
* *New England Journal of Medicine*, Vol. 340, No. 3, January 21, 1999.
* *New York Times*, pg. 1, April 20, 2000.

In spite of the historic 1999 and 2000 findings **conclusively showing the worthlessness of high-fiber diets (fruits and vegetables and bran)**, if you still desire vegetable fiber, eat celery. It has almost no sugar and few calories. Most processed carbohydrates (such as ready-to-eat cereals) do not provide significant fiber or other nutrients. **However, meat has lots of fiber**.

Go easy on dried fruits and fruit juices. The juice diets suggest you drink juice throughout the day to counteract the naturally occurring sugar low which follows an hour or two after drinking the juice. How can eating any natural fruit or vegetable be bad? None are harmful in small amounts, but most of the juices in the stores concentrate the fruit sugar and remove the fiber. If the first serving produced an undesired result, the second serving will only do it again! You won't crave nearly as much juice once your EFA balance is restored.

Fruit juice is a processed carbohydrate.

A pediatrician tells parents not to let children drink much juice. According to an article published in *Your Health* magazine, the doctor says, "What many people think is a moderate amount of juice isn't." She found that children drinking more than 12 ounces of juice per day are more than three times as likely to be overweight as kids who don't drink much juice! She has also found that it stunts children's growth.[27]

Our *Life-Systems* Engineering team suggests that adults follow this advice, too.

After you have followed the higher protein and natural fat menu (described a few pages back) for a couple of days, compare how you feel on the following menu:

Carbohydrate Time Bomb Menu:

Breakfast: Two bagels, jelly or any fat-free stuff (these products usually have increased carbohydrates and chemical additives to compensate for their lack of fat);

Lunch: Any kind of sandwich and french fries, with ketchup, a soft drink or iced tea with plenty of sugar;

Dinner: Anything you want as long as it has a good dose of carbohydrates (consult the carbohydrate list at the end of the book), such as pasta, rice, potatoes, and beans; with lots of bread, and, of course, dessert.

27 *Your Health*, March 4, 1997, page 10.

I had to ask you to experience this eating self-torture for yourself. Although the food might taste good at first, you probably won't feel good at the end of the day.

By contrast, if you follow your personal experiment of eating fewer processed carbohydrates while taking basic essence, you'll soon see that you don't gain weight. You'll also discover that eating a larger volume of high-carbohydrate food doesn't satisfy you as well as eating a smaller volume of low-carbohydrate food.

If you eat the high-carbohydrate menu above, you will probably feel stuffed, bloated, and listless – if you managed to eat it all. But, even in spite of the high volume of carbohydrates and high calories, you will feel hungry later.

A starving person living in a sub-standard economy may subsist with one small bowl of rice a day. It's cheap. In that case, carbohydrates can be considered useful. The problem is that you will still get a starving feeling around midnight, even after eating 3,000 carbohydrate-loaded calories during the day.

How you feel is important. Once your body has the basic essence it needs, hunger will begin to function as it should. Without the EFAs, you are running on incomplete low-grade fuel. Unfortunately, *most of us have no idea what it's like to feel really good.* Nor have we known what "eating well" really means.

No weight or cellulite control program can work successfully – long-term, without basic essence.

A bowl of spaghetti is virtually devoid of nutrients – even the natural fiber has been removed, along with the life-sustaining EFAs. *Basic Medical Biochemistry* (page 510) tells us that carbohydrates make us fat: **"Adipose tissue [bodyfat] can <u>store</u> fatty acids <u>only</u> when glycolysis is activated from glucose by eating [carbohydrates]**."

Many of us confuse the body's tolerance for nutritional abuse with good health, when, in fact, we are actually malnourishing ourselves. We may get by with this for many years, thinking we have good health, before becoming very sick.

Many illnesses may seem to appear "out-of-the-blue." Most really don't; we are not consciously aware of the ongoing damage from inadequate nutrition.

If your belly, thighs, or hips are too big, now you know what to blame — lack of basic essence.

People quit dieting programs when they are not working. Most require calories to be restricted by sheer willpower. The average person easily becomes disenchanted. It is even more of a financial drain when special foods must be purchased.

Some weight-loss clinics now add prescription drugs to their plans, because their programs have been so ineffective. By now, most of us have heard how risky those drugs can be.

Dieters will stay hungry and will have to deny themselves foods they like, without the basic essence connection.

When willpower is used to override the client's true food desires, these desires and cravings are not eliminated. They are simply buried in the subconscious. And it takes a lot of energy to keep them under "control." Even though they may be denied, they still exist. That's one reason why, within a few months or years, most people gain back all the weight they have lost. Often, they gain even more weight than they initially lost.

You may resist and you may fight, but you can't stop food cravings through willpower alone.

Dieting based on willpower is rarely successful in the long-term. It is another example of telling us: if the plan doesn't work, it's your fault – not the plan's. The people responsible for these programs don't understand how our life-systems work. When you give the body what it was designed to run on, it can then perform its job naturally. Sacrifice and suffering are not a requirement.

The body has its own wisdom, but it requires the right fuel.

Why have so many eating plans developed in this country? Let's assume we don't know how gravity works. If we tried to explain all of its effects without actually knowing the principles, our explanations wouldn't be very good. There would be numerous special situations where one thing works one time and something else works another time. You'd never really get to the heart of the matter. Instead of one basic equation, we could offer a string of numerous "specialized cases" in order to make different conditions come out right. Does this sound close to the current state of dieting theory?

This is precisely what resulted from the omission of the EFA-connection. Plan after plan of specialized instructions based on incomplete EFA knowledge cannot avoid contradictory theories. That's why it's true that about *the only thing the nutritionists can agree on is that other nutritionists are WRONG.*

Cravings will decrease and then disappear only when your body gets the basic essence it needs. There is simply no other way.

It appears that diabetes will become even more prevalent. Why? Because food processors keep reducing fat and adding more carbohydrates and synthetic chemicals to simulate the taste and texture of fat.

Because your body has to work so hard to process these big overloads of carbohydrates, a condition called "insulin intolerance" (or "insulin resistance") often develops over time. Most children have no problem eating all the carbohydrates they wish because they are growing and burning calories so fast. For some people, snack foods and fast foods don't cause excess fat until years later. It's as if the body finally starts to tell us, *You've abused me too much, and now I can't respond adequately anymore.* Many of us are running on borrowed time.

Just twenty years ago, there were few obese children, but not so today. The biggest change in nutrition in the last 50 years is the proliferation of processed food. Today, children live on these processed foods. And just look at the results.

People sometimes joke or complain about children increasingly becoming overweight "couch potatoes." There is nothing funny about children developing diabetes. In a regional diabetes referral center, there was a 10-fold increase in children developing type II diabetes over just a 10-year period![28] This disorder was once seen only among adults; hence the name "adult-onset" diabetes.

The *Journal of Pediatrics* published these findings of dramatic rise in juvenile diabetes in 1996.

There is a worldwide epidemic in diabetes.

The Centers for Disease Control and Prevention (CDC) and the World Health Organization estimate that *125 million people worldwide have developed diabetes!* It's expected to double by 2025.[29]

What can this increase mean? By consuming huge amounts of processed carbohydrates and starting to do so at earlier ages, we accelerate the rate at which the pancreas and related *Life-Systems* are overloaded and prematurely fail. Unfortunately, the blame has been misplaced on lack of physical activity, and not on eating too many low-fat foods.

With less carbohydrate to trigger insulin's fat-storage function, you have a better chance to burn excess bodyfat. But you won't be able to maximize this potential until your body has one more tool – an adequate supply of fat-burning basic essence. Without it, you'll still have the desire to eat too much.

It is widely claimed that you need various "proper" ratios of carbohydrate, protein, and fat for best health. The fact is, for the vast majority of people, **no processed carbohydrates are needed for proper functioning**. In today's world of supermarket convenience, you can't help but get loads of carbohydrates. They are everywhere! Most of us will regularly get more than enough carbohydrates – even if we try to avoid them totally.

Now, with adequate basic essence, your body won't crave excessive carbohydrates. Your body knows what it needs to

28 "Unsettling onset: Grown-up diabetes and school-age kids," Susan Flagg Godbrey with Laura Goldstein, *Prevention*, March 1997, page 42.

29 "Overweight population blamed for sixfold increase in diabetes," *Houston Chronicle*, October 31, 1997, 4A. Note: Although the official estimates are a 6-fold increase, the actual number is much greater.

function best, but without basic essence, your body has no choice but to insist you keep feeding it. Since there are virtually no EFA-containing foods, your body is driven into a feeding frenzy.

Early man probably didn't eat every day. There were no supermarkets back then. His body feasted when he had food and fasted when he didn't.

One of my *Life-Systems* associates thinks that *man learned to eat grains in order to ensure rapid bodyfat accumulation for surviving times of famine.* Thousands of years ago, there were "feast and fast" cycles. These are well documented. Any excess beyond the daily needs of the body would be stored as fat in case the next meal wasn't available for a while. We may not require such an efficient mechanism today, but we are stuck with it.

Partly because of the numerous high-carbohydrate drinks, including many processed fruit "beverages" and soft drinks promoted today, the amount of sugar in the typical diet has substantially increased from years ago. After eating basic essence for just a few months, most people don't find these drinks as tasteful anymore. I drank a soft drink the other day, and it made me physically sick. It should. Our body is expecting something usable, and along comes this stuff, forcing huge amounts of insulin to be spit out so that the processed sugar can be eliminated from the bloodstream. There are few vitamins, minerals, or other useful nutrients in most of these drinks.[30] Your body goes nuts trying to get rid of something which is unsuitable. Now, with basic essence, you can offer your body some compassion and relief.

What is a processed carbohydrate, such as a bagel or pasta: paste. That's right, paste! When I attended grade-school, we used flour and water to hold paper together. Prisoners used to be kept barely alive by feeding them a diet of bread and water (paste). Would you even consider eating a plate of plain spaghetti without sauce, olive oil, or butter on it? Most of us probably wouldn't even think of eating it. Likewise, with the bagel. Without jelly, butter, cream cheese or other topping, we don't have a taste for it – especially

30 Worse, the phosphoric acid, common in colas and some other brown soft drinks, leaches calcium from the bones.

once our taste-appetite system functions properly, with the Foundation of Radiant Health nutrients.

The next time you eat a bagel or a big plate of spaghetti, because you have been told how "good" they are for you, realize it's paste that you are eating. That's why you'll have the "lump in your stomach feeling," too. Your body doesn't want this as fuel. It can't make good use of it.

Flour and water make *paste*.

How well does the high-performance human body run on paste? As you would imagine, not very well, at all!

Fats and oils

With the Foundation of Radiant Health, your body can make good use of natural fats and oils, improving your health too.

The 1988 *Surgeon General's Report on Nutrition and Health* concluded that:

More than two-thirds of the deaths in the U.S. involve nutrition.

Isn't this incredible? Vitamin sales have never been higher. What nutrient is missing the most? Could EFA deficiency rate the top of the list?

As Leo Galland, M.D., an eminent physician specializing in treating undiagnosed and difficult-to-treat illnesses, clearly states, "EFAs are absolutely critical to good health."[31]

Women's coronary risk is linked to *particular kinds of fat* – not to the amount of dietary fat.[32]

A *New York Times* feature story detailed a new study which concluded that *trans*fatty acids (chemically distorted fats)

31 "How to Be Healthy," Leo Galland, M.D., *Bottom Line*, December 15, 1997.

32 "Women's Heart Risk Linked To Kinds of Fats, Not Total," Jane E. Brody, *New York Times*, November 20, 1997, page A1.

consumed were much more related to causing heart disease than the total amount of fat the women consumed. The researchers of this 14-year study of 80,000 nurses included the Harvard School of Public Health, and was published in the prestigious *New England Journal of Medicine*. The study also concluded that monounsaturates, which are prominent in olive oil, offer only a small benefit.

Dr. Walter Willett, co-author of the study, said *the problem with low-fat diets is that people replace fats with carbohydrates, primarily sugars and refined starches which can have adverse effects on coronary risk, particularly on people with more sedentary lifestyles.*[33]

One can imagine the controversy the results of this new study are causing, because it is so "politically incorrect" to criticize low-fat eating. We will learn that this study's results are completely consistent with how our body works and that consuming *natural* fats are what Mother Nature intended – that's why we have a great taste for meat, cheese, eggs and butter.

The medical community is beginning to recognize a different perspective concerning fats and cholesterol.

> **"*Trans*-unsaturated fat, as the man-made stuff is called, is *14 times more potent as a disease risk factor* than the saturated fats the public has been warned about for years – the kind in marbled beef, butter, and cheese."**[34]

From the same article, Dr. Willett, who is with the Harvard School of Public Health, continues:

> **The percentage of total fat in our diet probably doesn't make much of a difference. It's about time we discard that recommendation altogether and focus on what is really important, which is the *type* of fat.**

The article concludes with co-author Dr. Frank Hu:

"Here we're talking total fat being almost irrelevant to heart-

33 "Women's Heart Risk ...

34 "'Bad' fat connected to heart attack risk," *Houston Chronicle*, November 20, 1997, page 2A. Source: *Boston Globe*, Richard A. Knox.

disease risk and emphasizing the type of fat. I think it's going to be very controversial in that respect."

As we will learn, this conclusion has been precisely predicted by a *Life-Systems* Engineering analysis, based on how the body works. Remember, it often takes 25-50 years for the medical and nutrition fields to incorporate new knowledge into their recommendations.

When you eat *natural* fat, the fat goes directly into your lymphatic system – not the bloodstream. A protein is placed around the fat before it enters your bloodstream. *There is no loose fat running around in your bloodstream.*

The stomach provides a highly acidic environment where foods start their conversion into basic components. This is one reason it's clear that the common myth of "fat goes to fat" (adipose tissue) is false. The fat gets broken down into basic structural components.

Here's a bit of shocking history. In 1950, Sir Charles Dodds, appearing before the Royal Society of Medicine in London, threw a monkey wrench into the well-established low-calorie theory for losing weight. He tested both men and women who had kept their normal weight for years. He then had them eat two to three times more food than they were accustomed to. All of them stuffed themselves, yet none gained weight. As is so frequently the case, this new idea was not easily accepted. The doctors in England did not like to give up their established ideas that becoming overweight is caused by overeating and that the way to correct it is to count calories and eat less. Doesn't this type of thinking sound familiar? It's the same even 47 years later, in 1998!

In the U.S., Doctor Pennington stated the same thing: "People can burn only small portions of carbohydrates – and any excess is turned into fat. Carbohydrates are the fat person's poison!"

Back then they didn't know that EFA-removing industrial food processing made everyone crave these carbohydrates, but they did know of the damage the carbohydrates caused.[35]

35 *Gayelord Hauser's Treasury of Secrets*, pages 382 - 385.

Once Doctors Kekwick and Parvan published their highly accurate scientific test of this diet, carried out in London's Middlesex Hospital, the medical establishment was forced to accept that "The composition of the diet can alter the expenditure of calories in obese persons, increasing it when fat and proteins are given, and decreasing it when carbohydrates are given." Translated: Fats and proteins take more energy to release their inner nutrients so you lose excess fat – fat burning increases naturally.

Here are some details of the testing of Doctors Kekwick and Parvan:

> In the 1950s Doctors Kekwick and Parvan in England published the results of a study showing that, with a diet of less than 1,000 calories a day, and 90-percent of them from fats, the patients lost significant weight. When these same patients were put on a 90-percent carbohydrate diet with the same calories, they lost no weight. We aren't told of the patients' initial states of health or weight, or whether or not they remained hungry on these particular diets.

We might have expected an increase in weight if they ate such a large amount of carbohydrates. There's a simple explanation why they didn't. First, there wasn't as much food-processing. Second, when you eat this little (close to starvation), you won't gain weight. But eating 1,000 calories a day of carbohydrates will keep you hungry. In contrast, eating 1,000 calories of fats will keep you feeling quite satisfied.

I'm not suggesting a high-fat diet. We'll discuss some of the possible negative health implications from eating excess fat later. But when it comes to losing weight, natural dietary fat can actually be quite helpful.

Keeping adequate basic essence in your system will ensure that you lose only excess fat and not muscle. Many diets or eating programs aren't really well-balanced, so you lose muscle and water along with the excess fat. This is not what we want.

Only with adequate basic essence will excess bodyfat — not muscle — be lost.

I'd like to share with you some little-known information from an article about women from Okinawa. The article is from the September 1996 issue of *Health* magazine.

"The Healthiest Women in the World"

- The island of Okinawa has been a large pork producer for hundreds of years. Pork is this country's meat staple.
- Researcher Kazuhiko Taira states: "Okinawan cuisine is very healthy – and very, very greasy."
- Leftover lard from the pork is used liberally in their food.
- Okinawans eat three times more meat than the Japanese do.
- Japan's Institute of Health and Nutrition recently stated that the Japanese "make too much of the staple food, steamed rice."
- Okinawans have far less heart disease and fewer strokes than their Japanese neighbors.
- Okinawan women have the longest life expectancy in the world: 84-plus years.

Okinawa also has minimal food processing. This is one more case where high levels of meat and fat are eaten in a particular culture and positive effects are seen.*

Most people have tremendous difficulty losing that final five to ten pounds of excess bodyfat. Exercise didn't help me lose mine, and *exercise won't help if your food intake is unbalanced.*

You will actually lose more fat, maintaining adequate basic essence and minimizing processed carbohydrates with moderate exercise than you will by vigorously exercising all day long without basic essence

Exercise plays only a minor supporting role in weight loss and cellulite removal. Exercise may help in fat loss because growth hormone is released as a result of the additional stress from exercising. It's not that a lot of calories are burned up from exercising – they aren't. Only 300 calories per hour are burned by walking, about 600 with aerobics. One pound of (exess) bodyfat has 3,500 calories, so about 12 hours of walking or 7 hours of aerobics (including warm-up and cool-down times) are required to lose just one pound of excess bodyfat, *if* you could access it immediately. Many of us don't have enough free time to seriously consider doing a lot of vigorous exercise. *Because of EFA deficiency many of us are adding more bodyfat than exercise can burn* – we can't exercise the fat away as fast as we are piling it on!

* Hormone-treated meat is harmful. The European Union has **banned** American hormone-treated beef and won't eat it. Source: *New York Times*, March 23, 1999, Section C1.

Exercise won't help eliminate cellulite, either. An entire chapter of this book is devoted to explaining what cellulite really is and how only basic essence eliminates it.

If you can't exercise a lot, don't worry. Simply make sure you take basic essence every day.

When taking EFAs, it is important to obtain a properly balanced blend. Some brands of EFA supplements use fish oil as their source of Omega 3 EFAs. It's a cheap source. We have three primary concerns regarding fish oil.

- First, fish concentrate their toxins in fat like we do. Water pollution is rampant, so you could easily be consuming lots of toxic heavy metals, PCBs, and other pollutants at the same time. A chemical pollution-removing process might remove some of these impurities, but such a process would ruin the quality of the Omega 3 and would raise the cost. This is such a significant issue that California's Proposition 65 specifically targeted fish oil manufacturers with environmental toxin levels above those allowed by law. Activists sent nineteen suppliers a letter warning them about illegal levels of DDT and DDE.[36]
- Second, how do you juice a fish? A fish doesn't lend itself easily to extracting the oil from its fat. We don't want any other part of the fish except the Omega 3. Because chemicals are required to extract the oils, nutritional value is compromised.
- Third, processed fish oils contain more than just parent Omega 3 EFA. They also contain other Omega 3-derived substances which our bodies naturally produce from the parent Omega 3. Fish oil has a preponderance of the derivatives EPA and DHA. From a *Life-Systems* Engineering analysis, this unbalances the system, because the body now has more of these by-products than it required. Once again, the system becomes artificially unbalanced. We don't need this.

36 "Prop 65 Activists Target Fish Oil," *Nutrition Science News*, Boulder, CO, November 1997, Vol. 2, No. 11, page 537.

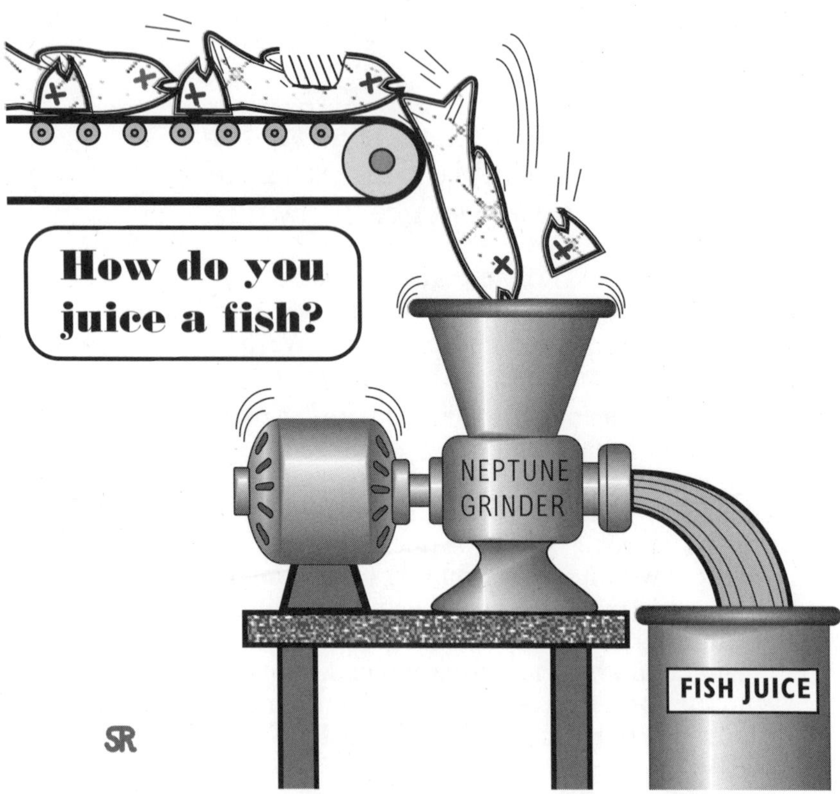

Well, you **start** with rejected fish, and then you *process* them . . .

Some manufacturers use GLA instead of parent Omega 6. GLA may be used successfully in specialized therapeutic applications such as headaches, but for a daily supplement, our *Life-Systems* team prefers parent Omega 6, because the body easily makes GLA from Omega 6 as needed, when it has the parent EFAs available. With basic essence, *you get GLA's protection from headaches, automatically.*

There is a controversy regarding the quality of synthetic infant formulas. It focuses on the use of DHA, a derivative of EFAs. This is one of the special temporary cases where a derivative of EFAs may be as important as the parent EFA. Even so, the mother's EFA deficiency directly affects the health of her child. Newborns need this derivative from their mother during their first months of life until they begin to produce it themselves. Newborns were meant to be breast-fed.

One researcher used fish oil in the formula in an attempt to provide DHA, but it didn't work.

Another researcher advised that DHA levels have dropped in mother's milk over the last 40 years. However, he says there is no sign that younger generations are less intelligent because of this deficiency, so the infants may not need it.[37]

Why are school test scores decreasing year-after-year, and why are students in the U.S. so academically poor that they aren't even mentioned in world-wide academic excellence surveys anymore? How many young cashiers at retail businesses can calculate correct change when the electronic register malfunctions? Not many. If the mothers had adequate basic essence in their diets, their newborns should really thrive!

Our *Life-Systems* team prefers *an EFA blend from 100% freshly juiced, organically grown and organically processed seeds* – without heat, fish oil, solvent-extracted oils, or derivatives.

Here's how important unadulterated fats and oils are:

The 1982 Nobel Prize for medicine was presented to Professor J.R. Vane for his work with prostaglandins. It is now known that prostaglandins help prevent heart disease. EFAs are the raw materials for prostaglandins.

As early as 1929, it was known that omega 6 promoted naturally "thinner blood," along with increasing energy levels.

"Thin blood" isn't really thinner like milk is thinner than cream. "Thin blood" means that the blood flows more easily because platelets don't stick together in the bloodstream. This is very important for protecting against heart attack and stroke. Omega 6 assists in this function to naturally maintain platelet fluidity.

Few of us are aware of these and many other important facts concerning omega 3 and omega 6. Sadly, we are deluged with story-after-story promoting carbohydrates and implying that fat in

37 "FDA Considers Changing Formulas," *Associated Press*, February 23, 1997.

our food is an evil villain. *Natural* fats keep the lipoprotein molecules from clumping together in the bloodstream, because their molecular charges repel each other. It's like two magnets of the same polarity. They can't stick – they push away from each other – naturally preventing arterial blockage. Is it the **EFA deficiency** causing the problems? This could certainly explain the American lack of cardiovascular disease in the first half of this century. Mother Nature designed us to eat meat together with natural fats and oils, including EFAs. That's why a rib-eye steak is so satisfying and fills you up for 6-8 hours, too! We have attempted to replace nature's design with imaginary ideas, and the results speak for themselves – rampant obesity, ill-health, and fatigue.

Molecular Biology of the Cell states, "The key to every biological problem must finally be sought in the cell." There's a lot of insight in that, but there's much more. Starting on page 478 of this medical textbook: "The lipid bilayer has been universally established as the universal basis for cell-membrane structure." ["Lipid" means "fat."] "Lipid molecules constitute about 50% [half] of the mass of most animal membranes – nearly all of the remainder being protein." The book further says, "The most abundant are phospholipids. These have a polar head group and two hydrophobic ['water-repelling'] hydrocarbon tails. One tail is unsaturated fat [EFAs] and the other tail is saturated fat."

Fats and proteins are the building materials for all of our cell membranes.

There's no mention of carbohydrates at all.

Notice the fact that cell membranes contain lots of EFAs and saturated fat – the "dreaded saturated fat" we've been told to avoid at all costs!

The scientific and medical truth is the opposite of what we often hear day-in and day-out. This medical textbook is among the most authoritative ever published. Let's look at who wrote it. *Molecular Biology of The Cell* is authored by: Bruce Alberts – Ph.D., Harvard, and Professor of Biochemistry and Biophysics; Dennis Bray – Ph.D., M.I.T., and medical research fellow at Oxford; Julian Lewis – Ph.D., Oxford; Martin Raff – MD from McGill; Keith Roberts –

head of Cell Biology at John Innes Institute; and James D. Watson, Nobel Prize-winner for discovery of the structure of DNA.[38]

Most nutritionists and dieting specialists maintain that it's not all the food that makes you fat, but just the fat that makes you fat. It sounds so logical on the surface that we are easily led to think that it should be correct, but it is not correct. The body isn't designed this way. *This theory doesn't hold up to real-life experience.*

Others will maintain that it doesn't matter what you eat, it's how your body processes it. There is only a seed of truth here. Give a car the wrong fuel, and there is no adjustment you can make for it to run well. Period.

Without this fundamental knowledge about basic essence, no successful long-term solution for cellulite and weight-loss is possible.

A nutritional theory had better work for me, and it must work for you, too, or it is incorrect. It must work every time. That is the bottom line. One difficult issue for researchers is the variances between individuals. For example, one would expect some degree of metabolic difference between a "couch potato" and a world-class athlete. Basic essence is one of the absolutely essential requirements for all of us, and its importance must be recognized by anyone attempting to understand nutrition.

A scientist looks at the outcome of an experiment, then tries to explain why the particular result occurred. When current theory (guesses) don't predict all of the results, sometimes a new, even radical, theory is needed. In the early 1920s, work in quantum physics followed this pattern. Strange results occurred when physicists tried to explain how electrons acted. Conventional theory couldn't explain it, so a new theory had to be developed. This theory seemed very, very strange, but it worked 100 percent of the time and predicted exactly what was seen.

38 We have not personally consulted with these authors concerning *Life-System* Engineering views.

A Case study: an all-meat diet.

There was a famous study done in 1929 and 1930. Two explorers, Vilhjalmur Stefansson and Karsten Anderson, returned from the Arctic with a surprising report. Innuit people (Eskimos) could live on almost nothing except caribou meat, including natural fats, all winter with no adverse effects. In fact, the Eskimos had tremendous energy. The explorers were intrigued enough to volunteer to eat a high-meat, high-fat diet for a year under supervision at Bellevue Hospital in New York. They consumed 75 percent of their calories from meat and fat, consuming about 2,500 calories a day. The results? After one year, the men lost about five pounds each. They had normal cholesterol levels and other related blood-chemistry levels. They were in fine shape.

My wife used to crave a favorite ice cream from a local shop. After just three months of eating basic essence, her taste changed so much that she couldn't believe she once liked it. Her new favorite is an all-natural vanilla. Unlike the old brand, which was full of additives, this brand uses no additives or artificial flavors. She prefers the all-natural brand now, but she only wants about a quarter of a serving. Plus, in just 90 days, her cellulite decreased by more than half and she dropped a dress size, too.

A low-fat diet did not reduce my love handles. As a personal test, I lived on a diet of more than 40 percent fat for 90 days and lost most of my love handles! Recall all of our information which shows that dietary fat *does NOT* turn into excess bodyfat.

Protein

No one should suffer protein deficiency – there's no shortage of meat, fish, poultry, eggs or cheese in this country. Yet, many people suffer a protein deficiency as a result of their quest for low-fat foods. Natural fats are a significant part of most natural protein. Mother Nature designed it that way. By avoiding foods that contain natural fats and oils, you may unknowingly cut out some critical protein, too!

If protein has gotten a bad rap, it is probably because protein is usually associated with fat and we have been led to believe that fat is bad for us. If you mention eating a juicy steak to someone, they are likely to remark about "all that *bad* fat." Furthermore, our protein requirements are playing second-fiddle to the highly promoted king, carbohydrate. Inadequate protein leads to system imbalance. **A 150-pound person requires a full pound of protein per day for normal bodily processes* — much of this requires dietary replacement.** Let's make a *Life-Systems Engineering* assessment of your needs.

With a protein shortage, you won't die, but your body can't rebuild itself, so degenerative diseases set in, and grow progressively worse. Continued ill-health is your reward.

From protein, we get amino acids – the building blocks of muscle. Amino acids are vital to many other bodily functions, too, including all enzymes (which aid in the digestion of foods), the production of energy, the building of new tissue, the tearing down of old tissue, making hemoglobin (the iron-containing substance of the red corpuscles), hormones, and even DNA.

Proteins also help prevent the blood and tissue from becoming either too acid or too alkaline. They are important in blood clotting. Proteins even form antibodies, which combine with and render harmless the bacteria, bacterial toxins, and other foreign materials that act as poisons in the blood. When proteins are not supplied to carry on these many functions, the body is susceptible to sickness and even premature death. About fifty percent of our body weight is protein. Significant dietary protein is critical to our well-being.

We aren't just burning protein for fuel; we need it for cellular structure.

Just like basic essence, *Basic Medical Biochemistry* (page 7) tells us that **amino acids are used in the cellular structure and don't go to excess bodyfat — in fact, carnitine (a non-essential amino acid) is required for fat-burning.****

There are twenty amino acids. The human body can produce only eleven of the twenty. That leaves nine which are called "*essential*

---

* *Basic Medical Biochemistry*, page 648.

** *Essentials of Biochemistry*, page 220.

amino acids," because they must come from the food we eat.[39] Amino acids, the building blocks of protein, along with EFAs, are the basis of life. Amino acids are much easier to obtain from foods than EFAs, because quality protein is readily available in lots of foods – even some processed products.

The *essential* amino acids

Histidine	Isoleucine	Leucine
Lysine	Methionine	Phenylalanine
Threonine	Tryptophan	Valine

Our body uses protein for muscle manufacture and muscle maintenance. It is important to eat sufficient protein, *especially when you do physical work or vigorous exercise.* Your body requires protein to maintain or increase the size of your muscles. Eat more protein a few hours before going to the gym or running and see how much better you feel compared to the high-carbohydrate approach.

Food bills will actually go down – even though protein may cost more than carbohydrate. With basic essence you need less food.

There's another important bit of information you should know. Not all proteins are created equal. Outdated analyses focused on measuring the amount of protein consumed ignoring how much was absorbed.

Protein absorption is clearly a more meaningful measure. This measure is called the Biological Value (BV); it measures the amount of protein retained in the body in relation to how much is eaten. A whole egg is rated as 100. Brown rice and beans are 59 percent and 49 percent, respectively.[40] Therefore, *the utilization of the protein in rice and beans is only approximately half of the protein utilization from eating an egg.* AND *there is not very much protein in beans and rice.*

To obtain meaningful levels of usable protein from these vegetable sources requires that you eat tremendous amounts of

39 *Molecular Biology of the Cell*, page 74.

40 "The Protein Primrose Path," Dr. Michael Colgan, Ph.D., CNN, *All Natural Muscular Development,* May 1997, page 34.

them. The downside? They are loaded with carbohydrates and will send your blood glucose (sugar) levels soaring! Plus large amounts will add to excess bodyfat. The conclusion? Humans are meant to live on a diet that includes meat.

Vegetarians can easily become protein-deficient.

They often develop high blood glucose levels relying on the traditional *theory* of mixing foods such as rice and beans to make a "complete" protein. Surprise — Most niacin in cereal grains has low bioavailability (it can't be used).*

Many nutritionists will tell you that eating lots of protein with few carbohydrates will cause health problems. We are told that, with higher protein and lower carbohydrates, the body then starts converting muscle tissue to glucose for energy, and it will hurt your kidneys by overloading them with so much protein. But does that really happen once EFA-deficiency is eliminated? No, not at all. New research has proven this old myth incorrect. Protein is fine for your kidneys. Glutamine (protein-derived) removes toxic ammonia from your blood so you don't die, and an impeccably performed 1995 study proved it.[41**]

Here are two more reasons why we need more protein and less carbohydrate:

1) Virtually everyone in the US today eats lots of carbohydrate, so this muscle cannibalization can't occur. With carbohydrates being so plentiful, it's virtually impossible for anyone not to eat enough of them. In fact, just two apples will give you most of the carbohydrates you need for the entire day.
2) Basic essence eliminates the short-circuit that could cause muscle cannibalism.

With the Foundation of Radiant Health, your taste works properly with your hunger. You can eat whatever your body wants. Don't let anyone tell you what they think you need. *With the proper nutrients, your body will tell you what it wants.*

Any bodybuilder will attest to how difficult it is to build extra muscle. I trained in the gym for years under professional guidance. Bodybuilders have my utmost respect. Does it make sense that the body would so quickly cannibalize this muscle that was so difficult

41 *Protein Power*, Michael Eads, M.D., and Mary Dan Eades, M.D., Bantam Books, New York, 1996, page 188.

* *Basic Medical Biochemistry*, page 16. ** *Basic Medical Biochemistry*, page 653.

to create when it has access to stored bodyfat? No, it doesn't. If this process does happen, a Life-System is drastically screwed-up. The problem can arise only if there aren't enough EFAs in the system. Basic essence eliminates the short-circuit in the body's natural control system, by satisfying the appestat.

Is a condition called "ketosis" something we should be concerned about? No. Ketones are produced when fat breaks down for use by the body. This is a completely natural and required process. You should be more concerned about a shortage of ketones! Many health writers completely misunderstand this topic, and they may have done great damage with their misinformation. The heart prefers ketones to all other fuels. By not feeding the heart enough of its preferred fuel we may be contributing to its premature failure.

Is lack of ketones resulting from low-fat diets adding to the dramatic rise in heart disease? A *Life-Systems* Engineering analysis says YES.

Dr. Lubert Stryer, Professor of Biochemistry at Stanford University, and the author of a biochemistry textbook used in many medical schools, states: "Ketones are normal fuels of respiration and are quantitatively important sources of energy."[42] This fact is rarely mentioned by popular health writers.

Unless you are a type I diabetic producing virtually no insulin whatsoever, or you have some other compromising condition, ketosis cannot occur unless you eat meat or fish to the exclusion of everything else.[43] You'd feel terrible eating like this day-after-day. When I tried to eat nothing but protein while taking basic essence, my body wouldn't let me do it. I simply didn't feel well. The Eskimo (Innuit) cultures don't get ketosis on their higher-fat, higher-protein diet, but they also don't eat zero carbohydrates. They eat few carbohydrates.

Your body's natural hunger won't allow this type of imbalance to continue. While eating basic essence, you would use up all your fat stores first before your body would cannibalize your muscle.

---

42 *Protein Power*, pages 195-196.

43 A diabetic with extremely high glucose levels (400-500), lacking insulin, will enter a state of ketosis, but this is a highly non-typical systemic state *caused by a hormone deficiency.*

Indeed, only if you ate no fat whatsoever (extended hospitalization could deplete fat reserves), or if you were an untreated type I diabetic, could your body cannibalize its muscle for energy. An average person in today's modern society doesn't have a chance of this happening.

It has recently been discovered that, if you eat massive amounts of protein to the exclusion of everything else, your insulin will increase, because your body doesn't want huge excesses of amino acids, just as it doesn't want excess carbohydrates. Once again, basic essence comes to the rescue. You simply won't have food cravings to eat this way anymore.

We are sometimes told that high-protein diets cause you to lose weight, then gain it all back. How much is considered high protein? Is it 20 percent, 50 percent, 90 percent, or what? One thing is certain:

With adequate EFAs, it is more difficult to overindulge in any food group, because *your body's feedback naturally instructs you not to.*

Eating pure protein without any natural fats and oils won't satisfy your appetite for long. Mother Nature designed us this way. A protein-filled breakfast of bacon and organically raised eggs, fried in organic butter, with one slice of toast, is a delicious, welcome replacement for the cereal and milk which so many of us quickly wolf down each morning. That is, if you even have an interest in breakfast anymore after eliminating your EFA deficiency. The bacon and eggs take a bit longer to prepare, but are much more satisfying and won't pack on the weight.

A dinner of chopped steak with mushrooms sauteed in butter wins hands-down to a bowl of spaghetti and a roll. *You can eat spaghetti, but now you'll desire a much smaller portion.*

Many people are familiar with the notion that "too much" protein causes harm to the kidneys. This mistake appears to have been based on analyzing diabetic patients and drawing a wrong conclusion. The real cause of their problem was high glucose (sugar) levels causing proteins to become surrounded by glucose molecules (glycosylation). This causes abnormal protein spillover into the urine. Normally, the blood proteins are repelled by the kidney's pores and don't overflow into the urine.

Move over, "Food Pyramid"
Enter the Foundation of Radiant Health

The Food Pyramid, inspired by the cereal industry, has become a familiar sight since its introduction.

This "politically correct" Food Pyramid is clearly a complete nutrition failure as experienced by the majority of us. We are struggling with obesity and ill-health, because the pyramid does not provide the results we wish to achieve.

Life-Systems Engineering is the science of maximizing desired results by working cooperatively with the natural processes of living systems. Real-life results must be accurately and consistently explained. Our new understanding shows us that the Foundation of Radiant Health is really what we need. It looks like this:

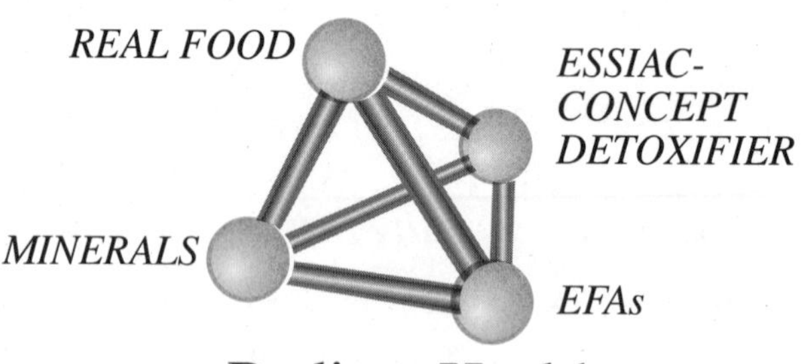

Radiant Health

With the Foundation of Radiant Health, we can eat what we desire and our body will offer feedback if we need other nutrients. Our hunger and taste finally work together, as they were meant to.

Special information for vegetarians

It is important to understand three points concerning amino acids, the building blocks of proteins:

1. You need each of the nine essential amino acids in the quantities correct for proper building of the body.
2. An excess of one of the essential amino acids won't help replace a deficient amino acid.
3. *Without enough total "complete" protein* consumption, even if you obtain enough of each essential amino acid, many of the essential amino acids will be sacrificed because they will give up their nitrogen for other life-system needs.

Concerning utilization of protein from animal vs. vegetable (plant) sources, the bioavailability (our body's ability to use them) of plant-based protein is much lower – usually about 40% less than animal-based or fish-based protein sources. Plant-based protein is naturally combined with indigestible cellulose. Our body can't use the cellulose, so much of the protein goes right through us!

A non-vegetarian gets more than enough of all the essential amino acids from a combination of two eggs, four oz. of cheese, and one-third pound of chicken or equivalent per day.

> ***Surprise!* An egg's yolk contains more protein than the white (16% for the yolk and 11% for the white). This is 50% more than the white! We keep getting just one side of the story from the "low-fat, high-carbohydrate" defenders.**

A vegetarian has a much harder time obtaining his or her essential protein requirements. For proper growth, a *Life-Systems* Engineering analysis suggests we take three to four times the RDAs.[44] RDAs are only meant as a life-sustaining amount – not an amount for radiant health. Furthermore, protein isn't 100% bioavailable to the body, no matter how good its quality – no food is. *Eggs are the highest in protein bioavailability* so they are considered as 100% *for comparison with other foods*. Other high-protein foods are as low as 50%! Because of the cellulose/protein-inhibiting factor, a vegetarian should consume at least four times the RDAs of essential amino acids. This is one step that is essential for radiant health.

Real dairy cheese is an excellent source of the essential amino acids. Cheese is high in natural fat, and it goes a long way in protein content, too. Two eggs give you about one-quarter of the essential protein for a day. A quarter-pound of cheese is good for almost a third of your requirements. A third of a cup of tofu will only give you 10 percent of most of the essential amino acids, but at least it is with very little carbohydrate. Three ounces of mixed nuts will give you about 15 percent. A quarter-pound of wheat pasta will give you 10 percent, but close to 1,000 calories of carbohydrate (metabolically equivalent to 50 tsp. sugar). Three-quarters cup of

44 These levels are still well below what most nutritionists consider "mega-doses," at above 10 times the RDAs.

rice will give you five-percent of the essential amino acids but with high carbohydrates. Sunflower or sesame seeds are a good source – just two ounces give you about 10-percent with only 50 carbohydrate calories. EFAs derived from seed will help supply these essential amino acids, although not in significant amounts.[45]

It is very difficult to obtain enough of these nine essential amino acids each day without animal-based sources.

Rice and beans are actually a terrible way to get your protein. Three-quarters cup of white rice and three-quarters cup black beans gives you a whopping 800 calories of carbohydrate and only 20-percent of protein requirements.[46]

Rice and beans have been called "complementary" proteins because rice is low in lysine and beans are much higher in lysine. Overall, the combination is significantly lower in essential amino acids than any meat and fish combinations.

"Complementary" does not mean adequate. If you choose not to eat meat, fish, cheese, or eggs, then please read the *Food and Nutrition Encyclopedia* to get a more realistic understanding of what you're up against. As you will see, obtaining the essential nutrients from exclusively vegetarian sources is not easy.

We frequently hear vegetarians tell us the longer they go without eating meat, the more their system reacts when they do eat meat– stomach discomfort, indigestion, etc. Some attribute this change to some form of beneficial personal transformation.

While researching the metabolism of proteins, we learned that the more protein deficient one is, the more impaired the digestive system becomes. In fact, **when one is deficient in essential amino acids, it is very common to experience digestive upset when protein is eaten in any significant quantity.** *The body's need is still there; it's just that the digestion function has been impaired and the needed protein must be reintroduced gradually to avoid destabilizing the system.* Shortage of essential protein may also account for a shortage of enzymes the body uses in digestion.

> No matter what your source of protein, your body still depends on essential nutrients in the Foundation of Radiant Health.

45 *Bowes & Church's Food Values*, 1997.
46 *Bowes & Church's Food Values.*

Is Cholesterol A Scapegoat?

> *"It is far more important to increase intake of unsaturated fats than to decrease intake of saturated fats."*
>
> Michael F. Oliver, M.D. Source: *American Journal of Clinical Nutrition,* " Fats and Oil Consumption in Health and Disease," October 1997; 66: 4(S)

"... because the students had been taught how to learn by rote from books and lectures, without any understanding.... The students had learned a list of facts, but *had no idea what the facts really meant, and no understanding....*"[1] [emphasis added]

" ... Details that could throw doubt on your interpretation must be given, if you know them. If you make a theory, for example, and advertise it, or put it out, then *you must also put down all the facts that disagree with it, as well as those that agree with it.*"[2] (emphasis added)

These are principles that all researchers should follow. Too many researchers neglect to mention all of the evidence in conflict with their pet theory. **This analysis by Professor Feynman, a Nobel Prize-winner, helps to explain why cholesterol is broadly misunderstood by so many in the nutritional communities.** Professor Feynman would have been delighted to read our STAT-SMART chapter giving you the tools so *you can evaluate a study's reported conclusions for yourself.*

"Technology Follies" in the *Journal of the American Medical Association* (269:3030; 1993) states, "Much, if not most of the contemporary medical practices still lack scientific foundation." This problem explains the "Great Cholesterol Hoax."

Listed below are some examples of the many studies about cholesterol, diet and heart disease:

St. Mary's Hospital Trial (1965)
London Research Committee Trial (1965)
Norwegian Trial (1966)

1 *Richard Feynman, A Life In Science*, John and Mary Gribbin, Penguin Books, New York, NY, 1997, page 144.

2 *Richard Feynman, A Life In Science*, page 217.

Anti-Coronary Club Trial (1965)
London Medical Research Council Trial (1968)
National Diet Heart Study (1968)
Finnish Mental Hospital Trial (1968)
Los Angeles Veterans' Trial (1968)
Framingham Study (1970)
Ireland-Boston Heart Study (1970)
St. Vincent's Hospital Trial (1973)
Diet and Coronary Heart Disease Study in England (1974)
Edinburgh-Stockholm Study (1975)
Minnesota Study (1975)
UCLA Study (1975)
Honolulu-Japanese Study (1975).

How many more studies do we need?

No vegetable oil or plant product has any naturally occurring cholesterol – cholesterol comes only from animals.

Don't be fooled by special claims and labels.

The margarine companies must really love it when the media trumpets the "no-cholesterol" aspect of their product. All sorts of products have "no-cholesterol" plastered all over their packaging. Actually, *since cholesterol comes only from animal sources,* ***any plant-based product will be cholesterol-free****!*

Some people think it's important, yet, it has been known for years that dietary cholesterol doesn't significantly influence the body's blood cholesterol. Your own body churns out 3,000-4,000 milligrams of cholesterol each day, no matter how much or how little cholesterol you eat. *So, should we really care about low-cholesterol foods?* Not from a *Life-Systems* Engineering view.

For many years, margarine's "no-cholesterol" label has distracted us from the issue of its possible harm. The vegetable oils in margarine are chemically processed and partially hydrogenated.[3] This process destroys many EFAs that could still be present. Also, how healthy are the various chemicals and additives in margarine?

3 "Hydrogenation" is the chemical addition of hydrogen to another chemical. When applied to oils, the process turns the healthy essential oils into dangerous transfatty acids, which are unhealthy for humans.

You can easily prove to yourself that dietary cholesterol has minimal influence on blood cholesterol levels once EFA-deficiency is corrected. Ask your physician about obtaining a blood cholesterol and triglyceride (blood fats) test. Afterwards, eat more of the higher cholesterol-containing foods while eating basic essence. Then get another test, three months later. The laboratory test is relatively inexpensive. There probably won't be a significant difference, or the HDL may increase (considered "good"). The triglycerides will probably decrease, too (also considered good).

Most of the popular nutritional buzz words focus almost exclusively on how foods affect us in one specific area. While this focus can be useful, we should be aware of how foods affect us in an overall *Life-Systems* fashion. Unfortunately, the weight of today's public and professional attention is targeted toward cholesterol reduction.

There is no finer example of the application of incomplete understanding than the intensity of monitoring dietary cholesterol and blood cholesterol levels almost to the exclusion of anything else.

Fat in our food (which supposedly leads to excess cholesterol in our blood) often gets a bad rap. Yet, how is the Innuit (Eskimo) "paradox" explained? The Innuit live on an extremely high-fat, high-protein diet. They may have higher blood cholesterol levels, too. Yet virtually no atherosclerosis (obstructive clogging) is found. Their arteries remain free of cholesterol buildup (plaque). Can this be explained by a genetic difference? While it is possible, there is a more plausible explanation.

Innuits eat much more raw, unprocessed meat than we do. Their food comes from the wild. Guess what they get in that wild meat and fish – *unprocessed EFAs.* **They also get no chemicals, hormones, steroids, or other harmful food additives.** Time-after-time we see this pattern when looking at a healthier culture or race. Remember the healthy, pork-eating Okinawans? Healthy EFAs are a common element with each of those cultures, and they have no significant heart-related problems. Could these cultures' exceptional health be based simply on the lack of food processing?

A *Life-Systems* Engineering analysis strongly suggests that it is an EFA-deficiency that results in cholesterol-related problems.

It is not caused by eating too much natural fat.

In recent years, cholesterol has often been blamed for heart attacks and strokes. Heart attacks are tragic events, and I am also deeply saddened every time I hear about another person who has a stroke. Although heart attacks and strokes are two different things, they are both related to problems with blood circulation.

At least 60% of people who suffer heart attacks do not have elevated cholesterol levels.

Here, once again, is a gross inconsistency. *Blaming cholesterol levels as the cause of the problem, when there is no correlation and no evidence of cause-and-effect relationship is an example of poor science.* Looking at this statistic and then even considering there might be a cause-and-effect relationship doesn't make any sense. We can only logically state that there are almost as many heart attacks in people with elevated cholesterol levels as there are with lower cholesterol levels. **We have to conclude that elevated cholesterol levels cannot be the cause of heart attacks.**

We will find, time-and-time-again, that properly conducted studies about cholesterol don't show cholesterol to be the direct cause of any problems. The problem is in how the companies who pay for these studies present the findings.

Let's look at what was said in the *Condensed Chemical Dictionary* over 20 years ago.[4] This is the "bible" of scientific chemistry. They had no political agenda or money to be made by promoting any specific viewpoint.

- Under "cholesterol": Dr. W. Stanley Hartroft is quoted, "It still has not been shown that lowering the cholesterol in the blood by this amount [20%] will have any protective effect for the heart and vessels against the development of atheroma and the onset of serious complications."

---

4 *Condensed Chemical Dictionary*, VanNostrad Reinhold & Company, 1977.

- Under "fatty acid": "There is still no conclusive proof that increase in body cholesterol as a result of high dietary intake of animal derived saturated fats or fatty acids is causatively related to atherosclerosis [clogged arteries]."

The chemical facts haven't changed since 1977, yet there has been an explosive growth of industries making incredible profits based on cholesterol measurement, low-cholesterol foods and cholesterol-reducing drugs.

This information isn't new, yet it is still not widely publicized. Back in 1973, research sponsored by the Food and Nutrition Board of the National Research Council confirmed that:

There is no significant link between cholesterol in the diet and cholesterol in the blood.

They advocated not restricting fat or cholesterol.

This fact has been known for more than 30 years! Here's the quote from *Martinis and Whipped Cream* published in 1966:

Question: Is it true that high-fat diets can cause hardening of the arteries and heart trouble?

Answer: **There is controversy that is still unsolved by the medical profession.** Cholesterol, a type of bodyfat, was discovered to be present in cases of atherosclerosis, a thickening of the walls of the arteries said to be an underlying cause of most heart trouble. It was therefore thought that high-fat diets caused these maladies. Immediately, the word went out to get artery and heart patients off poly-unsaturated fats. But *later observations showed that there were two types of cholesterol and the one that appeared to be the trouble-maker was not limited to foods, but was also produced by peoples' bodies.* It was also discovered that **levels of both types of cholesterol did not seem to have any relationship with diet**. All of this uncertainty is eclipsed by the unquestioned fact that **you will lose weight on a high protein, low carbohydrate diet, and weighing less will be good for you**. (emphasis added)[5]

Note: Between 1994 and 2000, numerous published (impartial) studies conclusively showed carbohydrates, not unprocessed fats, are indeed the culprit (see the timeline in the front of the book). Why haven't we been told?

5 *Martinis and Whipped Cream*, 1966 page 33.

This finding is still largely ignored. Fat and dietary cholesterol continue to be improperly blamed for arterial problems. Will it take another 25 years for the establishment to admit they were mistaken again?

Cholesterol can't be the cause of cardiovascular disease (CVD).

1. Cholesterol levels have remained relatively constant over the past 100 years while CVD has increased significantly.
2. The body makes the cholesterol it needs, no matter what the amount of cholesterol in your food. **The body must have it to function**.

The body maintains a relatively constant level of cholesterol according to its needs. This fact is rarely mentioned and is downplayed when it is mentioned.

More than one in three people have blood cholesterol levels between 150 and 200. William P. Castelli, MD, medical director of the Framingham Cardiovascular Institute, directed a study over a 16-year period. He reports that *twice as many people with life-long cholesterol levels in this range have heart attacks as do people with cholesterol over 300*![6] **Cholesterol, in and of itself, isn't a cause of heart problems.**

Dr. L. Maximilian Buja, dean of the University of Texas Medical School at Houston, agrees that there is more to be understood. He states, "There is no question that the inflammatory process in vessel walls is very important to the progression of atherosclerosis. **The question is what triggers it?**"(emphasis added)[7]

Even though cholesterol may be present, the essential question, "Why is it there?" is seldom asked and never really answered. Without understanding the basic essence-nutrition connection, cholesterol may continue to be blamed.

The LDL (low-density lipoproteins) carry critical basic essence EFAs to the cells.[8]

Without EFAs in our cells we'd die.

6 "Identifying At-Risk Population for Heart Disease," *Energy Times*, March 1997, page 10.

7 "Study Finds Apparent Trigger of Heart Attacks and Strokes," *New York Times*, April 3, 1997, page A13.

8 *Enter the Zone*, page 121.

Yet, we continue to hear about how "bad" the LDL transporter is and that it should be minimized at all costs.

Could this constant pressure to lower the LDL-based cholesterol be a direct cause of our massive increases in illness today, including: chronic fatigue, chronic obesity, and chronic diabetes levels? **A *Life-Systems* Engineering analysis says YES.** This is a good example of complete misunderstanding by the nutritional communities about how our *Life-Systems* actually work!

Consider these important facts about cholesterol:

- Cholesterol is produced by the body in large quantities relative to other substances.
- All cells contain it and all tissues make it.
- Cholesterol is so important that every cell regulates its own level internally.
- Cholesterol gives cell membranes their integrity and strength; without cholesterol, we'd be soft, flabby, and worm-like – about the consistency of a jellyfish hung on a skeleton.
- Cholesterol enhances the permeability-barrier properties of the lipid bilayer.[9] This is critical for proper cell nutrition!
- Bone would be hollow and brittle if it weren't for cholesterol and protein.
- Cholesterol has a major structural role in the brain, where it is found in high concentrations.
- Cholesterol enables nerve impulses.
- Vitamin D is made from the interaction between cholesterol and sunlight hitting your skin, so that calcium can be utilized.
- Bile, manufactured by the liver and essential for proper fat digestion, is produced from cholesterol.[10]
- Cholesterol is essential for the liver and intestines to function properly.
- Cholesterol protects the skin against absorption of water-soluble toxins.

9 *Molecular Biology of the Cell*, page 481.

10 A major portion of the body's cholesterol is used by the liver to produce bile salts. These salts are crucial in digestion to make sure that fats get broken down and that oil-soluble vitamins (A, D, E, and K) are utilized.

- It holds moisture in so we don't dehydrate. Cholesterol will give your skin a nice, naturally moisturized feel.

With so many major functions, how could one ever come to the conclusion that cholesterol is negative in any sense of the word? Without a lot of it, we would all quickly die.

A paper titled "Controlling Cholesterol" was published by the Physicians' Committee for Responsible Medicine. It was shocking that several points in *the paper and its recommendations were exactly opposite to established research.* This paper came out in the 1990s, so the authors should have been aware of the latest research. If they weren't, then they shouldn't be publishing recommendations. People are relying on accurate, current information. At the very least, authors should present the latest facts and let us decide for ourselves what we wish to do with the information.

Incorrect, misleading, or unfounded items in the report include:

- Claims that cholesterol is minimally important in only a few cell functions and is a very minor substance.

Not true. Cholesterol is abundantly produced and is one of the most important substances in your body. Review the list above.

- LDLs (low density lipoproteins) encourage the growth of plaque deposits.

Not true. They don't encourage anything.[11] LDLs transport cholesterol and the essential EFAs to the cell. This is a critical function. If something elsewhere goes haywire, it's not the fault of LDLs. There is no cause-effect relationship as implied in the report.

- Saturated fats should be avoided.

Saturated fats are required for proper membrane integrity. The *Condensed Chemical Dictionary* states that saturated fats give required rigidity and support to the cell wall. *Molecular Biology of the Cell* agrees. There is a natural

---

11 Current researchers now think that the cholesterol transported by the LDL mechanism becomes oxidized. This makes some sense. However, this is a different issue. It's like saying that spoiled meat can kill you if eaten, and, therefore, all meat is inherently bad. Except in rare situations, the bottom line is that cholesterol shouldn't require forced control. Nor should any automatically regulated life-system.

balance between rigidity and flexibility. You don't want one without the other. Too stiff makes the cell wall brittle and easily breakable. Too flexible and it always bends. One without the other doesn't work.

• Weight can be lost using a "low-fat" diet.

This method has already been shown to be harmful for two reasons. First, it causes an even greater shortage of EFAs. Second, the committee suggested eating more carbohydrates in place of fats, and we have already seen the problems with insulin and high-carbohydrate diets. Never mind that low-fat diets also clearly do not work – over 50 percent of American adults are now overweight, now that many of us have been relying on the low-fat concept for more than 15 years.

• Eat lots of small meals. They even cite a study with people eating seventeen snacks a day! This method is supposed to have lowered cholesterol levels compared to three-meal-a-day eaters.

They don't say how much the level was lowered. Whether it was a significant amount or not remains unanswered. This doesn't make *Life-Systems* sense. Most of us could not eat seventeen times a day. Furthermore, the continuous insulin-release from this frequent eating is extremely dangerous – over time you'll destroy your pancreas. It is better to eat as few times a day as possible to minimize the insulin response. A study like this can be meaningless, especially when significant details are missing. This is an example of looking at one issue (cholesterol levels) to the exclusion of everything else.

• Exercise raises HDL levels, yet may lower LDL levels.

How significant was the HDL rise? Why is one (HDL) absolute and the other (LDL) only a possibility? Exercise either lowers LDL or it doesn't. This point also assumes that HDL is desirable while LDL is undesirable.

• They say exercise doesn't have to be terribly vigorous.

How much is vigorous?

• They say a daily half-hour walk is helpful.

What does "helpful" mean – compared to what? What results can be expected?

Does their analysis leave you wondering? Perhaps it is this sort of report that prompted the writing of an article called "Technology Follies," published in the *New England Journal of Medicine*.

> "As noted by Pickering, medical education in the United States is, to a large extent, worship at the improbable shrine of useless knowledge. We produce 'scientific illiterates'...**who are not scientific in their approach to clinical questions or new technologies!**
>
> *...New is not synonymous with improved....*
>
> Twenty years ago, the well-being of the fetus late in pregnancy was measured by analyzing the woman's urine. **This was ultimately shown to be worthless**."[12] (emphasis added)

Before cholesterol can form plaque on arterial walls, something has to make it come out of its liquid state and solidify.

We can't assume cholesterol is responsible just because it is found at the site.

If I am at a crime scene, does it automatically make me guilty? No, it doesn't. Not any more than all the other people at the scene. It may make me seem suspect, but that's not enough to convict. If cholesterol did spontaneously build up by itself and form plaque, all our capillaries would quickly plug and we'd all die in a matter of hours. Arterial walls normally are very slick – like a non-stick coating. However, after a tear, scuff or chemical injury on the inner arterial wall, a cholesterol "scab" can form. This is similar to the scab that forms when you cut your skin – except it happens on the inside, and the way it happens is somewhat different.

Plaque buildup occurs as part of the protective healing process. Actually, the arterial buildup (plaque) is composed of fifteen or so different materials: calcium (yes, calcium), cholesterol, triglycerides, phospholipids, etc. What's obvious is that a major malfunction over several years has taken place in the body to cause this buildup. Buildups happen when artery walls have been

---

12 "Technology Follies," *New England Journal of Medicine*, 331:674, 1994.

attacked by insulin, Xanthine Oxidase (XO),[13] and other substances that are toxic to the artery wall. **Constant abuse of the artery walls causes excessive buildup.**

Obviously, we want to avoid injuries to our arteries. How can we ensure that the arterial wall doesn't develop an internal injury? Later, I discuss a remarkable nutritional drink – Essiac-concept tonic – that has a non-stick property and helps keep plaque from sticking.

The nutrition establishment is slowly coming around to the indisputable fact that cholesterol, in and of itself, doesn't cause cardiovascular problems. The American College of Physicians (ACP) stated in 1996 that regular cholesterol testing isn't necessary for everyone. According to its new guidelines, men under age 35, women under age 45, or persons over 75 don't need a test unless they smoke or have a family history of heart disease, high blood pressure, or diabetes. For healthy men 35 to 65 and women 45 to 65, testing is "appropriate but not mandatory." The American College of Physicians says there's little evidence that lowering cholesterol in such individuals helps prevent illness or death.[14]

The recent rage is to try and blame cardiovascular problems on a virus – in particular, chlamydia pneumonia. An article in *Newsweek* (August 11, 1997) states that, whatever their age, sex, or nationality, people with sclerotic arteries tend to show signs of infection. They say this bug never shows up in otherwise healthy tissue. Yet, as the article clearly states, "**Finding the bug at the crime scene doesn't prove it's a criminal**." (emphasis added)

The article asks the question, "Do fat and cholesterol make us sick by themselves, or only in the company of this bug?" *Hurrahs for the article's author, Geoffrey Cowley, for at least raising a question!*

A subsequent, more in-depth article appeared in the November/December issue of *Health* magazine.[15] The article starts by admitting that cholesterol, in and of itself, is not the cause of heart attacks because high cholesterol doesn't generate higher occurrences of real-life cardiovascular disease.

---

13 See chapter 9, "Milk: Does it *Really* Do a Body Good?"

14 "Cholesterol Controversy," *Your Health*, August 20, 1997.

15 "Could You Catch a Heart Attack?" Michael J. Mason, *Health*, November/December, 1997, pages 90-94.

ARTERY WALL
I DON'T CARE. SOMEONE'S GOT TO PAY! YOU'LL DO!!
BUT OFFICER! I'M NOT GUILTY! I WAS JUST TRYING TO FIX IT!
CHOLESTEROL
CHOLESTEROL
CHOLESTEROL POLICE

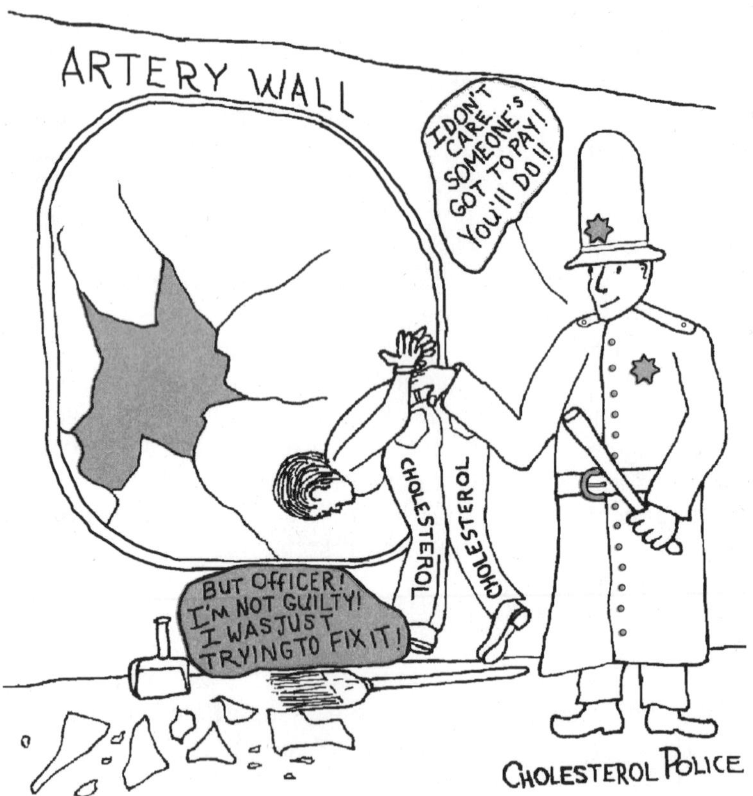

The article mentions a study where over half the cardiovascular victims carried antibodies to this virus. It refers to another study: "People with and without blocked arteries were likely to have antibodies to *C. pneumonia*, they found, but levels averaged 25 percentage points higher among the heart patients." From a *Life-Systems* Engineering analysis, this implies:

EFA deficiencies and mineral deficiencies weaken our immune system so that infection is more likely to occur.

An attack in the cardiovascular system is as likely as anywhere else in the body, but **because we are deficient in prostaglandins, the arteries may weaken quickly**.

In the article, epidemiologist Thomas Grayson states, "Of course, the association doesn't prove anything, either. The organism could be present without causing the disease." Paul Ridker, cardiologist at Harvard Medical School, states, "People are making a very big deal out of these observations. There are a dozen other plausible explanations."

Hurrahs for both of them – *they don't draw a cause-effect conclusion, because the evidence isn't strong enough*. The evidence here is on the order of cholesterol evidence – lacking in a definitive cause-effect relationship.

Another drug company bonanza may be in store. Margaret Hammerschlag, a chlamydia researcher, has a fear:

"I'm telling you, they are going to start putting azithromycin [an antibiotic] in the drinking water."

She fears widespread *use of powerful antibiotics could create drug resistance* in other germs that attack the respiratory system, even in *C. pneumonia* itself.

Do you fear the possibility of a new wave of "preventive" antibiotic drugs similar to the suggestions of "preventive" cholesterol-lowering drugs? Once again, the Foundation of Radiant Health comes to the rescue.

Prostaglandins, which our bodies make from basic essence EFAs, are one of the best protections against cardiovascular disorders on the planet, and Essiac-concept tonic can be an excellent protector against infection of the heart and arteries!

Eggs and cholesterol

Here's an interesting bit of information which could offer one reason why eggs were given such a bad reputation regarding cholesterol. For several years, we were warned of supposed dangers of eating eggs because of their cholesterol. In 1940 a study was conducted to explore the effects of dietary cholesterol in humans. Dried egg powder, instead of fresh eggs, was used in the study! The negative results of this study wouldn't have been caused by real eggs. The processing required to powder the eggs would cause chemical changes in the egg. Oxidized substances are harmful to the body, so, from a *Life-Systems* Engineering analysis one would rightly expect this processed material to cause problems.

Current research indicates that the problem with cholesterol was a result of oxidation-induced food processing methods.

Chemically, transfatty acids appear very similar to EFAs, yet our body can't make good use of transfatty acids. The processed, powdered egg has little nutrition compared to a real, fresh egg. With misleading findings such as this, no wonder, for half a century, eggs were inappropriately called "bad." This is another example of a half-truth. The adulterated cholesterol in the powdered egg would cause problems, but only because the cholesterol may have been ruined to begin with!

The results of a study relating blood cholesterol levels to either survival or hospitalization for coronary heart disease were quite clear. With 1,000 subjects, men and women over age 70, during a 4-year period, **there was no reported correlation whatsoever between blood cholesterol level and hospitalization.** That is, these people were no more and no less likely to be hospitalized with high cholesterol levels.[16]

In 1993, a report titled "Cholesterol Screening and Treatment" was released by the University of Leeds in England.

Drugs for lowering high cholesterol levels were given to a study's participants. *The patients whose cholesterol was artificially lowered with drugs developed heart disease just as frequently as the drug-free high-cholesterol group.* The drug increased HDL and decreased LDL (the supposedly "ideal" condition). *There were more health problems among the group taking the drugs!*

Its conclusions were:

- Apart from those with extremely high cholesterol levels (the top two percent), cholesterol screening can't be connected with individual risk of heart-related disease.
- Few people identified purely on the basis of cholesterol levels will benefit from drug treatment.
- Drug treatment only benefits those with additional risk factors, such as high triglyceride level or high blood-pressure.

16 *Journal of American Medical Association* : 272: pages 1335-40, 1994.

- The study *discourages general cholesterol screening.*
- Their overall conclusion: For the 98 percent with less than "lethal" (above 300) cholesterol levels, **there was no benefit from treatment**, and **drug therapy given to lower-risk patients was actually detrimental**.

Despite these findings, England's estimated number of prescriptions for cholesterol-lowering drugs is increasing by 20% per year.

Lowered LDL may mean the cells don't receive enough life-sustaining basic essence* – nutritionally starving us – the very opposite of what we wish to accomplish!

A dire warning was published in a 1995 study by two physicians, Thomas B. Newman and Stephen B. Hulley, at the University of California in San Francisco. They said widespread cholesterol testing for people under twenty years old should be abandoned.

Newman and Hulley are concerned that popular cholesterol-lowering drugs are being prescribed far too frequently – and often unnecessarily – for people who are at little risk of developing heart-related problems.[17] Remember the Phen-Fen disaster? This combination drug was dispensed to virtually anyone who asked for it. It produced life-threatening disorders, and now millions of people may suffer its long-term health consequences. A *Life-Systems* Engineering analysis explains why this happens.

Cholesterol-lowering drugs are prescribed ten times more often than just ten years ago.

Newman and Hulley are physicians concerned about the routine prescriptions for young people – who have no serious risk factors. Young patients are now being given these drugs with the expectation they will be staying on them for twenty to thirty years. *The long-term negative effects aren't known.* **Do you want to be one of the guinea pigs?**

The American Medical Association now wants to lower what it considers "acceptable" cholesterol levels even further. To meet these lowered standards, the AMA would have to propose to place

---

17 "Drugs to Lower Cholesterol May Cause Cancer, Study Says," David Perlman, *San Francisco Chronicle*, 1995; pre-pub. ref., *JAMA*, vol. 275, pages 55-60, 1996.

* LDL is *rich* in basic essence (EFAs). *Biochemistry*, page 700.

many more people on drugs. Does this make sense in light of what we have reviewed? No. Many physicians don't agree with this new policy.

9 million people now take cholesterol-lowering drugs in the hope of warding off heart disease ....[18]

A television newscast featured a story on the AMA decision to lower the "acceptable" levels. Directly after this television news feature, there was a major advertisement by a cholesterol-lowering drug manufacturer! Could there have been a connection between the two?

The traditional drug orientation of modern medical practice is decreasing in popularity.

There is a huge increase in people turning to alternative medicine.

The amount of money now spent on alternative therapies, including nutrition-based remedies to fight disease and dysfunction, is approaching the amount spent on conventional medicine!

Take note of the conclusions from a long-term study performed in Finland, where the researchers tried to artificially manipulate cholesterol and blood-pressure levels with disastrous consequences:

One thousand male business executives aged forty to fifty-three were physically well but had risk factors for developing heart disease. Half the group was medically supervised, whereas the other half wasn't. The results were surprising.

The supervised group was given a program of regular exercise, "strict" diet, and even blood pressure-lowering drugs. There were a shocking 240% more (nearly two-and-a-half times more) deaths from heart attacks in this supervised group. Lots of exercise, strict diet, and even blood pressure-lowering drugs apparently did more harm than good![19]

18 "The Heart Attackers," Geoffrey Cowley, *Newsweek*, August 11, 1997, pages 54-60.

19 *Journal of the American Medical Association*, Timo E. Strandberg, et. al, Vol. 266, 1991, pages 1225-1229.

These researchers didn't understand *Life-Systems* Engineering. Once again, we see that, when one thing changes, everything changes – and it's not always for the better!

"**We'd like to move beyond cholesterol testing**," commented Dr. Peter Libby, chief of cardiovascular medicine at Brigham and Women's Hospital. "**More than half the heart attacks out there occur in people who have normal cholesterol levels, don't smoke, and have few other risk factors**."[20] (emphasis added)

Our Life-Systems Engineering team applauds Dr. Libby and his colleague Dr. Paul Ridler, at Harvard Medical School.

The results of this study, published in the *Lancet* were based on 1,000 middle-aged physicians (participating in the 22,000-man Physicians' Health Study). Four hundred seventy-four (474) of the doctors went on to have a heart attack.

The study cites a probable cause leading to the heart attacks called ICAM-1 (Intercellular adhesion molecule, type 1). This substance makes certain inunune system cells stick to blood vessels. The inflammatory substance C-reactive protein has also been implicated as a possible cause of heart-related ailments.

In the previous chapter we learned how Prostaglandins (made from EFAS) help protect against harmful blood vessel adhesion.

> An analogy can be made between cholesterol in the blood and *fibrin* in the blood. When you cut yourself, fibrin (adhesive) causes quick clotting at the injury. Your blood is loaded with fibrin in its *un*activated form. Only certain conditions activate fibrin. *Life-Systems* Engineering analysis: Like cholesterol, it's there — but it's not a problem.
>
> *Enzymes,* pages 211-212

20 "Discovery may help battle heart attacks," Richard A. Knox (Boston Globe), *Houston Chronicle*, January 10, 1998, page 10A.

To know means to Know All.

Is there a different kind of gravity for feathers than bricks? Of course not.
To understand the apparent difference you must know about air friction too.
SR

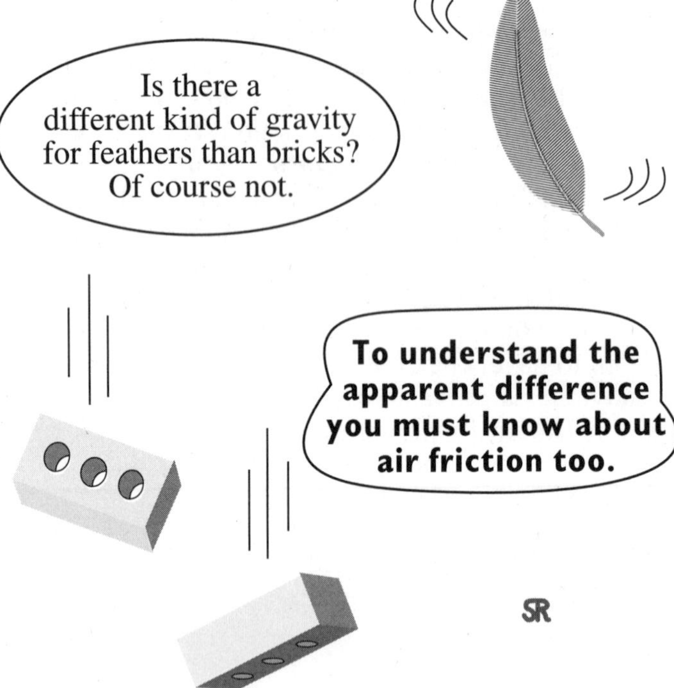

Not to know ALL is not to know. Incomplete knowledge is dangerous.

Surprise:

1) Triglycerides of VLDL (a form of LDL, which is often labeled "bad cholesterol") are produced mainly from dietary *carbohydrates.**

2) Basic essence (healthy *essential* oils) *naturally* decreases blood cholesterol levels.**

* *Basic Medical Biochemistry*, pages 25-26, 512.

** *Textbook of Medical Physiology*, page 873.

Exercise, Why Sweat It?

> *"Walking is man's best medicine."*
>
> Hippocrates — father of modern medicine

Truth in exercise

Depending on the channel and time, turn on the television and you can see endless "infomercials" selling the latest exercise machines. Typically, there is a great-looking couple, a man and a woman, demonstrating the device. From my years of bodybuilding training under two Mr. Olympia contest winners – the same contest Arnold Schwarzenegger won – and running for years while in college, I discovered three important truths about exercise:

1. ***There is no such thing as spot reduction.* Fat-burning occurs in all areas of the body.**
2. ***Bodybuilding (weightlifting) is the only way to build up specific areas.* Aerobics instructors with shapely figures lift weights – they just don't always tell you.**
3. ***The exercise devices being sold on television are not likely to give you bodies like those hosts.* Were those hosts hired because they were already attractive?**

You can gain muscle in specific areas with weightlifting – you just can't lose fat selectively! The spot-reduction myth was disproven beyond any doubt years ago, although equipment manufacturers are hoping you don't know. I can personally verify it doesn't work. My years of bodybuilding under the direction of personal trainers never reduced my love handles. I did hour-after-hour of crunches (effective situps), too. This didn't help at all.

Look at photos of concentration camp victims or anorexia patients. Their abdominal muscles were always well defined. These people were near-death and emaciated, but they had finely chiseled abdominals.

There is only one way to achieve really nice-looking abdominals: STARVE!

Severe dieting is part of the required training for all bodybuilders. Starting months before a tournament, they drastically cut their calorie intake. There is no other way to develop razor-sharp abdominals, or they would have found it. There is nothing physically and psychologically more difficult than starving at contest time to decrease bodyfat and water reserves, while not losing any muscle mass.

An expose' on television about the abdominal exercise equipment infomercials showed the deception was so bad that one manufacturer even used different people in the before-and-after photos. Disclaimers were spoken so fast as to not be heard. The models didn't use the machine to achieve their physiques. Private interviews were conducted with some people who had great abdominals to find out how much time in the gym was required to achieve this look. The average answer was at least 6-8 hours a week! This amounts to a part-time job that most of us don't have time for.

Do you really need razor-sharp abdominals? Why? What is your personal goal? Mine is to look good in a swim suit. Personally, I don't care whether my abdominals show or not, but I certainly don't want a paunch, love handles, a flabby chest, or skinny legs.

With today's highly processed foods, many people have such a lack of vigor and vitality, or are so much overweight, that strenuous exercise isn't a real option. Most of us don't have the time or dedication to make a major effort going to the gym every day. That expensive exercise equipment bought from a store or through a television ad usually ends up as an expensive floor decoration.

For the majority of us, exercise equipment or going to the gym is not a realistic solution to our weight problem.

With the Foundation of Radiant Health discovery, lots of vigorous exercise is no longer required.[1]

1 The *Peak Performer*™ portable exerciser is an ideal inexpensive exercise solution for the busy person. It weighs less than a pound and is easy to use. See listing in Appendix.

Strenuous exercise often drives you to EAT MORE. For a person deficient in EFAs (the vast majority of us), this is a natural reaction to the demands placed on your body from a big exercising workout. You don't burn lots of calories, but, without enough EFAs, your appetite increases a lot. Bodybuilders consume a tremendous number of calories each day. During my 3 years of intensive training, I was an eating machine, yet I was always hungry. The more muscle you build, the more you will typically eat.

When your appetite increases and you are EFA-deficient, you typically eat even more of the same fat-depositing foods you ate in the first place. I gained muscle but did not lose all the excess fat I wanted to. This proved to me that gaining muscle doesn't automatically decrease excess bodyfat, as I was led to believe it would. Even with constant exercising, my excess fat wouldn't disappear. I would have given anything to have known about the EFA-connection back then.

There are about 3,500 available calories in one pound of bodyfat. A 200-pound man with a healthy 15% fat level has about 30 pounds of bodyfat. Not all this fat is available for energy, though, because the body needs a certain amount of fat in its structure. All cell membranes are composed of EFAs. EFAs are used throughout the body including the brain. Bodyfat is used to cushion various organs, and so on. In this example, the 200-pound man with 30 pounds of fat has about 25 pounds of fat available for direct conversion to energy. This is a tremendous amount (25 times 3,500 calories = 87,500 calories). Remember, just 2,000 calories of energy is stored in the liver and muscle as carbohydrates (glycogen).

A *Life-Systems* Engineering solution tells us how to access this 87,000-calorie fat warehouse.

It makes sense in today's world that we don't need this high level of fat storage to sustain us through feast-and-famine times of centuries past.

The 2,000 calories of stored carbohydrates will provide about a day's worth of energy for most people. By overloading on carbohydrates, we never access and burn the stored fat. EFAs in the cellular membranes and cellular mitochondria – cellular energy extractors – enable the stored fat to be accessed and used. Without EFAs, you can exercise all day long, cut back on calories (until your cravings make you cave in), and still not get rid of those impossible-to-lose pounds. A deficiency of EFAs will greatly inhibit your cellular oxygen transfer, so you'll also be sluggish and tired after exercising, and recuperating from the workout will take longer.

When the body doesn't have the raw materials (EFAs) to help convert fat (its preferred energy source) into energy, it settles for using its store of carbohydrates. We are designed to rountinely run on our stored fat. Our carbohydrate reserve is intended for physically stressful, or emergency siuations.

Never forget that **Carbohydrates Make You Fat!** EFA deficiency drives us to eat processed carbohydrates with constant cravings. Let's trace the source for the idea that so much exercise is now "required." Everyone needed a scapegoat to explain why we are still overweight, especially after diligently following heavy carbohydrate eating programs.

The natural exercise of regularly moving and walking around is sufficient to maintain our health when we have met our nutritional requirements. This *Life-Systems* Engineering discovery is based on natural balance – not lots of vigorous exercise.

Radiant health is our natural state, and all that is required to obtain and maintain it are:

1. the proper nutrients Mother Nature designed us to have, and
2. the natural moderate exercise of moving from place to place.

Pets don't require a gymnasium. They don't become overweight when properly fed, and neither should we. My 14-year-old cat has a voracious appetite – he eats a lot of food twice a day – but he maintains an ideal weight. The key is *what he eats*– almost all protein and natural fats.

Hippocrates, the father of modern medicine, advised us centuries ago that "walking is man's best medicine." The average person shouldn't have to exercise vigorously to stay thin and healthy. If we want to speed up the path to radiant health, we can put *Life-Systems* Engineering to work for us.

Vigorous exercise is not required to speed up the metabolism. We have been grossly misled. Studies show a full 80-percent of the benefit of intense exercise can be obtained with just 20-percent of the effort, **if you have the proper nutrients**. I have been fortunate to have been personally trained by two Mr. Olympia winners.[2] Both professional bodybuilders agreed that nutrition was a full 80-percent of a bodybuilder's success criteria. **Professional bodybuilders consider nutrition to be 4 times more important than the physical training.**

The main reason exercise became so popular is that many of the nutritional programs are failures. If you have 100 pounds to lose, losing just 5-10 pounds doesn't mean much, because you don't notice much of a physical difference. There are several methods that most of these eating programs rely on to quickly drop small amounts of weight; but you don't lose just the fat.

To lose just bodyfat and keep it off permanently, you need more than opinion. It was unfounded opinions that led us into the obesity epidemic and ill-health in the first place. The Foundation of Radiant Health is based on science, not opinion. Fewer people were overweight just 30 years ago – long before this massive explosion of new exercise and health clubs on every corner.

Just "Speed Up the Metabolism"

It seems like most people open their conversation with me with the question, "How do I increase my metabolism to become thin?" This is the wrong question. But few understand that it is the wrong question, and that is why so few people are successful at losing excess bodyfat. We don't really want to increase the metabolism. Here's why. **Whether functioning regularly or irregularly, the body is always seeking a state of equilibrium.** When one thing is changed, another corresponding thing changes somewhere else. This change must be anticipated.

We would say that a bodybuilder has a great metabolism, right? After all, their muscles are huge and they have great muscular definition. But a bodybuilder is an eating machine! I've been around them. I've been one. In order to keep feeding this metabolism, *they spend more time eating than they do training*. Bodybuilding stimulates growth hormone production. Bodybuilders train so much, growth hormone increases compensate for extra eating. So, do we really want to increase our metabolism so that we need to eat MORE and become fatter quicker? Of course not!

2 Lee Labrada and Samir Bannout.

Drugs, especially amphetamines, un-naturally distort our metabolism and, in the process, take away our appetite. Do we want to control our appetite with drugs, so our body wastes away due to loss of appetite? Of course not; we want to be thin and healthy.

We wish to *maximize the efficiency* of our metabolism. Simply speeding it up is too naive an approach and one of the reasons why past results have been so poor. **The real question is: how can we burn more fat?**

On the surface, it may seem simple enough to exercise the excess pounds off. I spent several years training like a crazy animal in the gym, three times a week, and ran at least once a week, too. Yet. I couldn't lose my side love-handles or decrease my belly noticeably. Because this much effort still wasn't enough, I questioned the role that exercise is supposed to play in weight loss. Some people enjoy exercising, but not many people today have enough free time to make exercise a second job. I got sick of having to do so much of it – not to mention the minimum results from the tremendous effort.

It would take ten hours of walking, or five hours of aerobics, to burn just 1 pound of fat (3,500 calories worth); **if fat stores were accessed immediately. But they aren't**! That's a lot of work just to lose a pound of fat. But this is only half of the story. None of those infomercials mentions the medical fact that your appetite increases significantly with vigorous exercise.[3] The increase in appetite makes us eat much more, which negates much of the supposed fat-burning effects – especially when we eat carbohydrates. It's no accident the equipment is usually designed to fit under the bed.

Also realize that few of the infomercial models got their physiques using just that piece of equipment. They spend 10-20 hours every week resistance-training in the gym and running, plus they are constantly starving themselves. But, remember, it is their job to look this way, and they're well-paid for it. This isn't the case for most of us.

No amount of exercise will ever solve a nutritional deficiency.

That's the problem in a nutshell.

3 Your appetite increases directly with physical exercise. The greater the exercise, the greater your appetite increases.

There is one thing that everyone should be aware of: a person burns at least 10 times as much glucose doing anaerobic exercise (like weightlifting), compared to the same amount of aerobic exercise (like running). That's right. **If you are going to do limited exercise specifically for fat loss, then lift weights or do isometrics** – at the gym or at home.

This analysis comes from calculating how much energy (ATP) is extracted from the Krebbs cycle compared with straight glycolysis. Anaerobic energy extraction from glucose is inefficient compared with oxidation, but if you are diabetic or desire to burn maximum fat, you always want the lowest possible insulin levels. You can make this inefficiency work for you so that more glucose is used. **Then your body's natural *Life-Systems* automatically mobilize and burn stored bodyfat to replenish the glucose.** *Life-Systems* Engineering produces desired results.

So, weightlifting is an excellent way to decrease blood glucose levels. Just make sure you don't "load up on carbs" either before or after your workout. That would be counterproductive.

Weightlifting causes the number of glucose receptors to increase, too, meaning that your insulin will be used more efficiently. If you are diabetic, this is excellent. If you're not, it's still good for you, because it will help keep the blood glucose levels down even if you still over-indulge on processed carbohydrates. Weightlifting also triggers the release of growth hormone. Growth hormone has lots to do with fat-burning. The *Textbook of Medical Physiology* states, "Growth hormone increases protein synthesis in all cells of the body, increased mobilization of fatty acids from adipose (bodyfat) tissue, and increased use of fatty acids (coming from excess bodyfat) for energy." It states that glucose utilization is decreased, but that's what we want here, because we want to burn stored bodyfat while exercising.[4]

In the final analysis, weightlifting gets excess glucose out of our system, inhibits potential diabetes problems, and even protects us against osteoporosis. The growth hormone, which weightlifting stimulates, causes the stored fat to be used as fuel.

Many people exercise in an effort to control their weight. Here's what the *Textbook of Medical Physiology* says about the role of carbohydrates in exercise: "... thus *an excess of carbohydrates* in the diet not only *acts as a fat-sparer* but also **increases the fat in**

4 *Textbook of Medical Physiology*, page 936.

the fat stores. In fact, **all the excess carbohydrates** not used for energy or stored in the small glycogen deposits of the body **are converted to fat and stored** as such." [5] (emphasis added)

> The more glycogen you store, the more bloated you become. Every single pound of excess glycogen adds three pounds of water![6]

My wife recently commented that few people she has seen exercising or attending countless aerobics classes over the years looked much better after all that effort. Now you know why. Carbohydrates are short-circuiting most of Mother Nature's natural fat-burning effects!

How much carbohydrate in the diet is considered an excess? Recall that *we don't require any carbohydrates for body structure*, and the answer becomes quite clear. Very little carbohydrate constitutes an excess: Just a few hundred calories a day.

About 2 containers of soda, or a few servings of chips can make the difference between fat-burning and fat-gaining for the entire day.

How long does it take for a runner eating lots of carbohydrates to start really using those fat stores? Once again, let's refer to the *Textbook of Medical Physiology*. On page 1064 it says, "For a real endurance event, one can expect fat to supply more than 50-percent (half) of the required energy after about the first three to four hours. Yes, it takes hours! The body starts off using mainly glucose/glycogen for energy and *only gradually shifts to increased fat-burning*.

How many of us have spent years sweating our tails off, running miles each week, thinking that we were burning lots of fat? I was getting up at 4:30 AM and jumping on the treadmill because I was told that is the time of the day when your carbohydrates reserves are lowest, so you'd get the most fat-burning then. Well, I never got any results from the full year I did that routine. Nor did I decrease excess bodyfat from all the running I did. Finally, I know why I didn't, and why few others do.

---

5 *Textbook of Medical Physiology*, page 871.

6 *Nutrition For Fitness & Sport*, Dr. Melvin H. Williams, Brown & Benchmark Publishers, Dubuque, IA, 1995, page 106.

The misinformation is even worse. *The more carbohydrates you eat, the longer it takes for fat-burning from aerobic activity to start.* According to the *Textbook of Medical Physiology*, if you eat mainly carbohydrates, like most people do today, then it takes over one hour of intense aerobic activity before you start burning just 25-percent of energy from fat.

Compare that to someone who eats about 20-percent (1/5) carbohydrates and the remaining 80-percent (4/5) – the bulk of the diet – from protein and natural fats. After just 10 minutes of aerobics, this man or woman is burning about 50-percent (1/2) of energy from bodyfat stores – a full 25-percent (1/4) more, almost immediately. No additional effort – just more *Life-Systems* Engineering understanding. Keep up the running or aerobics, and by the end of the 1st hour you're burning about 65-percent (2/3) from excess bodyfat – 40-percent more than if you eat mostly carbohydrates. So a carbohydrate-based diet even keeps an athlete fat longer. This is the medically-based scientific truth.

Carbohydrates stop fat-burning cold — even in athletes!

You may ask, "But what about 'carbo-loading' that we hear about so much? Many athletes do this. Isn't there some scientific reason for it?" There is a reason for it, but I want to make this perfectly clear: what is required of an elite athlete just before a competition has little to do with the rest of us. My concern here is to help the average person, not to address the one out of ten thousand who runs long-distance races or competes in professional bodybuilding tournaments.

When we want to maximize *Life-Systems* placed under extreme limits, we can make several modifications to a typically healthy diet. If you run a 26-mile marathon, your metabolic rate can increase as much as 2,000-percent (twenty times)! You could expect that, operating at this level, there would be some additional things that would help increase efficiency. If you are doing a lot of aerobic activity, such as marathon running, then you want as much stored glucose, in the form of glycogen, as you can get stored in the muscle – bursting at the seams, so to speak, during the marathon. You aren't concerned with fat-burning at all. You want every bit of energy for the task at hand, quickly feeding the muscles.

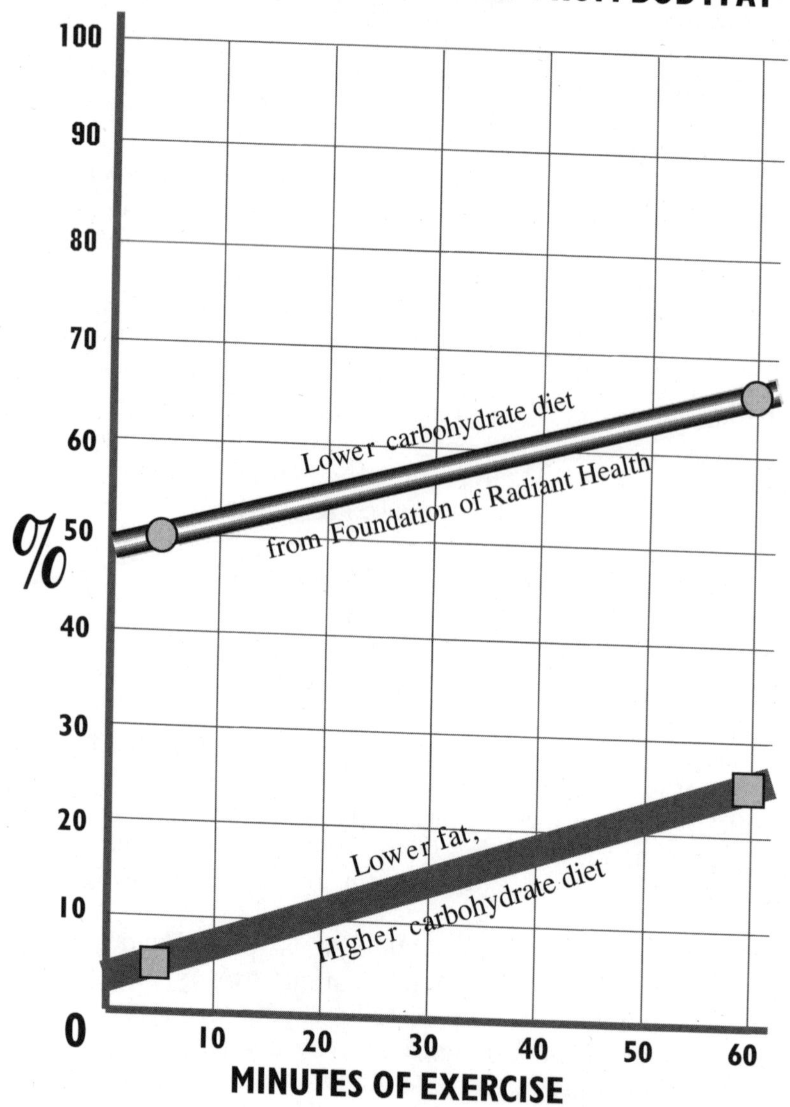

So for running a marathon, it makes sense not to restrict carbohydrates in the 12-24 hours before running. In this case, eating an excess of carbohydrates can be useful. Again, this is only for elite athletes and is an isolated case. There are many ways to enhance performance for professional athletes, but this is not the place to describe them. Most of us never have to think about this.

Carbohydrates are important for prolonged endurance events – *those lasting more than one-and a-half to two hours!*[7] How many marathon races are you running? Most of us aren't running at all, let alone running for over an hour-and-a-half at a time.

The energy content in an eight-ounce glass of orange juice provides enough chemical energy to enable the average man to run about 1 mile![8] If you aren't using this energy, guess what your body does with all the sugar it produces from the juice? You probably guessed it, more bodyfat!

How much carbohydrate does the body require per day? You have never heard anyone diagnosed with "carbohydrates deficiency." Here's why, as *Nutrition For Fitness & Sport* clearly states on page 87:

> ... The National Research Council has not established an RDA [recommended daily requirement] for carbohydrates, probably because the body can adapt to a carbohydrates-free diet and manufacture the glucose it needs from parts of protein and fat.

However,

The body cannot adapt to either a protein-free or a fat-free diet.

We require essential amino acids from proteins, and we require the essential healthy oils from fats. Without both of these, we become ill and ultimately die.

Does carbohydrate loading immediately prior to short or moderate exercise periods increase performance? Contrary to product marketing, the answer is a big NO. As Professor Williams, author of *Nutrition For Fitness & Sport,* states, "Adding a gallon of gas to a full tank will not make a car go faster. The same is true of [adding] sugar to a muscle already filled with glycogen."

Many nutritionists aren't aware that muscles don't use glucose most of the time and that glucose is NOT the body's preferred energy source – contrary to what is so often repeated. We are told that we need carbohydrates because (they think) we need to keep our glucose levels up! But it's wrong, and the results speak for themselves – with a nationwide increase in obesity.

7 *Nutrition For Fitness & Sport*, page 95.
8 *Nutrition For Fitness & Sport*, page 59.

We are told to base our diets on the one substance our body doesn't require (carbohydrates) and told to minimize or even eliminate the two essentials (protein and healthy essential oils)!

As page 973 of the *Textbook of Medical Physiology* clearly states: only under extreme physical exercise does a muscle use glucose. Most of the time, muscle membrane is only slightly permeable (open) to glucose.

Throughout the rest of the day – the majority of the time – the muscle needs fats! It can't even use glucose!

The high-carbohydrates activists don't like this fact. That's why you may never hear it mentioned. *Even when the muscles need glucose, the body can manufacture it as needed from stored bodyfat.* So, **for maximum fat-burning, we want minimum glycogen reserves**.

The energy available from fat (in the form stored in the body) is six times more, pound-for-pound, than the available energy from carbohydrates. Another medical textbook makes it quite clear.[9] Most people think that the difference is about double: four calories from a gram of protein or carbohydrates and nine calories from a gram of fat. This is what is always published on food product labels, etc. while it is *technically correct for laboratory measurements of the energy released* **outside** *the body*, **it does not take into consideration different body processes and efficiencies**.

However, much of what is reported in the nutritional fields is a half-truth. *Those routinely reported numbers don't take into account the entire life-system and how the substance is stored and used in the body.* The body uses different amounts of energy to

9 *Molecular Biology of the Cell*, page 658: "Quantitatively, fat is a far more important storage form than glycogen, in part because its oxidation releases more than six times as much energy as the oxidation of an equal mass of glycogen in its hydrated form."

digest each of these components. Once the nutrients are broken down in the body, they are repackaged in the form the body needs.

Carbohydrates are an easy-to-use form of quick energy. The body keeps only a very small supply – about a day's worth – of ready-to-use glucose, in a form called glycogen. How much energy is stored in fat? At least 30 days' worth. In the "average" adult, of all stored fuel, three percent is glycogen and a whopping ninety seven-percent is bodyfat.

Gorging on carbohydrates short-circuits Mother Nature's automatic fat-burning design. So unless you want to spend hour-after-hour vigorously exercising, you need to understand *Life-Systems* Engineering – the science based on how the body is designed and how it actually works.

Nature loves efficiency, and we are meant to eat plenty of natural fats and oils.

Even though I enjoy exercise, I haven't done much of it during the past three years because, being a scientist, I must change only one thing at a time to examine the direct effect of what I am studying. I have to be certain that our discoveries are primarily nutritional – not dependent on exercise. Our nation's current state of obesity and ill-health, in spite of our obsession with exercise, has proven, over-and-over, that we can't overcome nutritional deficiencies with exercise.

I recently measured my blood pressure on a highly accurate machine, and it was 109/63. That's elite athlete level, even though I do virtually no special exercise – just the moderate exercise of moving around from doing chores, gardening and parking my car farther away in the parking lot, so that I walk more. I'm 41 years old. My cardiovascular system is in great shape.

During my athletic days of intense running, weight training in the gym, martial arts, and constant low-fat dieting, my blood pressure was never better than 120/78. Nutritional improvements with the Foundation of Radiant Health gave me more benefit than lots of vigorous exercise by itself ever did. I feel much better than I did as an 18-year old elite athlete, and I have much more free personal time, too. My Stanford University-trained cardiologist told me after my EKG, "I wish I had your heart!"

Life-Systems Engineering produces maximum results in minimum time.

Quicker recovery from physical stress

A personal example:

After a three-year layoff from training in the gym, I resumed weight training. I had been taking the Foundation of Radiant Health for approximately 6 months. I was no longer eating many processed carbohydrates, because my desire for them had significantly decreased.

I went to the gym with my wife. She had continued going twice a week during my layoff. I resumed my training with almost the same level of weights that I had attained 3 years prior! Needless to say, my wife was surprised that I completed my entire workout. I was in no pain and I didn't feel exhausted or sick. In the past, I always "needed" to run to the smoothie shop and get a large one to "recover" after the workout. This time I didn't "need" or even want one. We were both amazed. My wife expected that I'd have to be carried out of the gym on a stretcher from exhaustion because of the long layoff and the high-intensity workout. What was even more interesting was that I hadn't eaten anything for 12 hours before the workout! Many exercise coaches and nutritionists would have said that this was impossible. They would have said that eating was needed prior to expending all this energy.

After that workout, I resumed working the entire day as usual, needing just five-and-a-half hours sleep that night as usual. Previously, I would need 10-12 hours of sleep to "recover" after a gym day. I had no pain the next day (unless I pressed against a muscle I had worked). The second day after the workout was pain-free, too.

I would have paid plenty of money to have known about this discovery years ago. The pain, exhaustion, high sleep requirements, and cravings associated with exercise are now all a thing of the past with the Foundation of Radiant Health!

You'll be able to tackle evening and weekend projects without becoming exhausted!

Which exercises give you the most benefit?

I'm always amused when the aerobics trainers come on television singing the wonders of aerobic exercise. For cardiovascular strengthening, aerobics can be helpful, but for bodyshaping, aerobics doesn't help much.

To shape your body by building bigger muscles, you'll want to focus your efforts on weight lifting or isometric exercises.

For overall health, and simplicity, walking or swimming provide excellent choices.

But I don't want too much muscle

I get a kick out of women refusing to engage in weightlifting because they don't want to become too muscular. A woman's hormones simply won't allow much muscle to be packed on – even if she trains in the gym every day. The women who have a significant amount of muscle are either extremely rare (the one-in-ten-thousand), or they may have taken steroids somewhere along the line.

I trained very diligently in the gym, under expert guidance, two to three times a week for two years. I followed the professional bodybuilders' diet, and still couldn't gain all the muscle I would have liked to. It is very difficult to build extra muscle – even more so for a woman.

Why does a muscle increase in size? Because a heavy load was lifted a certain number of times during a certain period. Doing many repetitions with a light weight won't change the size or strength of your muscle much. We need a big change from normal to achieve the stress needed to stimulate muscle growth.

Even if a woman were to gain too much muscle in a specific area, all she'd have to do is stop training that particular part of her body for a few weeks, and it would shrink automatically.

If I gain muscle, when I get older won't it turn to fat?

No, muscle can't turn to fat. Fat cells are structurally different from muscle cells. Muscle will decrease in size a bit from lack of stimulation, but once fat grows over the muscle, you simply don't see the muscle underneath. A walrus has lots of muscle, yet it needs lots of fat to insulate it against the frigid waters, so you never see its muscle. This myth – that muscle goes to fat – *came from the fact that exercising increases appetite.* Even after you stop the constant exercise, your appetite will stay high – unless you are getting the EFAs you need. You'll gain plenty of excess bodyfat, *especially when you eat lots of carbohydrates.*

If you wish to reshape your body by gaining muscle in particular places, nothing beats bodybuilding.

If you wish to lower your blood glucose (sugar) levels quickly, nothing beats weightlifting. Have a diabetic measure her blood glucose before, and again 60 minutes after training for an hour. It often drops significantly. If you are diabetic and wish to obtain low blood-sugar levels quickly, then lift some weights at home or at the gym. But this effect won't last for long if you consume too many carbohydrates.

Osteoporosis takes a hike!

Nothing will stop the onset of osteoporosis in both men and women like bodybuilding.

Bodybuilding (and eating more protein) – not more calcium – is the most effective way to prevent and reverse osteoporosis!

Osteoporosis is caused by problems with the protein-based bone matrix with which the calcium combines. This matrix structure gives bones their flexibility and structural integrity. Shortage of calcium causes flexible bones – like in the deficiency disease called *Rickets*. Sufferers from osteoporosis have brittle bones, from an impared bone matrix, due to lack of protein in the structure.

Calcium supplements offer little real benefit to most of us, and can even be harmful. Read more about this in Chapter 10.

Running and walking

Is running better than walking? This depends on your personal goals. Running can harm all the internal organs, joints, and feet. Walking is safer. But hour-for-hour, routine walking won't give you the fat-burning or the aerobic effect of running. But, with the Foundation of Radiant Health, the moderate exercise from walking still gives you great benefit. This is illustrated by the results of Harvard Alumni Study.

My father was thin all his life. As a postman he walked his tail off for 15 years. But he still needed a major triple-bypass operation at age 62, and that forced his early retirement. Is either walking or running the answer for a healthy heart and arteries (the cardiovascular system)? A *Life-Systems* Engineering analysis suggests it may help, but it isn't enough – not by a long shot.

With the Foundation of Radiant Health, just a few minutes of daily walking or moderate exercise is all it takes for a strong and healthy cardiovascular system.

If you don't have time for lots of vigorous exercise, you will still receive positive cardiovascular benefits from the nutrition of the Foundation of Radiant Health. Remember, nothing can take the place of solving a nutritional deficiency except eliminating the deficiency.

Therapeutic Hatha Yoga

Years ago, I learned the "positions" of Bikram-style Hatha Yoga. I was very surprised at the value of this particular style. If I was looking for an exercise program and could do no other form of physical exercise, I would pick this discipline as the best payback for my time. Few instructors are available in this particular style, but Bikram's book is available through bookstores. There is no comparable exercise method that provides this high level of muscle strengthening (not increased size, like weightlifting develops), stretching, blood flow slowdown and therapeutic flushing action for the organs. It takes about an hour a day.

The bottom line

Even if you start an exercise program, there is no assurance that you will reshape your body the way you'd like to. *Without utilizing the EFA-connection and the Foundation of Radiant Health, you aren't likely to benefit from the full potential of any exercise program.*

Runners and aerobics enthusiasts may tell you that performing their particular exercise regimen is the reason they stay thin. Here is another example of an inaccurate cause-effect relationship. Exercise alone seldom burns enough calories to obtain significant effects.

Significant weight loss will only occur after many hours and many miles worth of strenuous physical activity, and then your appetite will drive you to eat! We must look **beyond** the calories burned while exercising. *With an optimized EFA cell structure, fat-burning potential is maximized naturally*. Then, **you will burn more calories with any form of exercising!**

We desire the fastest natural metabolic rate as long as it doesn't increase our appetite. Here's an important tip: the greater the natural oxygen utilization, the faster the body can burn fat. Only basic essence gives you this combined effect. *Oxygen is about eight times more soluble (translation: usable) in EFAs than in water.* But, beware, chemically-altered and distorted EFAs reduce your oxygen usability.

When you combine exercising with adequate EFAs, you have created the best possible fat-burning environment.

Remember, too, that oxygen utilization is critical to active fat-burning. EFAs provide each cell with the means to optimize precious oxygen transfer. If your muscles can't fully utilize oxygen, you become sluggish, even drowsy. That's another reason why EFAs significantly increase your vitality – often within just 90 days. Cell membranes containing *trans*fatty acids (which are often produced by food processing) begin to get replaced by fully functional EFAs.

You may even need less sleep, because your body becomes so much more efficient at metabolizing food and increasing oxygen utilization.

Exercise enthusiasts can easily demonstrate that carbo-loading is inferior to taking basic essence. Simply take some basic essence half-an-hour before your workout, and no other food or supplements. Whether it be weightlifting, running, jogging, aerobics, or anything else, you'll perform better and FEEL BETTER. You'll burn more excess bodyfat, because your blood-glucose levels will decrease, and then your body's natural fat-burning metabolism will take over.

Q: I've read that it takes 6 hours of running to lose a pound of bodyfat. Is that true?

A: No. Your body doesn't burn fat first. It burns stored carbohydrate (glycogen) first. **On a high carbohydrate diet,* it takes *about 40 days of running an hour a day* to burn just a pound of bodyfat!** With a high carbohydrate diet, you access bodyfat stores just 15% of the time! When you are *Beyond The Zone*, it only takes about **9 days** of running to lose a pound of bodyfat — a significant improvement — **average fat-burning increases by 40%!** That's why the calorie "theory" of exercise is misleading and why lots of vigorous exercising — especially using a high carbohydrate diet, has failed to keep us lean.

Americans, showing great willpower to do the "right thing," have forced their bodies to adapt to a high-carbohydrate diet. Even under maximum adaptability, **the body *can't* use more than 4-5 ounces of carbohydrate* – just a cup of bread crumbs or 2 bagels** – the excess goes quickly to new bodyfat. A properly functioning human being, not forced to endure *the great carbohydrate experiment,* is **designed to have just half of this amount of carbohydrates!** How much damage have you unknowingly caused your body this week?

"Specific sugars are not required in the diet. Glucose can be synthesized from certain amino acids found in dietary protein."* So much for the great carbohydrate as king!

* *Basic Medical Biochemistry,* pages 24, 394.

With recommendations like this is it any wonder that exercise hasn't helped? Nancy Clark, M.S., R.D. recommends that when exercising, "a 180-lb man should consume 540 to 900 grams of carbohydrates per day." ***Life-Systems* Engineering translation:** This is the equivalent of 108 to 180 tsp. of sugar! You learned that, scientifically, insulin STOPS FAT-BURNING COLD! With recommendations like this, no wonder exercise hasn't reduced the obesity epidemic.

Men's Health, Dec. 1999, page 80.

***Trans*fatty acids!**

[the opposite of "cis" fatty acids]

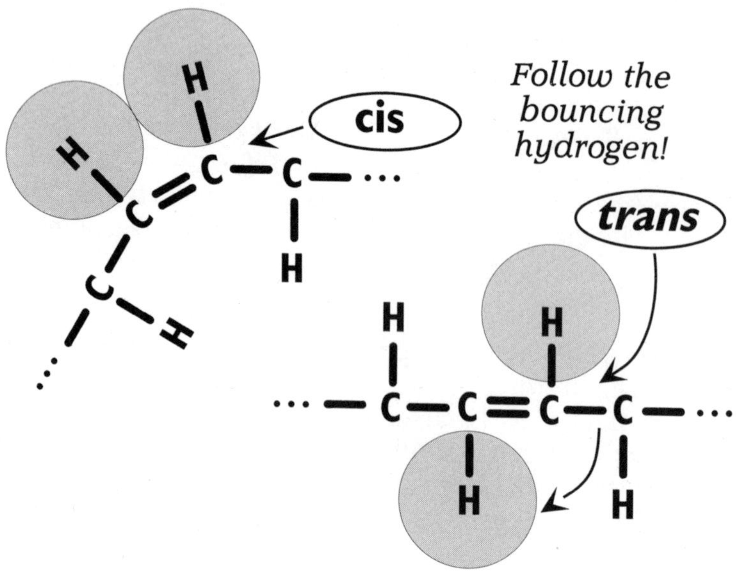

The only difference between **cis** and ***trans*** is a hydrogen shifted from one side of the molecule to the other. The food processing industry considers this "no big deal."

Note: For comparison, the chemical difference between starch (a digestible food) and cellulose (purified sawdust) is only a slight rotation of one half of the molecule.

*This may be no "big deal" except –
it changes the biological properties.
You can't digest cellulose!
It is metabolically worthless.*

What You Don't Know Can Hurt You

> *"Perfection of means and confusion of goals seem – in my opinion – to characterize our age."*
> Albert Einstein – Nobel Prize-winner

Hippocrates, perhaps the best known doctor in history (fourth and fifth centuries B.C.), and noted for the Hippocratic Oath, certainly knew the value of food.

"Let food be your medicine, let medicine be your food."
(Hippocrates)

One of our *Life-Systems* Engineering team's favorite medical sayings is: "Cooking is a branch of Medicine."

Is organically grown and processed food better?

"Organically grown and processed" – meaning without pesticides, additives, hormones, steroids, preservatives, or chemicals – usually yields superior nutritional content of the food. Organic is nearly always superior to traditionally raised and processed varieties of meat, fish, and crops. Even though most organically grown wheat flour has the important wheat germ removed, it is still more beneficial (more natural vitamins and minerals) than commercially grown and processed wheat flour that also has the wheat germ removed. Organically grown and processed food doesn't contain health-degrading additives such as man made preservatives.

Free-range eggs reportedly have 35 percent higher vitamin values, and more EFAs in them, too. Because free-range (non-caged) chickens are less stressed – getting regular exercise and outdoor light and air – their eggs even taste better than regular eggs.

You don't want chemicals, pesticides, steroids, antibiotics, or chemically-altered EFAs in the food you eat.

Eat organically grown and processed food whenever possible.

What about liquid "meals?"

Let's read the ingredients. When it comes to liquid "meals"[1] they are all **nutritionally lacking** from a *Life-Systems* Engineering analysis. They are made of a lot of "stuff," including some vitamins and minerals, in the hope we will think that everything a body needs is in the drink. If we analyze these liquid, supposedly "complete foods," we find they are often loaded with hydrogenated vegetable oil, sugar, and chemicals.

Read the information on the can or carton. You may be surprised.

These drinks often contain 5-7 teaspoons of carbohydrate (sugar)!

Each twenty calories of carbohydrate is metabolically equivalent to a whole teaspoon of common table sugar. There is no difference how the body reacts to it![2]

Calorie deprivation is the method by which the liquid drink manufacturers may hope we will lose weight. The idea is to keep us feeling full by adding bulk with fiber and gums, so we'll eat less. The problem is that these products aren't real food and their nutrients aren't well-used by the body. Their advertising can be highly misleading. Because of their high sugar content and the insulin connection, these products won't keep anyone full for long.

The manufacturers of these liquid drinks started by selling to hospitals. Their drinks provide "nourishment" to hospital patients who can't have or can't digest solid food.

---

1 Fruit drinks are not included in this category. Our *Life-Systems* team aren't impressed with fruit drinks or juices. They are loaded with carbohydrates. They often contain chemical additives, but at least they don't contain distorted EFAs, too.

2 *Textbook of Medical Physiology,* page 856.

After the hospital market was developed, sales efforts were then expanded to the healthy elderly. Maybe the manufacturers of these drinks think that older people don't cook anymore or that they can only drink through a straw.

Major advertising dollars are now being spent to attract a much younger clientele. Maybe the manufacturers think the younger generation can't cook, either, or that they have no time to cook. Analyzing their sales shows their advertising has paid off extremely well.

I monitored a relative during her hospital stay while she was on one of these liquid foods. She had a mild diabetic condition. While taking one of these liquid products, her blood glucose (sugar) readings rose consistently – well over 300. The average glucose reading for a non-diabetic is about 80. For a diabetic, maintaining a glucose level under 150 is mandatory. The nursing staff couldn't control her glucose level while she was being fed these high-sugar drinks.

With a high blood-glucose level, the body can't heal itself.

When I expressed concern to her physicians, they were aware that a high glucose level was harmful. Unfortunately, no matter how they changed the liquid feeding, the glucose levels remained too high. To counteract the sugar, she was given insulin. Too much was administered and she almost lapsed into a coma.

Liquid nutrition manufacturers routinely include lots of carbohydrates and sugar in their drinks. Don't let technical names fool you. Maltodextrine, sucrose, fructose, dextrose, corn syrup, corn syrup solids, and even honey are still virtually 100% sugar.

Most harmful organisms thrive with higher glucose levels. Reducing carbohydrates make it harder for "bad bugs" to live in your body.

Although the word "EFA" was acknowledged, the nutritionist I spoke with just lumped them into the overall category of "fat" and counted their calorie content right along with the harmful and metabolically inactive hydrogenated *trans*fats and oils from these liquid drinks. They didn't want me giving basic essence to my relative because, in their opinion, she had received enough fat already and they didn't want her caloric intake to be excessive. Translation: No *Life-Systems* Engineering understanding whatsoever.

The body is an amazing machine. For a short time, it may tolerate some gross deviations from what it needs, but not forever.

These drinks may help as an "inexpensive and quick" solution to keeping a comatose or near-death patient alive in the hospital. Used long-term, however, they may be harmful.

A *Life-Systems* Engineering analysis leads to the conclusion that obesity, arterial diseases, and overall poor health are long-term consequences of eating highly processed foods.

These liquids are highly processed. Because they don't require refrigeration, ask yourself how good the protein or fats in them can be? Someone may make processed fats and oils that don't need to be refrigerated, but they, most likely, are using processed oils instead of natural ones. It's very different from the original food source. Most of these drinks are made with hydrogenated oils, with little, if any, basic essence left in them, and are high in carbohydrates.

In fact, far from being healthy and "nutritional," these drinks may be *harmful*.

Instead of being the "best possible food", they may be among the worst. The long-term effects of these liquid foods have not been adequately studied. Will they ever be? Who is interested in funding such a study? Certainly not the manufacturers. Do you want to pay for being their guinea pigs?

Ask yourself whether our digestive systems are able to thrive on liquid food. Is there enough real fiber and bioactive nutrients in them, such as is found in real food? Do they give you diarrhea?

How do you feel after drinking them? Are you hungry soon afterwards? This type of drink was originally designed for the nearly dead and dying. Why aren't you eating unprocessed food?

What about "food bars?"

They are also promoted as "sports-bars," "energy-bars" and "nutrition-bars." "Complete meal" bars are claimed to be "healthy," but look at how much carbohydrate is in them.

If you want to lose bodyfat, avoid them. They are typically loaded with processed carbohydrates — with as much as seven teaspoons of sugar each.

A product sweetened with fruit juice will still typically contain lots of carbohydrates, and their fats and oils are often chemically distorted. *Read the labels.*

If you are running marathons and are *not interested in losing excess bodyfat*, these bars may be all right. For anyone interested in losing excess bodyfat and achieving radiant health, a *Life-Systems* Engineering analysis says, avoid them. Do your body a big favor. Eat real food instead. Read the labels to see for yourself what they contain.

What about carbohydrate gels?

Here's a case of more misunderstood information. Carbohydrate "gels" were developed recently for long-distance marathon runners. Unfortunately, gels already are being inappropriately used by non-marathon runners. Mag Donaldson, director of marketing for Gu (a gel manufacturer) states she has used the product in her office to get over the 3 o'clock lows and that the company has received letters about people who stir it into their coffee or use it as a spread on bananas (which are also a high-carbohydrate food).

Non-marathon runners will get a "high" while the body tries to get this toxic sugar out of their systems, by converting it to bodyfat. One more thing. Many of the gels contain caffeine, too. Could this be why the product is really being used?[3]

3 "Long-distance runners tear down walls with help of carbohydrate gel," Chris Magerl, *Houston Chronicle*, October, 27, 1997, page 2C.

What about "fortified" breads and cereals?

Cereal manufacturers are fond of calling their product "good" because they say it may be linked to cancer prevention, and they have "added" some vitamins and minerals. Cereal is generally made from processed carbohydrates, refined sugar, and *trans*fatty oils. Do these cereal manufacturers let you know about their possible role in feeding the diabetes epidemic? Read the label of any of them and you'll quickly see how high the carbohydrate (sugar) content is. Do they mention the bioavailability (how much really gets used) of their added vitamins and minerals? Be skeptical of believing any manufacturers' claims that their processed food is good for you. Chances are, it isn't. It's more often a question of minimizing how badly it will harm you.

What about artificial sweeteners?

Artificial sweeteners containing *aspartame* are sold under brand names including NutraSweet and Equal. One of the problems with *aspartame* is that it tends to remove chromium from the body. Chromium is a trace mineral that most of us need in our diet. Maybe one of the reasons many of us are chromium-deficient is because so many of us today now use these sweeteners in an attempt to reduce calories. We don't need much chromium, but we certainly don't want what little chromium we do have needlessly sucked out of our systems.

Aspartame, the main ingredient in many sweeteners, is chemically synthesized. One of *aspartame's* components is **methanol** *(wood alcohol)*. An excess of methanol can cause blindness and even death. Heat increases the rate of *aspartame*'s conversion back to methanol, so be certain to keep any products containing *aspartame* cool. Don't store them for very long either, because they break down into methanol and other possibly unhealthy components.

Aspartame-based sweeteners are now used extensively in yogurt, ice cream, fruit drinks, cereals, gelatin desserts, soft drinks, and even vitamins and medicines. *Aspartame* is also used in flavored coffee and some baked goods; think about that in light of what we just told you about *aspartame* and heat! Often, we won't know it's in there, either. Even so, it's still important to read the labels on the products you use.

After drinking a typical can of soft drink containing *aspartame*, you could be consuming almost twice the Environmental Protection Agency's daily limit for methanol![4]

It is reported that *aspartame*-related problems account for more than 80 percent of all of the FDA food-related complaints. Guess how many products now contain NutraSweet? Over five thousand (5,000).

One more point – *aspartame* triggers the appestat as though "real food" is coming. **It stimulates appetite**. Now you know why you feel hungry after drinking diet drinks.

Is sugar really all that bad?

Since heart disease has become such a prominent killer, Let's examine the food-heart connection from a *Life-Systems* Engineering perspective. A condition called "*hyperinsulinemia*" means an overreaction to insulin production. We have already discussed how eating too many processed carbohydrates will cause a significant increase in insulin production. Barry Sears, in his book, *Enter the Zone*, details some of the chemical mechanisms involved. The key to understanding these mechanisms is to know that **excessive insulin production is solely a response to an imbalance among carbohydrate, protein, and fat**.

Dr. Sears goes on to say: research indicates that hyperinsulinemia is the best predictor of heart disease. He suggests the people who have this condition make up the majority of those who suffer heart attacks. If this is true, then basic essence intake is even more important. With basic essence, we desire far fewer carbohydrates, and the potential problem of hyperinsulinemia is effortlessly reduced.

Basic essence naturally decreases our desire for carbohydrates (especially processed ones) so that our bodies will pump out less insulin. Less insulin means fewer problems!

Dr. Sears tells of rabbit tests in which essential fatty acids were injected directly into a rabbit's bloodstream. Nothing happens.

4 *Your Body Knows Best*, Ann Louise Gittleman, M.S., Pocket Books, New York, 1996, page 41.

Excessive **cholesterol** was injected into the rabbit's bloodstream. **Nothing** happened. When arachidonic acid (which comes from the eicosanoids that are triggered by **insulin**) was injected, blood clots formed, causing the rabbit's **death** within 3 minutes! Arachidonic acid is unique in that it is abundant in brain cells as well as other cells.* Once again, insulin is the culprit.

Remember, I cautioned that we should not jump to conclusions based on animal studies. Let's look more closely at these results. We know that essential fatty acids in humans don't clog arteries – in fact, EFAs decrease arterial clogging. We know cholesterol input doesn't cause a significant response in humans, either. So the rabbit test could be consistent with how a human would respond. We can't perform experiments on people with arachidonic acid – the risk of death would be too great.

Pharmacists will tell you that insulin-related conditions are rapidly rising among the U.S. population. Regardless of the arachidonic acid issue, if we eat too many processed carbohydrates, we will, with great probability, sooner or later develop insulin-related problems. The real-life facts have shown this result over and over.

How do fats and oils move around in the body?

Most fats and oils inside the body are packaged in a form called a triglyceride for easy transportation around the body. Oils in our body are often packaged together with two saturated fatty acids outside and one EFA inside. To protect important and fragile EFAs, saturated fats are required. We rarely hear anything positive about saturated fats, yet these fats serve an important function – to protect the EFAs! When most fats and oils are eaten, they are taken into the lymph system – not into the bloodstream![5] Your body makes sure that most fats do not directly enter your bloodstream. Because oil (fat) and water don't mix well and because blood is mostly water, fats and oils can't travel unescorted in our bloodstream. First, in the lymph system, an oil or fat molecule is attached to a protein. Surrounding the fat with a protein (which does mix well with water) enables fat to travel through the bloodstream. This protein-fat molecule is called a lipoprotein.

---

5 Short chain fats [found in butter] are water soluble. They can enter the blood directly.

* *Smart Fats*, pg. 51.

When bodyfat is transported via "free fatty acids"

The body converts your stored fat into free fatty acids. At any given time, there is only about 1/60th of a teaspoon of them in the entire circulatory system.[6] This isn't very much. Mother Nature designed us to keep burning our bodyfat stores every few minutes. Can this substance cause blockage? No, because it is surrounded by a protein which makes it resistant to sticking.

High blood pressure

High blood pressure (hypertension) is another common problem. This condition causes damage from overexertion to either the arteries or the heart. If blood vessels are rigid – instead of flexible, like they were designed to be – they are easier to damage. The vessels also need to expand and contract easily to be able to respond quickly to system changes. When arteries are more flexible, blood pressure decreases, too![7] EFAs in the cell membrane make it more flexible. Just as your skin responds well to unadulterated EFAs, so do your arteries.

Shortage of EFAs stiffens arteries, making them easier to damage, and increases blood pressure.

Insulin stimulates the sympathetic nervous system, causing the heart to pump faster, and constricts blood vessels, which further increases your blood pressure! Type II diabetics who eat excessive carbohydrates put themselves on the path to hypertension (high blood pressure). Type I diabetics who require large insulin doses to counteract carbohydrates are on the same path.[8] If you aren't diabetic, should you care about this? You bet you should. Overloading on carbohydrates causes insulin release, which can put you on the path to hypertension, too.

Excess carbohydrates can lead to high blood pressure.

6 *Textbook of Medical Physiology*, page 866.

7 The more rigid your arteries, the higher the systolic (the top number) blood pressure from the pumping of the heart; likewise with the diastolic (the bottom number). EFAs decrease the stress on your heart.

8 *Dr. Bernstein's Diabetes Solution*, page 319.

Salt and hypertension

Most people cut back on salt, because salt is often said to be a significant factor in raising blood pressure. The truth is, even if you overload on salt, the body's automatic equilibrium systems go into action to counteract it. This includes the "atrial naturietic factor" (ANF) which triggers the kidneys to dump sodium. Human cells contain almost 1% salt-based nutrients. Sodium is the #1 extracellular nutrient."* **Sodium (salt) is *required* for sugar (glucose) transport into the cell — particularly the kidney and intestine.** Stomach acid requires chloride from the salt!**

An international study called "Intersalt" included more than 10,000 people in 32 countries. The results, reported in 1988, concluded "salt has only small importance in hypertension.[9] The *Textbook of Medical Physiology* agrees. For the vast majority of people, salt's role in raising blood pressure is insignificant compared with other factors. The cause of hypertension must be sought elsewhere. Even in patients with severe hypertension where salt intake can make a difference, doubling the salt intake (a huge difference) only made a marginal difference.

The research of John H. Laragh, M.D. and Mark S. Pecker, M.D. at the Hypertension Center at Cornell University Medical Center, shows **there is no evidence that avoiding salt would ever prevent hypertension or cardiovascular disease.**[10] The supposedly damaging effects of salt have been elevated to the same high visibility as the supposedly damaging effects of dietary cholesterol.

However, there is one effect, concerning salt, that does warrant looking at. Distorted EFAs allow sodium to enter the cell in concentrations far above normal. Recall the gaps in the cell membrane that distorted EFAs (*trans*fatty acids) have. Cells with an abundance of *trans*fatty acids have to work extra hard to keep this extra sodium out. Researchers looked at the effects of *trans*fatty acid concentration on rats. They found that a diet of just four-percent of these distorted EFAs caused the mitochondria (the

9 *Dr. Bernstein's Diabetes Solution*, page 318.

10 John Laragh, M.D., states "The majority of people with high blood pressure *do not have a salt factor* and do not need to avoid the normal range of salt intake which can promote good health. A *minority of patients* are salt sensitive, so that avoidance or reduction of salt will reduce or normalize their high pressure. We always identify them and advise appropriate salt reduction or diuretic therapy."

* *Basic Medical Biochemistry*, page 142.

** *Body Fluids And Electrolytes*, pages 20-22.

cell's important energy-generating mechanism) in rats to swell two to three times their size! This effect can be likened to an enlarged heart, trying to compensate. The mitochondria don't just increase in size. Their function is inhibited, too.

The tissues of these rats contained up to 14-percent of these distorted EFAs.[11] A little of them caused a big problem in the cells. It doesn't take many *trans*fatty acids to cause great damage! How much of these *trans*fatty acids does the average American eat? Guaranteed, it's a lot more than just four-percent of our diet.

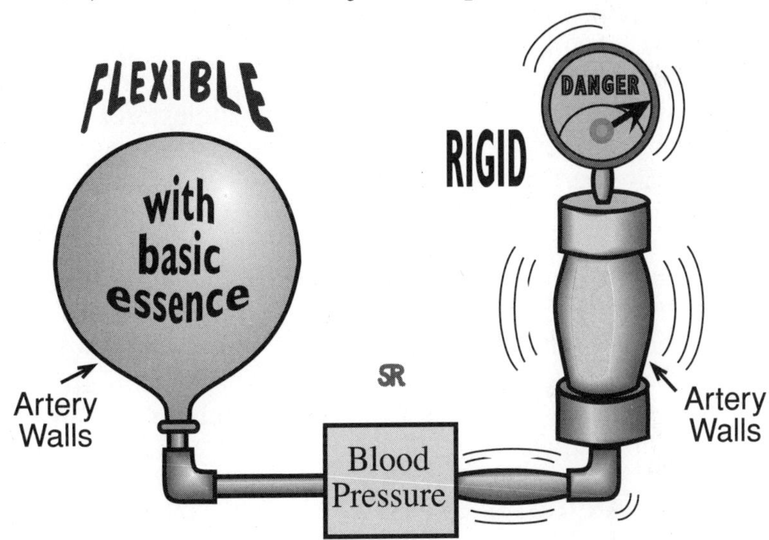

Blood pressure is lower with more flexible arteries, because they can expand.

Blood pressure frequently decreases when you have sufficient EFAs.

This happens because your cell membranes function better. You are less bloated at the cellular level.

EFAs also allow excellent fluidity in the bloodstream. EFA molecules carry a slight negative charge, due to their double bonds. Two EFA molecules behave like little magnets with the same pole pointing toward each other: They naturally repel each other.

11 *Sunlight*, page 101.

This is the same characteristic that keeps the blood platelets from sticking together in your bloodstream.

More EFA info

In addition to keeping cell membranes flexible, EFAs help increase surface activity of cells. This effect enables biological systems to remove toxins. EFAs even help govern the movement of chromosomes during cell division.

Lecithin, a phospholipid, is sometimes called "nature's edible detergent." Lecithin keeps fats and cholesterol suspended (technically "dispersed"). Detergent works the same way to remove the oil & grease from your dishes and clothes. Water alone won't remove grease – a dispersing agent must be used. What does lecithin have at its core? – the essential fatty acid omega 6!

EFAs are hard to study because they are highly reactive and are easily destroyed. Because they are very sensitive, we can understand why many nutritional researchers haven't noticed this missing link between EFAs and ultimate *Life-Systems* efficiency.

You have heard of buffered aspirin and how it has fewer side-effects than plain aspirin.

EFAs buffer excess acids and bases, too.

This is an extremely important function, because buffering assists in optimizing & controlling numerous chemical reactions throughout your body.

The great debate: butter vs. margarine

Here's a fact you need to know. Butter is used directly for energy. Butter is a short-chain fat, and is burned directly for energy. Butter never enters the lymph system because, even though it is a fat, it is reasonably water-soluble. It doesn't need to be surrounded with a protein for transportation because of its water solubility. Moderate amounts of butter can't end up as adipose tissue (fat) on your thighs.

Against Butter

Here's the *biggest negative* against butter. Unless it's organically-produced, butter can have more pesticide residues than other natural oils. Unless organically-raised, cows are routinely given antibiotics to keep them healthy. Some of these antibiotics are passed on to us through the milk. Long-term antibiotic use has been clearly shown to be detrimental to both humans and animals. The negative effect on our bodies from these antibiotics is far-reaching.

Hospitals now face new bacteria strains resistant to every antibiotic. Drug-resistant strains don't develop just from an individual's short-term over-use of antibiotics. An individual's occasional use simply isn't significant enough to generate such a widespread problem. A *Life-Systems* Engineering analysis suggests that the widespread problem must originate from a widespread source, such as long-term use by large populations. Is this grave condition accelerated by our constant ingestion of antibiotic residues in meat and dairy products? Our *Life-Systems* team thinks so.

Butter has few EFAs to start with, so there is little to ruin by processing. Making butter is mainly a natural process, yet, if you don't purchase organically-processed butter, then additives and chemicals are likely to be in the milk without your knowing it. If you purchase organically-processed butter, which is easy to do, you can be sure there are no additives.

Against Margarine

Margarine has few active EFAs left after processing. Even if it were to start with lots of them in the seeds the oils are pressed from, they are destroyed or altered by chemicals and heat in the processing. Margarine also has *chemical by-products* as a result of the process – partial hydrogenation – used to manufacture it. Even if they are not fully toxic, these remnants take the place of active EFAs. Margarine is partially hydrogenated to make the liquid oils semi-solid, so that the product will spread smoothly without running. We get convenience in exchange for an additional health risk.

Nickel, cadmium, and aluminum are frequently used as catalysts in margarine's production. Catalysts make reactions work or speed them up. Margarine's partial hydrogenation reaction has unpredictable intermediate stages. Many of the by-products from partial hydrogenation haven't been classified. The process can determine the final form – a semi-solid meltable mass – yet, the process doesn't fully control by-products. Some of these chemicals have not been evaluated for harmful or long-term side-effects. Margarine may also be a significant source of aluminum and nickel from the catalysts used in the manufacturing process.

A plastics engineer would call margarine "plastic food," – meaning that margarine's molecular structure resembles a low-grade plastic.

Margarine has tremendous amounts of harmful distorted EFAs called *trans*fatty acids.[12]

Margarine is polyunsaturated, and by itself that might be good news, yet to call margarine "good" is a misleading half-truth. Many of margarine's polyunsaturated fats are highly adulterated, unnatural, and chemically altered. **Their danger was described in medical journals as far back as 1956.**

Udo Erasmus' book, *Fats that Heal, Fats that Kill*, gives organic butter an overall score of minus 1, commercial butter a score of minus 3.5 and margarine a score of minus 10.5! Our *Life-Systems* Engineering team agrees with this relative rating. Butter made from organic milk is fine to eat.

Margarine has water in it, which, over time, slowly breaks down its chemical structure, causing additional by-products to multiply during its shelf-life.

Butter often has water in it, too, but because butter is naturally saturated, water doesn't react with or damage the butter. Nor does butter break down, even when heated to normal cooking (sautéing) temperatures.

Butter is used directly for energy by the body. It is classified as a short-chain saturated fatty acid. The body uses both short-chain and medium-chain saturated fatty acids to produce energy as a priority – these fats are not converted to bodyfat as commonly suggested.[13]

---

12 *Fats That Heal, Fats That Kill*, pages 103, 105.
13 *Textbook of Medical Physiology*, page 843.

Margarine is cheap to manufacture. This leaves plenty of money for massive advertising geared towards making you think that it's a great food.

Trans-Fat Margarine Co.
Executive Dining Room
ONLY TOP BRASS ALLOWED
Notice: Because we care about you and your health, we only serve REAL BUTTER
SR

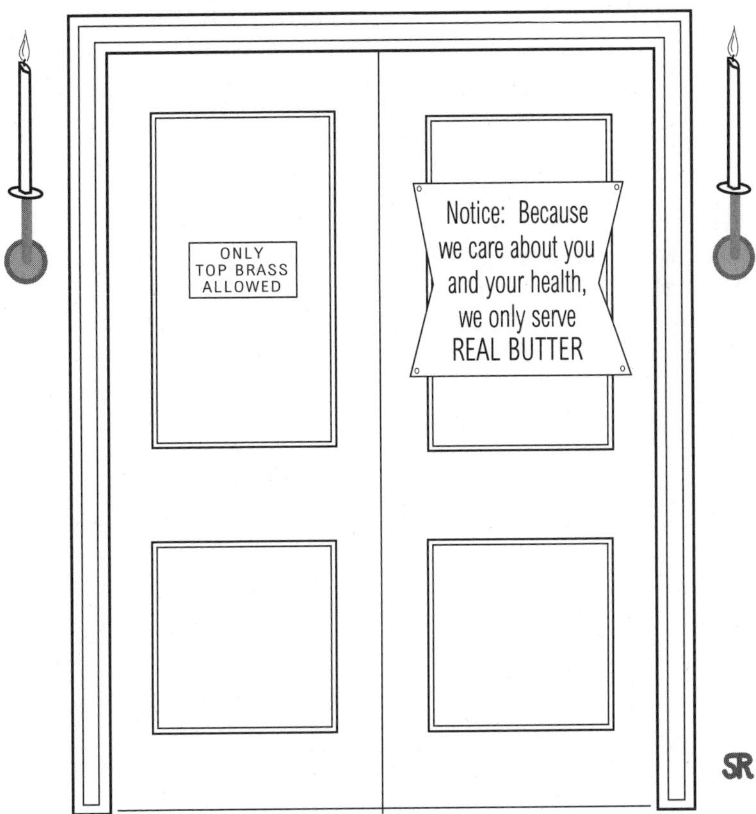

Because we've been misled into believing that all saturated fats are bad, we have been led incorrectly to conclude that margarine is healthier than butter.

If margarine were a new product, it would most likely fail to be approved under current "safe-certification" procedures.

The marketing of hydrogenated oil has been so effective, the manufacturers now have a liquid coffee "lightener." Some restaurants keep this on ice just like "half and half," which is made with real cream. There is absolutely no need to refrigerate this non-dairy "lightener" – it doesn't spoil at room temperature. Its ingredients include water, hydrogenated (highly processed) vegetable oil, sugar, and a host of added chemical stabilizers.

It's sad how many people willingly consume this stuff – all because they have been deceived into thinking that fat is bad. *They fail to ask: how much worse is its replacement?*

Butter & tropical oils ...

Let's look at frying. A saturated oil can withstand high heat without breaking down. The high temperature of frying quickly burns most natural (poly)unsaturated oils that haven't been chemically altered to resist these high temperatures. For deep frying, coconut oil is best, followed by peanut oil. These oils aren't easily degraded by high heat, because they are naturally saturated fats. Try some for yourself. They taste better, too.

When it comes to frying, we aren't choosing these oils for their nutritional benefit. We are concerned with how to minimize an oil's potentially harmful qualities. For frying, contrary to the popular views, a saturated oil such as butter, ghee or a tropical oil (such as coconut oil) is best. Here's why: since these oils are naturally saturated already, there's no reason for commercial oil processors to chemically distort (hydrogenate) them.

This is another prime example of how bad something isn't – rather than how good something is!

Saturated fats are extremely stable. This means they don't easily break down (become rancid) and produce troublesome by-products. Try frying in unprocessed coconut oil. Our *Life-Systems* Engineering team does, and the results are spectacular. You can even filter these oils through cheesecloth, refrigerate them after opening their containers, and re-use them again later on.

There are a lot of movie theaters across the country. Multiply their number by the number of batches of popcorn each theater sells each week. It's a very big number. Until the 1990s, coconut oil was used by theaters to pop their popcorn. Most of it has been replaced with hydrogenated canola or some other highly processed oil. Are these oils better? No. They are even *more harmful* because they have had lots of processing. Because these oils aren't saturated, the processing creates *trans*fatty acids. Who financed the "study" to show that coconut oil is bad?

Contrary to the misinformation that tropical oils (coconut oils and others) are bad, nothing could be further from the truth!

George Blackburn, M.D., a Harvard researcher, stated tropical oils [like coconut oil] don't raise cholesterol levels.*

A way to help *inhibit* cancer?

In the 1920's, another Nobel Prize-winner, Dr. Otto Warburg, discovered that decreasing oxygen to human tissues (cells) just 35 percent encourages the growth of cancer. EFAs are directly involved with oxygen transfer throughout the body. EFAs greatly increase cellular oxygen transfer. Conversely, shortages of EFAs reduce the oxygen transfer. Taking them is an easy way to gain an added dose of cancer immunity. Shouldn't we ask whether cancer could often be a result of EFA deficiency? The significant increase in U.S. cancer rates has followed the significant increase in food processing, so it is a good question.

Could EFA deficiency be a big reason for the tremendous increase in cancer?

* When no more than five-percent of calories come from them and overall fat is less than thirty-percent.

Cancer loves oxygen-deprived environments. EFAs are among the best oxygenators we have.

A way to *encourage* cancer

Many of us lump everything together, without differentiation. Cancer takes years to develop because multiple genetic cell mutations are required. A statement such as "all fats and oils are bad," is an example of this lack of insight. First, basic essence is a healthy essential oil, so the statement is medically and scientifically untrue. When we analyze fats and oils, we must be precise in what we deduce and why we think the deduction is true.

The facts clearly show that the distorted fats (transfatty acids) cause significant damage. Commercial food processing is at their root, because they don't occur in nature. In the chapter "Sunlight and Cancer," of the book *Sunlight*, numerous studies implicate these distorted (vegetable) fats under far greater suspicion than animal fats in causing ill-health![14] These two problems help explain our twentieth-century increase in ill-health.

We are getting a "double whammy":

1. We aren't getting enough basic essence.
2. We eat too many harmful *trans*fats.

A way to prevent Alzheimer's?

Alzheimer's disease has become an epidemic. By 1997. **there were at least 4 million Americans in some stage of Alzheimer's.** By the middle of the next century, it is estimated that 14 million Americans will become afflicted.[15] Two hundred-forty million dollars ($240 million) was spent on its research in 1996. Is everyone looking in the wrong places for its solution, too? Let's look at the facts.

---

14 "Experimental Evidence of Dietary Factors and Hormone-Dependent Cancer," K.K. Carroll, *Cancer Research* 35:3374, 1975; "Gastrointestinal Cancer and Nutrition," O.Gregor, *Gut* 10:1031, 1969; "Dietary Fat and Cancer Trends," M.G. Enig, et al, *Fed Proc* 37:2215, 1978.

15 "AMA endorses Chinese herb to slow effects of Alzheimer's," *Houston Chronicle,* October 22, 1997, page 5A.

Alzheimer's is a degenerative disease. Once it starts, it keeps getting worse. Studies show that by age 85, up to 40 percent (40%) of the population gets Alzheimer's. This statistic is similar to cancer rate statistics – more of us are becoming victims! The brain of Alzheimer's victims shows significant inflammation.[16]

The brain is supposed to be loaded with EFAs, but it may be deficient in EFAs, because commercial food processing either removes them or chemically distorts them. Basic essence EFAs are natural anti-inflammatories. Minerals are involved in all *Life-Systems*, but we are deficient in essential minerals because of overfarming the same soil.

This fact is stated in an Internet article concerning Alzheimer's disease.[17] In a section about the causes of the disease: "The major target for research on the genetic causes of the much more common late-onset Alzeheimer's disease is the apolipoprotein ApoE. ApoE normally plays a role in the movement and distribution of cholesterol for repairing nerve cells during development and after injury." EFAs maximize apolipoprotein ApoE's positive effects.

A *Life-Systems* Engineering analysis concludes that The Foundation of Radiant Health is one of the best nutritional Alzheimer's preventatives, because the Foundation of Radiant Health naturally enables your body to overcome many of the deficiencies commonly found in Alzheimer's patients.

Viruses are everywhere

Few of us are aware that we each harbor many viruses, but there has to be a critical number of them to do actual damage. If you have fewer than this critical quantity, your immune system maintains a balance.

When a relative of mine was in the hospital with pneumonia, I was shocked to learn that the physician couldn't tell me if her pneumonia was getting better. He said, "The mouth cultures show the 'bug' is still there."

So I asked, "If the bug is still there, then she isn't getting better, is she?"

He said that most of us would always show some presence of a pneumonia virus if a mouth culture was taken, so this meant little.

Published research verified this to be true.

16 "AMA endorses ...," page 5A.
17 *Ask NOAH About:* Alzheimer's Disease (Well Connected).

The big reason most of us aren't always sick with numerous ailments is because we have a strong immune system.

EFAs are among the best immune boosters we have!

I tell people all the time, "I can't get sick anymore." I've gone three years with only two mild colds since I started regularly taking basic essence, Essiac-concept tonic, and the nine minerals lacking in the soil.[18] Unless I abuse my body by not getting enough sleep or rest, I have become virtually "unstoppable."

Modern medicine has a tendency to rely heavily on drugs. Often, this is fine. Antibiotics are tremendous assets to assist physicians. But sometimes, drugs aren't appropriate. For example, when a drug is used to bring down a fever, it can often compromise the body's natural defenses. Temperature should usually be allowed to rise naturally to allow the body to fight more effectively – unless one has a temperature over about 101 degrees F. Yet, how many of us even realize that heat is an ally in fighting a virus – we just reach for a pill, which actually does the opposite of what we need by hampering our body's natural defenses!

Cholesterol – a bit more

I have already discussed the great cholesterol hoax with you, but there is even more to tell. Re-evaluate the "bad" and "good" LDL/HDL ratio numbers that the press (newspapers and magazines) print stories about. When viewed in a *Life-Systems* Engineering analysis, the terms "bad" and "good" often lose their traditionally accepted meanings.

Every cell membrane needs EFAs. They produce flexibility in the cell membrane, balancing the stiffness of cholesterol. These two opposing extremes are required for *Life-System* balance in the cell membrane. Recall that, in any *Life-System*, a balance is required between opposing extremes. LDL is the transport mechanism which brings life-sustaining EFAs and cholesterol to the cell. Therefore, LDL cholesterol should be expected to increase in the bloodstream once EFA blood levels increase and become adequate.

18 Previously, I would get colds and flus 3-4 times each year. Also, I'd get a bad sore throat almost every airline trip because I have a continual post-nasal drip. Now I don't need to get corrective surgery to eliminate the post-nasal drip. It's still there, but I rarely get sick from it anymore.

Did you know that insulin production caused by eating carbohydrates raises levels of cholesterol and harmful triglycerides!?

Basic Medical Biochemistry, pages 475, 566

When enough EFAs have been utilized by the body, especially in the cell membranes, a new "balance-point" is reached. Then, cholesterol levels may decrease because the EFA-deficiency has been eliminated. Because EFA and mineral deficiency are so universal, few nutritionists have taken this mechanism into account.

The body constantly produces tremendous amounts of cholesterol, compared with other essential biological components, regardless of what we eat. Artificially reducing the cholesterol level in a red blood cell will actually cause its membrane to break down. A broken membrane means a dead cell. Too little cholesterol available to the cell causes serious problems.

Cholesterol is even integral to hormone production in your body!

Without adequate amounts of estrogen, a woman's hormone system quickly becomes imbalanced and impaired. Without cholesterol, men's reduced testosterone production quickly produces dire consequences. Even adrenaline is based on cholesterol. Cholesterol production requires EFAs, too. Could an EFA deficiency cause defective cholesterol?

Artificially lowering cholesterol levels with drugs disrupts the body's automatic control system. In response, other bodily systems shift out of balance. That's why we often see a multitude of negative side-effects in other areas when taking any drugs. That's why you may wish to read the drug's "package insert," so you can be aware of the possible side-effects. Why must we be so frequently reminded that we can't fool Mother Nature?

The one thing that comes through, time and time again, is that there is no proven cause-effect relationship between "high blood cholesterol" and poor health.

It will likely be shown that any "problem" associated with cholesterol is based on distortion of EFAs in the cholesterol. Yes, even cholesterol uses EFAs!

It's often difficult to pinpoint the precise cause of a problem in complicated *Life-Systems*.

A drug that decreases cholesterol could have side-effects that increases health problems in the test subjects. Such a side-effect could indirectly influence ill-health from other causes, even if the drug did decrease cholesterol levels. We can't draw any cause-effect relationships from these limited results.

HMG CoA reductase is an enzyme that controls cholesterol production in the liver. In *Enter The Zone*, Dr. Sears states that all enzymes, including HMG CoA reductase, are under the control of insulin and glucagon. Glucagon inhibits enzyme production, and insulin increases its production. Therefore, glucagon will indirectly affect cholesterol levels in your bloodstream. What will increase glucagon? **Less carbohydrate.** What automatically gives you the desire to eat less carbohydrates? Basic essence. In other words, an adequate supply of basic essence should lead to a new cholesterol balance point.

Drug manufacturers use direct marketing

Parade,[19] a national magazine, carried a prominent advertisement for the drug Zocar. It's interesting that Merck, the manufacturer, paid to advertise directly to the public, since only a physician can prescribe Zocar. Marketing drugs directly to the public has become commonplace.

The advertisement states:

- The drug lowers LDL cholesterol. The ad doesn't mention how much it lowers LDL cholesterol. How significant is this lowering? We aren't told. It also implies that this is a desirable change.

- The advertisement cites a five-year "study" (no details are given) in which patients having both heart disease and high cholesterol demonstrated "dramatic" results. There were fewer heart attacks. How many fewer? The numbers aren't given. During the five-year period, there were 42-percent fewer deaths from heart disease. The ad doesn't say how many people were in the study or how many died. Also, we must realize that, just because you didn't die, doesn't mean you are well. Your heart could still be

19 *Parade*, August 11, 1996.

in poor shape. Should you put much belief in this advertisement? Certainly not – we aren't given the information we need. The manufacturers realize most of us don't ask these questions. Many of us seem to be happy with shallow promises and easy-sounding answers. When you read the STAT-SMART chapter, you'll see why we red-flag the claimed 42-percent reduction.

- The ad admits, "of course, not everyone gets the same results." How different are the results? If the results are inconsistent, then there's a good chance that the drug didn't cause those results! This automatically challenges the drug's effectiveness.
- Here's a shocking twist. The ad says, "in clinical studies one percent of patients experienced liver dysfunction." One percent may sound insignificant, but with 3.1 million people taking the drug, at least 31,000[20] may now have liver dysfunction as a result of the drug! We aren't told whether this dysfunction is permanent or whether it is temporary while taking the drug. The liver controls numerous bodily processes. Is the risk of dysfunction worth the supposed positive benefit of the drug? That certainly is your decision, but you're given little useful information on which to decide.
- The advertisement goes on to say, "*don't take the drug* if: you have liver problems, are pregnant, breast-feeding, or are allergic to its ingredients, and tell your doctor if you feel muscle pain or weakness while taking this drug." (emphasis added)

One result of this direct-to-the-consumer drug advertising method is that the patient tells the physician what drugs he wants because he read about them in a magazine. Some physicians may welcome this change because it's quick and easy. It also shifts some of the responsibility to the patient. From the drug company's point of view, it's a brilliant marketing system.

Newsweek magazine has instituted a pharmaceutical advertising campaign. The magazine features medical cover stories and

21 One percent of 3,100,000 = 31,000. But we don't know that these 3.1 million are taking the same dosages under the same conditions. The actual number of those developing liver problems may be higher.

medical editorials. The drug manufacturers get to place their advertisements strategically in the magazine. *Newsweek* likes this idea so much that they even took out a very expensive full-page, four-color advertisement in the *New York Times* to attract drug companies: "Rx Partnership. Your pharmaceutical TV campaign can't survive without it."[21] The media certainly knows how to influence our opinions to buy their advertisers' products.

For your information, the reason we now see television advertisements aimed at allergy suffers, is because of a drug advertising regulation. The drug manufacturers now get to name either the prescription drug or the illness treated – not both – unless they give you all the known health risks, too. *They certainly don't want to list the risks on television or have an announcer read them.* The FDA has eased up and will soon allow drug manufacturers to simply mention "major" side-effects. What will FDA's definition of "major" be? Probably, not yours or mine.

A *New York Times* article stated that pharmaceutical companies spent nearly $600 million ($600,000,000) in 1996 advertising prescription drugs, bypassing doctors, directly to their patients![22] This is 10 times the amount they spent in 1991 and double what they spent in 1995. The article states that drug companies spend an estimated $12 billion ($12,000,000,000) a year on advertising and promotion. In 1998 $**5 billion** was spent for pharmaceutical sales reps, and **$1 billion** for physician "events."

While I was a guest on a radio talk show, in Springfield, Massachusetts, on May 6, 1997, a newsflash came over the wire – Massachusetts just had their first Phen-Fen related death! The timing was amazing. This happens while I'm speaking about how our Foundation of Radiant Health discovery can frequently eliminate the need for diet drugs. The next day an article appeared in the local newspaper quoting Dr. Lewis Rubin, director of pulmonary and critical care at the University of Maryland Medical Center in Baltimore as saying, "**There is no question that either drug alone can produce pulmonary hypertension (PPH)**. *What we don't know at this point in time is the magnitude of the risk of taking the drugs together.*"[23] (emphasis added) Rubin co-authored a

21 *New York Times*, October 14, 1997, page C9, January 11, 1999.

22 "Drug Companies' Sales Pitch: 'Ask Your Doctor,'" Abigail Zuger, New *York Times*, August 5, 1997, page B9.

23 "Diet: Woman's death spurs probe of drugs," *Union-News*, Springfield, MA, May 7, 1997, page 1.

paper in the prestigious *New England Journal of Medicine*. The study found a 2,300-percent increase in PPH among those who took appetite suppressants. In the STAT-SMART chapter, you'll learn why, even though this is important, there may be more to the picture.

Animal studies show that high doses of the diet drug Redux destroy brain cells considered vital for mood and other functions.[24] Redux users often had to resort to higher and higher doses to get any effect from the drug. Is that what you want? And these drugs were often being handed out in wholesale fashion. Before the basic essence-appetite discovery and the Foundation of Radiant Health connection, the health profession was often without (non-drug) hope.

With the basic essence / Foundation of Radiant Health discovery, drugs are often no longer needed to satisfy the appetite and to become lean for life!

Ask your pharmacist to show you an old "package insert" for the diet drug commonly called REDUX. It was recalled in September 1997. The manufacturer was forced to state that the drug's effect is, at best, only good for losing a fraction of a pound a week, and the drug is, at best, of questionable value to begin with. This is directly from the manufacturer. After a few weeks, Redux wouldn't even work anymore, unless you kept increasing the dosage. Its side-effects were terrible, too. That's why the FDA had to ban it. This portion of the Phen-Fen combination is often now replaced with Prozac.

Mayo Clinic report reinforces a diet drug manufacturer's package insert admission of marginal effectiveness![24]

The Mayo Clinic reported this surprising information concerning diet drugs:

1. The medications don't work for everyone – at least a third of those taking them get no results from any diet drug.

24 *Mayo Clinic Health Letter*, October 1997, page 6.

2. There's a limit to how much weight you can lose. Most weight loss occurs in the first 6 months – and it's usually limited to just 10% of your initial bodyweight. [If you start at a weight of 300 pounds, then the best results you can expect are a reduction to 270 pounds 6 months later. If you weigh 200 pounds, you may "reduce" to 180 pounds. This isn't very significant, especially given the associated health risks of all diet drugs. Also with these drugs, important muscle is lost along with bodyfat, – it's not all fat loss!] (comments added)
3. Finally, when you stop taking the drugs, you start regaining all the lost weight. [Translation: Taking diet drugs could be a lifetime proposition.] (comment added)

A quick physical predictor of heart-related problems:

A crease in your earlobe is an indicator of a possible future heart- or artery-related problem.

Army physicians back in the 1950s were the first to suggest this link. Back then critics were skeptical. Nothing more was made of it. Afterward, cholesterol-related issues received the bulk of discussion to the virtual exclusion of anything else.

You should be aware of this visible indicator of possible coronary-related problems. The reason this crease develops may be that the carotid arteries in the neck feed the ears as well as the brain. If there is an arterial obstruction or decreased blood flow, the earlobe responds with this crease. This doesn't automatically mean that if you don't have a crease, you have nothing to be concerned about. But *if the crease is visible, you should take immediate action to reverse the condition.* A quick and painless carotid artery ultrasound scan can easily detect any degree of arterial blockage. Ask your physician's advice.

A diabetic's best friend

Diabetics will greatly appreciate the results from taking more EFAs. With a reduced desire to eat processed carbohydrates, they will eat less of them, and therefore reduce their insulin requirements.

Diabetes is the single greatest cause of kidney failure in the U.S., and diabetes leads directly to numerous life-threatening diseases.

High blood-glucose levels place excessive stress on the kidneys.

High blood glucose levels cause numerous problems. One of them is that this extra glucose surrounds (encapsulates) the proteins. These glucose-encapsulated proteins enter the kidneys, forcing your *Life-Systems* to maintain equilibrium by drawing extra water into the bloodstream. Hence, more work for the kidneys, increased blood pressure, and increased blood flow through the kidney.[25] This is why consistently high glucose levels often cause premature kidney failure in diabetics. Now we can stop that problem cold! All diabetics should monitor their glucose levels once they start taking EFA supplements, because insulin requirements typically decrease. Don't just keep taking the usual amount of insulin. If you are taking any medications, keep your physician informed of your changing glucose levels. Remember, when one thing changes, everything changes.

Just like too much alcohol kills the liver, too much carbohydrate kills the pancreas and kidneys.

The horror of insulin resistance

This is an urgent topic, because we are eating ever-increasing amounts of (processed) carbohydrates. Increased insulin is required to counteract this increase of processed carbohydrates in our diet. The body doesn't want much sugar in its bloodstream and the response to these carbohydrates is more insulin.

The more carbohydrates we eat, the more insulin the body generates. If we eat frequently, like four-six small meals a day, then at least four-six insulin shots a day are generated to rebalance the system. If there is an overabundance of carbohydrates at each of these small meals, as is often the case, then the amount of insulin must be proportionately larger. Remember, when we overload on

25 *Dr. Bernstein's Diabetes Solution*, page 316.

carbohydrates, we also experience the inevitable sugar low driving us to eat more carbohydrates just a few hours later. A vicious cycle is created. More insulin per meal is required. More insulin is needed throughout the day. More sugar lows feed this cycle and sap our energy, too.

The neurotransmitter, serotonin, is released when we eat carbohydrates.

Serotonin is a natural sedative!

That partially explains why we often feel tired soon after eating.

By subjecting our bodies to constant carbohydrate and insulin stimulation, over time, more and more insulin is released, but the body gradually loses its tolerance, so that less and less glucose gets metabolized. Over the course of many years, our excessive diet of processed carbohydrates will drive many of us into insulin resistance.

Insulin resistance occurs for the same reason that a bodybuilder has to keep increasing the amount of weight he or she uses to keep stimulating muscle growth.

Our bodies quickly get used to a stimulus. All types of addictions illustrate this. A cigarette a day quickly increases to two or three a day. Can any regular soda drinker drink just one a day?[26] More and more stimulus is required to obtain the same effect.

The *Foundation of Radiant Health* naturally diminishes your desire for processed carbohydrates.

Some people may lose some weight with high-carbohydrate diets, but they are being lulled into a false sense of security! When people are on a high-carbohydrate diet, their triglyceride levels tend

26 We analyzed a can of soda for aluminum content. The result was 6 milligrams per liter. A liter is a little more than a quart. No amount is considered safe for toxic metals. If you are concerned about aluminum, glass containers may be safer.

to rise. High triglycerides are a strong warning signal that something is seriously out of balance. As a rule, triglycerides (fats in the blood) decrease as we lose bodyfat, and they definitely decrease as fewer carbohydrates are eaten. They typically decrease with basic essence consumption. Recall my personal experience on an extremely high-fat diet while taking basic essence: my triglyceride levels dropped 25 percent! Before that, I had been on a high-carbohydrate diet for years.

One may ask: what if I am on a high-carbohydrate diet and take basic essence and the Foundation of Radiant Health, too? Won't the effects counteract each other? Good question. The answer is yes, they will, but with basic essence, our desire for carbohydrates significantly decreases. Processed carbohydrate overload short-circuits the Foundation of Radiant Health's natural fat-burning effect. If we now continue to force ourselves to eat more carbohydrates than our bodies are telling us they want, we are willfully overriding our bodies' natural responses. With the Foundation of Radiant Health, taste and hunger finally work together. Why not achieve maximum benefit?

Does this mean we'll never want a hamburger, a piece of cake, or fried fish? No. It only means we won't want them as often, or in such large portions as we used to. We may not eat all of our hamburger bun or we will eat just a few bites of cake, or half the bagel. Our sense of taste significantly increases once EFA levels become balanced. Food tastes better and you won't need or want nearly as much.[27] It's wonderful how, with basic essence, the body naturally responds to what is best for it.

To accurately monitor the system effects of insulin and blood chemistry, it makes sense to study persons with diabetes. Our team did this, and it was wonderful to see how, with basic essence and minerals, the desire for processed carbohydrates significantly decreased. Less carbohydrates gives a more consistent blood-glucose level with a lot less insulin required. Recall, only carbohydrates (sugar) force the body to produce lots of insulin, converting the sugar to triglycerides, and storing the triglycerides as bodyfat.

27 This sounds like a contradiction, but without basic essence and the Foundation of Radiant Health, our hunger system is "short-circuited." Once it works properly, you receive more satisfaction and pleasure with much less food — the way our hunger-taste system was designed to function.

Calorie restriction

Life extension through calorie restriction has become a popular topic of discussion. A *Life-Systems* Engineering analysis gives us insight. Using the same reasoning of restricting calories, we could erroneously generalize that restricting our breathing would make us live longer, too (if we didn't pass out from oxygen deprivation). Using an organ less does not ensure that it will last longer.

Today's typical diet has a lot of processed carbohydrates (sugar), so, if we eat less food, we get less processed carbohydrates. This means less insulin is produced. And that means less probability of insulin-related problems.

If we eat less, we consume less toxins from food processing. Positive results attributed to calorie deprivation may show that, in today's diet, we are overwhelmed with an excess of toxins. This *Life-Systems* Engineering analysis may be the true basis of the calorie deprivation concept and its relationship to better health.

Salad and sugar lows

Is eating a large salad as a meal good for you? You may re-evaluate your answer when you understand the insulin-connection. Here's why: Most salad is cellulose along with a lot of water. **Cellulose cannot be digested by humans***, but it fills your stomach. Vegetables contain up to 97% water! When something enters your stomach, your pancreas produces some insulin in anticipation of food. Normally, this presents no problem because most foods have some amount of carbohydrate in them. But in the case of indigestible cellulose, like salad, there is little significant food value compared with proteins and healthy essential oils. That's why eating just a large salad for lunch or dinner – in the hopes of tricking your stomach into thinking that it is full – doesn't really work. You'll get a sugar "low" after eating the salad by itself. Now you know why it happens. *Humans aren't meant to dine on just salad – no matter how good a diet consultant may say it is.*

What the brain likes

The brain is composed of a high percentage of fat. There is a chemical barrier to the brain, commonly referred to as the "blood-brain" barrier. This barrier lets in oxygen, most water-soluble

---

* *Essentials of Biochemistry*, page 185.

nutrients, and most lipid-soluble (fat-soluble) nutrients. But it won't let in large-chain proteins. Drug manufacturers have an extremely difficult time influencing the brain directly with drugs, because most drugs rely on a protein-based structure.

Here's an analogy: We don't want sloppy workers moving our important household furnishings and keepsakes. Sure, the truck and your belongings arrive at the final destination, yet sloppy packing results in lots of damage.

What is the best carrier of lipid-soluble structures? EFAs. So we see that basic essence, containing EFAs, is vital to carrying nutrients to the brain.

Brown "age spots" take a hike, too

Age spots, frequently called "liver spots," are indicative of degeneration within the body. Our *Life-Systems* team has seen these spots become lighter or even disappear altogether once basic essence and the Foundation of Radiant Health is added to the diet.

Increased oxygen

Here's another important piece of information we can use. Increased oxygen in the cell is one of the best ways to prevent disease. Most harmful organisms exist primarily in anaerobic (no oxygen), or low-oxygen environments. These organisms love mucus in the body, where oxygen is minimal. Guess what is a great cellular oxygenator? Basic essence (EFAs). Each of our cell membranes contain a large proportion of EFAs. One of the main functions of a cell membrane is to control oxygen transfer into the cell. With a healthy membrane structure, cellular oxygen transfer is maximized. This produces an environment where harmful organisms don't grow well. With real EFAs, the immune system becomes the warrior it was meant to be.

Sunlight is healthy

Even the sun, often blamed for giving us skin cancer, has taken an unwarranted bad rap. The sun is a natural life-giving source of energy. Many people in "developing" countries spend considerable time out in the sun and don't get cancer from it. A *Life-Systems* Engineering analysis would say that humans need sunlight for radiant health and that, contrary to what we are constantly told, the sun should be very good for us. So where does the real problem lie?

These developing countries don't have the high levels of nutrient-destroying food processing that "developed" countries do. When skin's cellular structure has the integrity it is meant to, the body's natural protection from ultraviolet radiation is increased. Am I saying it will now be OK to burn yourself like a piece of toast? No, but there is less need to fear the sun if the skin's EFA structure is intact. The skin will be protected from moderate sunlight – as it was designed to be. In fact, we need sunlight for our bodies to produce vitamin D!

An article called "Too Little Sun?" said this about vitamin D and sunlight:

> ...underexposure can dangerously lower vitamin D levels.... Vitamin D has inhibited the development and growth of many different cancers in both test-tube and animal studies. In humans, the risk of various cancers – notably breast, colon, and prostate, the three most common kinds in nonsmokers – is *substantially lower in sunny regions than in areas with less sunlight*, both around the world and within the U.S. One possible reason: The skin produces more vitamin D in sunnier climates."[28] (emphasis added)

Vitamin D (produced naturally from sunlight) significantly reduces risk of breast cancer![29]

A significant study performed at Northern California Cancer Center compared breast cancer rates of two groups of women: A) those from climates with the most sun exposure or who had moderate to frequent exposure to the sun; and B) those from climates with the least sun exposure. Group A, **those exposed to more sunlight, had the lowest risk of breast cancer**. Those in the southern climates have a lower death rate from breast cancer compared to women in northern climates.

Vitamin D is made by the body from the interaction of sunlight with the EFAs in your skin! Would the breast cancer rates decrease even further if the women weren't EFA- and mineral-deficient, too? Would detoxification with an Essiac-concept tonic have helped?

---

28 *Consumer Reports On Health*, July 1997, pages 78-79.

29 "Vitamin D from sun may fight breast cancer," *Houston Chronicle*, November 2, 1997, page 5A.

The researchers also looked at the effect of vitamin D supplements. Their comment: **"The role of vitamin D [supplements] from the diet was less clear."** [emphasis added]

If your EFA level is adequate, your skin will be loaded with EFAs, so the sun can interact as Mother Nature intended and form natural vitamin D. *The high rate of skin cancer from sunlight is another indication of the lack of unadulterated EFAs in our food.*

All members of our *Life-Systems* Engineering team have noticed a major change in their skin's response to the sun after taking EFAs for more than a year – no more painful sunburn! This verifies, through personal experience, another powerful benefit of EFAs.

Sunlight becomes invigorating instead of exhausting.

Here's a bit of personal verification about how important the sun is. I live in Houston, so I'm used to getting lots of sun. It feels really great, and I'm invigorated all the time. I can tell you that when I went to Massachusetts last winter with my wife, Debbie, it got dark at about 4:30 PM – and *we were both tired and ready to go to bed by 6:30 PM.* This happened day-after-day and it wasn't due to excess work, either mental or physical, or jet lag – simply less sun. In Houston, we normally retire between 11 PM and midnight. So here's yet another personal verification that sunlight makes a difference in how you feel.

At home, you can use light bulbs that simulate natural sunlight, called full-spectrum bulbs. They make a real difference when you spend a lot of time indoors. You will feel more energetic in their light. Gardeners call them "grow lights."

Here's where the "sun is bad for you" idea probably came from. Virtually everyone is deficient in EFAs and bioavailable minerals. These EFAs and minerals are critical to every cell in our body, including our skin. So wouldn't it make sense that we should see symptoms of this deficiency? So could it be that skin problems, and maybe even skin cancer, are closely related to EFA and mineral deficiency?

It was found, many years ago, that **eating distorted cottonseed**

oil (containing *trans*fatty acids) led to an increase in skin cancer from ultraviolet light. This was reported in the *American Journal of Cancer* in 1939![30] This fact is rarely mentioned today. This significant possibility has to be considered more seriously. Our team of *Life-Systems* Engineers is one of the few groups, today, who have examined this connection.

Our studies show that, once we have solved the nutritional deficiencies relieved by the Foundation of Radiant Health, even fair skin no longer burns as easily. Keep in mind that it takes several months – up to a year – for the body to fully achieve radiant health.

This is one of the long-term benefits. Even when exposure is extreme enough to cause a sunburn, it heals with incredible speed – without pain – rarely even sore to touch. I first noticed this when I went to a weekend art fair. I was out in a short-sleeved shirt for more than three hours and my arms barely turned red. I was amazed. My wife, Debbie, who is very fair-skinned, had the same results. She had always avoided the sun because she believed how bad it was supposed to be. Numerous others using the Foundation of Radiant Health have reported similar experiences.

We are designed by Mother Nature to enjoy the sun. Without it, we'd all die. By the way, in 1903, another Nobel Prize-winner, Niels Finsen, won the prize for applying sunlight therapy in the treatment of tuberculosis of the skin. Even the dreaded *E. coli* bacteria is killed by natural sunlight![31]

Many confirmed healthy practices of the past have been turned backwards today.

We are constantly told that sunlight is bad for us and loads of carbohydrates (sugar) are good for us. With the *Life-System Engineering* discoveries, the results suggest otherwise.

A natural prostate protector?

For a long time it has been known that men living in areas of the world with less sunlight have a higher rate of prostate cancer. One explanation for this higher cancer rate is that less vitamin D is produced by the body because of less sunlight there. Recall,

30 "The Effect of Diet on Tumors Induced by Ultraviolet Light," C.A. Baumann and H.P. Rusch, *American Journal of Cancer* 35:213, 1939.

31 *Sunlight*, Zane R. Kime, MD, World Health Publications, Penryn, CA, 1980, page 27.

Vitamin D is produced by the interaction of sunlight with cholesterol and EFAs in your skin. It has been shown that vitamin D inhibits the growth of prostate cancer.[32] A study performed at the University of North Carolina showed a decrease in prostate cancer requiring surgery among men who "utilize" vitamin D more efficiently. The researchers say these more-efficient vitamin D men have a "genetic" difference.

A *Life-Systems* Engineering analysis would predict this lower rate of prostate cancer. However, as we already saw, we would state that increased basic essence – not the vitamin D, is the direct cause of the additional protection because, without enough EFAs and minerals, your body can't manufacture vitamin D. In regard to the supposed genetic difference, could it be that some of the men in the group simply had more EFAs and minerals in their diet, and that was the direct cause of the vitamin D efficiency? We think so.

From any perspective, optimum health & peak performance require the Foundation of Radiant Health.

The world's best artery protector?

Why do we get arterial tears that cause buildup (healing)?

Let's start with the structure of an artery. We will examine 2 of its layers: the extremely thin inside layer of skin, which is surrounded by a thick muscular layer. Wrap your hand around a straw. The straw can be thought of as the inside skin, and your hand as the muscle.

We live with increased stress today, including the body's almost constant "fight-or-flight" stress response to the toxic overloads of carbohydrates. Could the thick muscular arterial layer be constricting much more frequently than in earlier years before commercial food processing? If this is the case, then the fragile, thin layer has much more stress applied to it much more frequently as well. Given our basic essence EFA deficiency, this skin is more readily harmed by the abuse from the increased stress and frequent carbohydrate overloads. So, it tears more easily.

32 "Prostate Cancer and Vitamin D," *Dr. Alexander's Health Gazette*, Vol. 20:7, August 1997, source: *Journal of the American Medical Association*, 277:201, 1997.

Adding to the abuse, our diet is crammed with high levels of food processing and a constant deluge of numerous harmful food additives. We can use all the help we can get to keep our arteries smooth on the inside.

Would you like to know about something that an associate of mine calls the "natural nonstick coating for the body"? It's called Essiac-concept tonic, and it allows arteries to remain slick and smooth. A slick, smooth surface makes it difficult for any substance to attach to the arterial wall.

Oil in your automobile engine allows the piston to travel up and down smoothly in the cylinder. Likewise,

EFAs are the body's natural lubricant in the bloodstream.

Minimizing a cut or a tear on the inside of an artery is fundamental to ensuring that no obstructions occur. If a cut or tear happens, healing automatically takes place, and this could cause the build-up of cholesterol, calcium, and other components, commonly called "plaque." A special herb from South America, called Cat's Claw (Uncaria Tomentosa), has significant anti-clotting properties (it is a natural platelet fluidizer). These properties add to EFA's beneficial ability to keep your blood fluid. Essiac-concept tonic plus Cat's Claw is a remarkable combination you'll want to know about, too.[33]

A word of caution:

If much of the material in this next section seems hard to read, that's because it is! The Krebbs Cycle and everything about the human physiology, especially the digestion and metabolism processes, are extremely complex and technical. Here you get a sample of the sources our team reviewed in order to find the material which we have sorted out and condensed for you. We think it becomes evident why so many in the nutritional field do not fully understand what they (and we) are dealing with here. There is valuable information here, but if it just seems too difficult, don't feel inadequate – you are in good company. Besides, we have extracted most of the important points and boxed or emphasized them.

33 Essiac has an interesting story. The author has reached an agreement to reprint sections of an informative booklet about its use, which is included as Chapter 14.

Cardiovascular disease takes a hike
(prostaglandins in the cardiovascular system)

Because cardiovascular-related disorders kill more than half of us, let's review how some recent Nobel Prize-winning knowledge of prostaglandins can allow us to escape this disorder. Here are some important findings from the "*5th International Symposium on Prostaglandins in the Cardiovascular System*," held in Vienna, Austria, in 1991 and the "*10th International Conference on Prostaglandins and Related Compounds*," held in Vienna in 1996. It is rather technical information, but there is no simpler way to discuss prostaglandin's very complex *Life-Systems* effects.

The editors of the 10th International Conference include in their preface: "The editors feel that this actual information might be helpful to all physicians and scientists working in this exciting area of vascular biology and medicine." [34]

The proceedings were published in *Prostaglandins in the Cardiovascular System.* I went to one of the nation's best medical booksellers to obtain it. The book was priced at $109.50. There was only one copy in the store. Marcus went to the main public library in Toronto, Canada and *couldn't even find one book on prostaglandins!*

Here are some of the 1991 proceeding's most significant findings: "Eicosanoids [prostaglandins] and cytokines play a role in the cardiovascular cholesterol homeostasis and **have a profound effect on cholesterol delivery and trafficking within the vessel wall**. It also appears that the eicosanoid pathway is linked to the cytokine network regarding modulation of the vessel wall lipolytic activities ... Certain dysfunctions which occur very early after the onset of hypercholesterolemia, including a marked loss of the ability to produce the eicosanoid prostacyclin (PGI2) and endothelium-derived hyperpolarizing factor (EDHF), provide evidence for this." [35]

Arterial plaque contains high concentrations of lipid peroxides, which are known to inhibit *prostacyclin synthase*.

34 *Prostaglandins and Control of Vascular Smooth Muscle Cell Proliferation*, edited by Karsten Schor, M.D., and Peter Ney, Ph.D., Birkhauser Publishing, Switzerland, 1996.

35 *Prostaglandins in the Cardiovascular System*, Birkhauser Publishing, Switzerland, 1992, page 321. The next two references are included in the book, as well.

What this means is that: Prostaglandins protect us, and we need EFAs to produce them!

More information we don't frequently hear about: "Atherosclerosis is a complex multifunctional disease which leads to excessive deposition of lipids in the vascular wall (Ross, 1986; Steinberg, et al., 1990). Even though the sequence of events leading to the formation of atherosclerotic plaque is still unclear, lipid peroxidation is known to be involved in pathogenesis of atherosclerosis (Tanko & Mineo, 1990)."[36] Cholesterol is not blamed for causing the plaque buildup. Indeed, these researchers are not sure what initiates the buildup except that it is related to prostaglandin dysfunction.

At the conference, it was suggested that "A combination of omega 3 and omega 6 is best."[37] [to prevent atherosclerosis]

The positive evidence about basic essence EFAs continues – only we don't hear much about it. This very important conference was held outside of the United States, and its findings aren't well-publicized or well-known here in the U.S. – even 7 years later!

Especially for WOMEN

Women taking oral contraceptives and exercising have a significantly higher risk of developing a prethrombic [blood clot] condition.[38]

36 "Identification of Oxidatively Modified Lipids in Atherosclerotic Lesions of Human Aortas," J. Belkner, R. Wiesner and H. Kuhn, Institute of Biochemistry (Medical School), Humboldt University, Berlin, Germany.

37 "Influence of Omega-3 Fatty Acids on the Prostaglandin-Metabolism in Healthy Volunteers and Patients Suffering from PVD," A. Gazso, D. Horrobin, H. Sinzinger, Wilhelm Auerswald-Atherosclerosis Research Group, Vienna, and Efamol Research Group.

38 "Increase in Endogenous Fibrinolysis and Platelet Activity During Exercise in Young Volunteers," Brixi Beisiegel, Norbert Treese, Gerd Hafner, Jurgen Meyer and Harald Darius II, Medizinische Klinik, Klinisch-Pharmakologisches Johannes Guttenberg - Universitat, Mainz, FRG.

This means the chances of acute venous and arterial thromboses [blood clots] occurring following strenuous activity has increased due to increased t-PA activity during exercising. Although the risk is low overall, a woman's risk is greater than a man's, especially if she is taking oral contraceptives. **Women who exercise really need the added protection of basic essence EFAs.**

Thromboxane A2 and *prostacyclin* are two main prostaglandins formed in the cardiovascular system. They influence the role of platelets in the pathogenesis of atherosclerosis [clogged arteries].

If you are short on EFAs, you are short on the prostaglandins PGE1 and prostacyclin. You can get constricted micro-vessels and intra-vascular aggregation (buildup). Is it any wonder that at least 75 % of us die with cardiovascular disease?[39]

EFAs are the "basic essence" and foundation of prostaglandins.

Arachidonic acid[40] is likely to be lost from cell membranes and converted to pro-thrombotic vasoconstrictor and pro-inflammatory metabolites. The loss of arachidonic acid will damage the membrane and lead to depletion of important components.

> "Antiplatelet and anticoagulant drugs are currently used as the standard treatment to prevent and treat thrombosis [blood clots]. While this approach is beneficial, it is not optimal."[41] Buchanan, et al, state that constituents such as prostaglandin PGI2, tissue plasminogen activator, thrombomodulin, and 13-HODE directly affect the vessel wall.
>
> Buchanan, et al, state: "Normally platelets circulate as discoid-shaped inert cell bodies which do not interact either with other blood cells or the vessel wall."[42]
>
> "Aspirin prevents the metabolism of arachidonic acid into

39 *Beyond Pritikin*, page 46.

40 We are frequently told that arachidonic acid is "bad." Once again, a *Life-Systems* Engineering analysis shows that there is no "good" and "bad" regarding *Life-Systems* — there are processes. To the cell membrane, arachidonic acid is critical. Elsewhere, it may not be as beneficial.

41 "Eicosanoids, Other Fatty Acid Metabolites and the Cardiovascular System: Are the Present Antithrombotic Approaches Rational?" M.R. Buchanan, S.J. Brister and M.C. Bertumeu, McMaster University, Dept. Pathology and Surgery, McMaster Clinic, Hamilton Hospital, Hamilton, Canada.

42 "Eicosanoids, ...

thromboxane A2 (TxA2). As a result, platelet function is impaired. It is well-documented that inhibition of platelet function by any 'antiplatelet' agent renders the platelets 'haemostatically defective,' thereby increasing the risk of bleeding side-effects."

Once you have arterial blockage, anticlotting (antiplatelet) drugs don't help, as evidenced in peripheral (involving arms and legs) vascular disease.[43]

"In fact, low-dose aspirin, which enhances platelet adhesivity, increases thrombosis (clotting) when platelet adhesion dominates as the response to injury![44,]**

In-body testing (in vivo) confirms that 12-HETE facilitates platelet adhesion, independent of aggregation. We have a *Life-Systems* balance. When we artificially alter the platelet aggregation, we inadvertently alter their adhesion properties. So, drugs preventing platelet aggregation can cause increased adhesion to the vessel wall.

The presenters state, "Thus a battery of evidence supports the concept that adhesion molecule expression necessary for cell adhesion, be it to the endothelia cells, platelets or other circulating blood cells, can be manipulated by altering the fatty acid [EFAs] milieu, in particular, by altering the relative amounts of lipoxygenase products derived from linoleic and arachidonic acids." Here again, we see the importance of basic essence.

These investigators found that the vessel subwall was not thrombotic – contradicting the other studies suggesting the wall was highly thrombotic (clotted). We stressed before the questionable quality of studies with EFA-deficient people.

For those people considering angioplasty (PTCA) to "un-clog" arteries, you need to know that **the average clog, that was 80%, "re-clogs" to about 60% blockage just 6 months after the**

43 12-HETE is produced in at least a 10-fold greater amount than TxA2. But the drug manufacturers have not concentrated on the 12-HETE pathway.

44 "Enhanced platelet accumulation onto injured carotid arteries in rabbits after aspirin treatment," M.R. Buchanan and E. Dejana, *Journal of Clinical Investigation,* 67:503-508.

** Reyes syndrome is caused by aspirin ingestion after a viral attack! *Basic Medical Biochemistry*, page 312.

procedure.[45] A *Life-Systems* Engineering analysis considers this a drastic failure. This procedure is routinely performed at thousands of hospitals. Temporarily, it may be a lifesaver, but alleviating symptoms temporarily without relieving the cause is not a long-term answer.

I still want to speed up the metabolism

The most frequent question I am asked by clients is: "How do I speed up my metabolism?" I ask them why they would want to do such a thing, because it will typically just make them want to eat more food. If you have extra bodyfat, your metabolism is already making you fatter.

Increasing your metabolism is asking your body to do the same thing it has been doing, but more quickly. If you are gaining weight, it would make you fatter, faster!

You don't really want this. What these folks are actually looking for is a way to burn off excess bodyfat.

We must understand what metabolic rate really means. The metabolic rate is the speed of the body's internal activity as measured by the rate of heat output during all the body's chemical reactions. The amount of oxygen consumption is measured and then, based on certain assumptions, converted to an equivalent measure of heat.

Over the course of a few minutes, during a high level of physical exertion, the body's heat output will increase as much as 50 times its normal resting state. This increase is a natural system response to the exertion – something like driving your car fast on the road. If we tried to stimulate this result with drugs, the result would be analogous to keeping your car stuck in first gear or racing your car's engine with the brake on in order to burn off fuel. Sooner or later, something would fail.

Is there a natural way to burn off our excess fuel (calories) stored in bodyfat?

45 "Effects of Ciprostene on Restenosis Rate During Therapeutic Transluminal Coronary Angioplasty," Harald Darius, Uwe Nixdorff, Johannes Zander, Hans-Jurgen Rupprecht, Raimund Erbel and Jurgen Meyer, Department of Medicine II, Johannes Gutenberg - University, Germany.

After we eat a meal, the metabolic rate increases, more or less, depending on the type of food eaten.[46] This is because of the *Life-System* processes involved: the chemical reactions of digestion, absorption, and storage of the food. This was well-known and published back in the 1950s by Sir Charles Dodds, Dr. Kekwick, Dr. Parvan, and Dr. Pennington, to name a few.

A mostly protein and natural fat meal naturally raises the resting metabolic rate 30% above normal, for three to 12 hours! A high-carbohydrate meal raises the metabolic rate by only about four-percent. Again, we see that carbohydrates (sugars) interfere with burning excess fat.

I discussed brown fat in a previous section. This type of fat contains large numbers of mitochondria. Here, they produce mainly heat without stimulating the appetite. The more efficient brown fat is, the more heat will be generated – raising your body temperature a bit – by burning excess bodyfat.[47] What can make brown fat more efficient? EFAs.

Increasing the efficiency of your body's brown fat and minimizing intake of carbohydrates (a natural benefit of basic essence), are the only natural ways to increase the body's metabolism. Be wary of so-called "metabolic enhancers." They either artificially knock your body's *Life-Systems* out of balance or they just won't work at all.

So How Much Food Do I REALLY need?

A simplistic answer to the question of how we got so overweight has traditionally been: "You eat too much. We become fat from taking in more energy than our metabolism can consume." Much more insight is needed to accurately answer this question. There wouldn't be so many overweight people if it was that simple. This assumption doesn't correlate with real life experience.

You must burn 3,500 calories to lose 1 pound of bodyfat. One might think that all you have to do is cut your eating by 500 calories a day and you'll lose 1 pound of flab in a week. Don't count on this happening! If you cut back proportionately on all foods, but your EFA and mineral intake is inadequate, your overall carbohydrate (sugar) levels will still be too high. Even worse, if you follow the traditional approach of limiting protein and natural fats, the

46 *Textbook of Medical Physiology*, page 908.

47 Technically, this is called an "uncoupled reaction."

proportion of processed carbohydrate will rise and you can easily gain more bodyfat. This is exactly what happened to me during my bodybuilding days. I couldn't understand why I didn't get the results I was promised. Now I do:

- All food is broken down into its basic components by the body. This takes varying amounts of energy depending on the type of food.
- Carbohydrates are more readily converted to fat than proteins, healthy oils and natural fats.
- Dietary fat is not the culprit – but the excessive processed carbohydrate is.
- The number of calories eaten is not enough to explain gaining excess bodyfat.

We explained how the insulin/glucagon connection offers insight into the missing fat-gaining factor. Once basic essence and mineral requirements are met, your daily calorie requirements will decrease dramatically! So you get a double benefit. Fewer calories from fewer carbohydrates and fewer total calories.

Recall the illustration on page 54 of Chapter 3, which showed your poor stomach with its EFA switch always in the "ON" position. All your stomach can hope for is that the next batch of food might provide these needed EFAs. Unfortunately, with today's processed food, this almost never happens.

EFAs increase the efficiency of the lining of the small intestines, so food is metabolized more efficiently. Your appestat is finally satisfied.

When you are in the Zone, calorie consumption is usually cut by as much as 50%.[48]

Could it be that we eat so much because our body is doing the only thing it can when it doesn't get the nutrients it needs? Staying hungry is the only way the body has to tell us to give it the nutrients it lacks, especially when our taste is distorted by excess carbohydrates (sugar).

48 *Enter the Zone*, page 51.

We have all had food cravings at one time or another. We do respond to them. Usually this means going for the hot fudge sundae, pizza, or other carbohydrate-loaded foods. This used to happen to me all the time.

The freedom from cravings is a great relief once the Foundation of Radiant Health becomes part of the diet.

Hunger may never be ravenous again. Hunger takes on a completely new, friendly form. This is hard to appreciate until it is experienced. The days of slavery to a voracious appetite are gone. Eating becomes a more natural function, much like breathing.

Once the body gets the nourishment it needs, through the Foundation of Radiant Health, your pleasure from eating takes on a new, enhanced dimension. The body no longer wants to overeat. Because the body has the nutrients it needs, we simply don't desire all the excess food we have been spending significant time and money preparing and consuming.

Don't worry about losing the pleasure from eating. We eat less but like it more. The total enjoyment remains the same or even increases.

The best part is that we won't be gaining weight by overeating. Nor will we be eating the same large quantities of processed carbohydrates (sugar), thus greatly reducing the problematic insulin-related effects.

Why Do I Need a Detoxifier?

We have seen that, frequently, when we are told something in the nutritional field, we later find it was wrong to begin with. Learning about product labeling (or lack of labeling) will surprise and possibly shock you. I'll start this section with a little-known area of food processing called food irradiation.

Do you want your food irradiated?

Most people don't know what food irradiation is or how commonly it is performed on certain food groups. Virtually all herbs and spices are subject to the irradiation process. We often don't know this process took place. If an irradiated food is used as an ingredient in a processed food, the irradiated item doesn't have to be identified on the label as being irradiated. So if you have irradiated oregano in your spaghetti sauce, there is no indication on the label.

If a manufacturer purchases an already irradiated item and uses it as an ingredient, the food won't be labeled as irradiated.

This same procedure holds for preservatives and other chemicals such as monosodium glutamate (MSG). If MSG is already added to one of the ingredients, there is no listing requirement. As long as the manufacturer didn't add the MSG directly to the mixture, there will be no indication of the MSG.

Ridiculous, you say? The ingredient gets into the mixture either way. It's only through a "technicality" that, with one method, the ingredient doesn't require listing. It's true.

If you were to examine the food or perform routine chemical testing, you would see no obvious visible difference between the irradiated and non-irradiated food.

Compare the difference between beet sugar and chemically synthesized sugar. There is no "chemical" difference between these two varieties of sugar, yet living bacteria immediately knows there is a difference between them. The bacteria avoid the chemically synthesized version.

The technical term for irradiated food is *radiometric*. The irradiated food isn't radioactive.

Just because it's not radioactive doesn't make it safe.

Irradiation extends a food's shelf life by *killing all living organisms*. Yet, **if the food is already spolled, prior to receiving radiation, the spoilage actually increases**.

A Canadian company planned to irradiate potatoes so they could be sold throughout the year, reducing the country's imports. The company didn't do their homework. If there was any initial damage to the potato, the radiation made the damage accelerate or changed the sugar content of the potato. In either case, the potatoes couldn't be sold, and the company went bankrupt.

Laboratory animals often become sick when given significant amounts of irradiated foods.

As Dr. Gibbs states, "It is the *interpretation* of the results of irradiation that has been the subject of debate for more than three quarters of a century."[49]

Proponents of irradiation will say how much food spoilage can be prevented by irradiation. Even if this is true, we must weigh the cost to human health. We have seen the same type of arguments used with pesticides and other synthesized chemicals. Unfortunately, the same chemicals which kill pests and other food-related diseases do harm to, and also kill people.

We saw the same type of ill-logic used with Phen-Fen until its use had to be forcibly stopped. How many people needlessly suffered, died, or will become ill in the future because they used Phen-Fen?

There are serious drawbacks to irradiated foods. Irradiation changes the food at the molecular level. The taste and smell of the irradiated food change. On a molecular level, it stops the natural decay process by killing the organisms that cause the decay... they are "frozen" so-to-speak. If a food is so dead that it can't even decay – would you really want to eat it?

Typical irradiation facilities produce a "burst" of radiation close to 100 times the amount required to kill a human. This amount is typically in excess of 1,000,000 (one million) times the amount of radiation you'd receive in a chest X-ray!

Can the changes produced by the radiation in the food affect us when we consume them? You bet they can. Ingesting irradiated food can compromise a cell's membrane. If the cell membrane is compromised in any fashion, its immunity to disease is decreased, and fat-burning potential is decreased, too.

Food irradiation works as follows:

High-energy waves bombard the food. Electrons are knocked out of their normal positions and create artificially charged molecules (ions). In this case, an ion acts almost like the dreaded free-radical.

---

49 *The Food That Would Last Forever*, Dr. Gary Gibbs, Avery Publishing Group, New York, 1993, page 5.

Once this ionization process starts, thousands of electrons are knocked off, and a "chain-reaction" starts.

The food's nutritional value is compromised, yet, that's not the worst. New chemicals are also a result of this ionization process. **Formaldehyde and benzene are formed; both are known carcinogens.**

The cell is virtually destroyed once it becomes ionized. Its DNA is altered, and cell division is stopped cold. All natural processes are stopped.

Naturally occurring sugars found in virtually all foods produce formaldehyde when bombarded with radiation as used in this process. This single dose of radiation causes noticeable detrimental effects!

How can the FDA allow such a process? It is said that, because the irradiation process changes only a few of the chemicals in food, these few changes aren't significant enough to ban the process. Does this make sense? Maybe not. If only one chemical produced from irradiation may cause cancer, we shouldn't want to be eating that food.

Here's what Dr. G.L. Tritsch told the members of Congress:

> "When food is irradiated, approximately six out of 10,000,000 chemical bonds are broken. For comparison, a quarter of a pint of water contains around 10^{25} bonds (one followed by 25 zeros). Water is a particularly relevant substance, since it constitutes about 80% of many foods. If just six out of every 10 million of these bonds are broken, a total of 10^{18} bonds are destroyed."
>
> In other words, says Dr. Tritsch, a million trillion highly reactive molecules would be produced in a quarter-pint of irradiated water. Although the percentage may seem small, *the actual number of molecules is huge.*[50] (emphasis added)

If someone asked how significant one part in a million is, we'd probably have to answer, "not very significant." What we forget is that a small number multiplied by a huge number becomes a huge number.

50 Tritsch, G.L.: Statement before the Subcommittee on Health and the Environment of the Committee on Energy and Commerce (House of Representatives) on House Resolution 956; June 19, 1987. U.S. Government Printing Office, Washington, D.C., 1988:97.

> "Certain chemicals, such as pesticide DDT, accumulate in the fatty tissues of the body. These bodyfat storehouses magnify the effect of the daily intake, so an intake as little as one-tenth of one part per million will result in a total storage of ten to fifteen parts per million (an increase of more than one hundredfold over time). While these levels may seem small, over time they can be deadly."[51]

Anything which interferes with cell structure will impede optimum fat-burning capability. Whatever benefits synthetic chemicals may offer to food processors, they usually have an adverse effect on biological systems. If we desire to optimize our *Life-Systems* to burn excess bodyfat, the last thing we need is a hindrance caused by food processing.

"The F.D.A. Says Process Is Safe, Approves Irradiating Red Meat."[52]

We must remember that food processing functions are profit-motivated. Yet food processors can only be partially blamed. We like convenience foods, so manufacturers are placed in a tough position. Most foods can be made with minimal processing or additives, but the costs increase because the products won't keep as long. Organically raised and processed beef may cost $8.00 per pound compared to non-organic at just $3.00 to $4.00 per pound. Mainstream manufacturers aren't interested in pricing themselves out of the market. They care more about uniformity and the lowest possible retail price of a product than about the food's nutritional content. In the past, so have most consumers.

Because many products must be shipped great distances, most crops can no longer be picked when ripe but must be picked early. Often, introducing certain gasses will slow down the ripening process to allow for the great shipping distances and processing time. That's why it's almost impossible to purchase a decent tomato anymore. If it's not from a local grower, the tomato will usually be tough, thick-skinned, and tasteless. How nutritional is it?

Take away a commercial farmer's pesticides, fumigants, synthetic fertilizers, and other chemical additives, and he will be virtually helpless. Unfortunately, these chemicals are often toxic to

51 *The Food That Would Last Forever*, page 51.
52 *New York Times*, December 3, 1997, page 1.

humans as well as to the insects, molds, and bacteria that they destroy. Farmers apply them in such a way as to maximize the effects on pests and to minimize the effects on humans. Commercial farmers have become dependent on these "tools" in order to meet high production quotas with minimal labor.

The Environmental Protection Agency (EPA) classifies the chemical, methyl bromide, as a Class I Acute Toxin, a category reserved for the most deadly substances. Regardless, it is routinely used as a soil fumigant, especially for strawberry crops. Countries around the world are stopping the use of this substance. The USA will (supposedly) stop its use by 2001. California was already supposed to stop its use, but this hasn't happened yet.[53] If you are a strawberry lover you may wish to consider spending a little extra money on organically raised berries.

Laboratory testing confirms that ingesting methyl bromide causes central- and peripheral-nerve-system damage, brain lesions, brain damage, and genetic damage.

It is our personal responsibility to know what we are eating.

There has been significant press regarding salmonella in the poultry industry. This bacteria flourishes mainly with improper sanitation during poultry-processing, yet the consumer is misled and made to think it is from lack of kitchen sanitation.

It is frightening that **about 20% of salmonella reported each year are antibiotic-resistant.**[54] This may come as a result of using antibiotics in raising poultry.

Approximately 40% of all antibiotics sold in the U.S. goes into feeds for cattle, poultry, and other livestock.

53 *Los Angeles View*, May 10-16, 1996.

54 "Petition of the Natural Resources Defense Council, Inc., to the Secretary of Health and Human Services Requesting Immediate Approval of the Subtherapeutic Use of Penicillin and Tetracycline in Animal Feeds", Ahmed, A.K., et al: November 20, 1984: 13-14.

Where do you think the antibiotic-resistant strains of bacteria develop? It's not possible that enough individuals overuse antibiotics. Few people take them every day as a "preventative," yet this is what industry would like us to believe. Human resistance to antibiotics is likely from constant long-term exposure to the antibiotic residues in animal meat. Antibiotic residue really does stay there – especially in the animal fat, where it is deposited so the body doesn't have to process it. Organically raised and processed meats minimize this risk.

Did you know that *the FDA only inspects fish-processing plants about once every 4 years*? *Fishing boats aren't usually inspected at all.* Don't expect much protection from the FDA, because their agency is severely understaffed.

It has clearly been shown that mercury impedes the functioning of many of our organs. Mercury is toxic, yet is a standard component in amalgam tooth fillings.[55] In 1988, the EPA declared scrap dental amalgam a hazardous material. Once a filling is removed, it is considered hazardous. So why isn't it considered hazardous while it is in your mouth? Mercury comprises 50-percent of the so-called "silver fillings." Mercury is well documented as a highly toxic substance.

You can see the types of toxic buildups we may develop in our bodies over a lifetime. Imagine many years of ingesting pesticide residues routinely used in farming, antibiotics routinely used in the meat and poultry industries, and irradiation from herbs, spices and other foods...to name a few.

In today's environment, a detoxifier is clearly a requirement for achieving radiant health. Be sure to read Chapter 14 describing Essiac-concept tonic. This detoxifier is something you certainly need to know about.

A bit of human physiology

- All cell membranes are composed of a very thin (five nanometers) double-layered continuous sheet of fat molecules in which protein is imbedded. The protein "floats" between the layers.

---

55 *International DAMS* (Dental Amalgam Mercury Syndrome) *Newsletter*, Albuquerque, NM, Summer, 1992, page 7.

- Your nerves are enclosed by fat, too. The structure is called the *myelin sheath*. If this structure is compromised by EFA deficiency, your entire nervous system suffers.

How does a restriction in an artery impair blood flow? For instance, if we have a clog half the width of a blood vessel, do we simply get half the flow out? Although this may be a first guess, the answer is not correct. We only get one-sixteenth of the volume out! It's not just a reduction in the "area" of the cross-section. However much we decrease the diameter of the artery, we multiply this number together four times to obtain the final decrease (e.g., one-half times itself four times = one sixteenth).[56]

Now we know why even a slight obstruction in an artery can cause such havoc.

> ***Life-Systems* Engineering analysis is so powerful, because it draws understanding from all the sciences.**

When the flow in a cylindrical vessel, such as an artery, is analyzed with physics, we find there are "layers" moving at different speeds. The flow at the center of the vessel moves the fastest, but due to friction, the speed and the flow decreases until at the walls there is virtually no flow whatsoever. This analysis involves the science of fluid flow and hydrodynamics.

This effect makes it clear that the idea of fat building up by itself inside the arterial walls is illogical. Because of the "vacuum-like" effect resulting from the big difference in flow at the center, your body is automatically keeping anything from sticking to the edges.

Even though flow is low at the inside surface of the arteries compared to the center, the pressure differential won't allow easy buildup. Something traumatic is required for a buildup of plaque to occur. We have previously reviewed some probable causes.

---

56 This is the basis of the famous Pouiselle's Law. A cylindrical area (like a blood vessel) changes as the square of the radius: r^2. In our example, this is the first 1/2 x 1/2 to account for the decreased flow. There is another issue to consider. Blood pressure = force of blood pumped by the heart /area of the artery. To make up for the increased resistance and pressure resulting from the clogging, if the force stays constant, the flow decreases again, in proportion to the area: r^2 again. If you don't care to know the physics, don't worry. The key information is: don't let your arteries get clogged, or you'll feel the formula's dire results from higher blood pressure, etc.!

Capillaries (arteries which have branched out and decreased in size) directly feed our organs. Capillaries are where the cell-level transfer of nutrients takes place. Oxygen and carbon dioxide are both oil-soluble (the same as fat-soluble), so guess what provides them one of the best substances for maximum transfer into cells? Basic essence.

The heart pumps out 2,100 gallons of blood each day – enough to fill a swimming pool, yet only about a gallon of blood a day travels through the lymphatic system.

What does the lymph system do? Besides transporting one type of white blood cell, it is the transportation highway for long-chain fatty acids (EFAs), most fats and triglycerides, along with cholesterol. Short-chain fats, such as butter, are burned for energy and are water-soluble, so they are transported by the bloodstream.

Artificial fat and sugar replacements

According to *Chemical Week*, there is a $4,000,000,000 annual food additive market in the U.S.[57] **Food additive sales projections for 1998 are double the growth rate of the entire chemical industry.** That means two things: food additives are chemicals and they constitute a hot market. Here are some of the article's high points:

- EDTA is sold as a color and flavor preservative. Sales of EDTA are growing by as much as 10% per year, in part, attributable to fat replacement. Low-fat formulations require increased water to replace the lost fat. Higher water content means more food degradation (decomposition), so *more preservatives are required.*

- Dow Chemical is attempting to increase its methylcellulose (indigestible "sawdust") sales to food processors. Previously, Dow sold this product primarily to construction and pharmaceutical markets. "Methocel gums" can be engineered to provide the proper mouth-feel in products reformulated to reduce fat or calorie content.

- ICI Surfactants is looking to expand its line of additives. They currently produce sorbitan esters, ethoxylated esters, and lactilates. These especially help "strengthen"

57 So, is it any wonder this magazine now devotes a section to food additives?

baked goods and prevent them from going stale. Now they want to develop biotech products for foods.

- The European market for food additives is far less active than the U.S. market. Europeans are culturally resistant to U.S. food trends. The European market for food additives is actually expected to decline in growth. However, *the U.S. market for artificial flavors and artificial sweeteners is expected to show the "healthiest" growth!* [58]

According to *Chemical Week's* Fat Replacements section (yes, this topic also warrants a section), sales of low-fat, low-cholesterol foods and beverages are expected to increase from $18 billion in 1995 to $40 billion by 2000! Here are some of the article's high points:[59]

- Carbohydrate-based fat replacements range from four dollars per pound to twenty dollars per pound. This explains why the cost of processed low-fat foods is so high – often much higher than natural foods.
- The global fat replacement market is growing at 15%-20% per year. **This helps explain why more of us are consuming greater amounts of carbohydrates than ever and possibly why diabetes has reached epidemic proportions.**
- The Calorie Control Council, a research firm in Atlanta, states that *fat-based replacements are growing fastest of all segments of the chemical market.*
- FMC, a chemical manufacturer, states that *most of its growth will come from providing fat substitutes in foods* with the highest natural fat content – processed meat and dairy products, processed fish, and poultry products. The company is also targeting ice cream and yogurt markets. [Fat substitutes will be found in more foods than ever before.] (comment added)
- Because of the positive response to Olestra (one of their brands of fat substitute), Proctor and Gamble is building

58 "Reformulation Continues to Stoke Growth," Rick Mullin and Brian Davis, *Chemical Week,* June 11, 1997, Food Additives: pages 29-30.

59 "Low-Fat Market Beefs Up," Kerri A. Walsh, *Chemical Week*, June 11, 1997, Fat Replacements, page 31.

a plant to support 20-percent of the entire world market for snack foods like crackers and chips. The plant will have a capacity for $500 million in Olestra sales and already has 12 contracts with food formulators. They are planning to enter the popcorn market by replacing the fat in butter flavoring with Olestra. Popcorn is already one of the worst carbohydrates for raising blood-sugar levels. Now your appestat won't be satisfied at all, because there won't be any natural fat with the popcorn. Olestra-based popcorn will stimulate cravings even more, causing even higher blood-sugar levels among theatergoers and popcorn consumers!

- Demand for protein-based fat replacement has peaked, but *demand for carbohydrate-based fat replacement is growing steadily.* Processed carbohydrates are used to substitute for the natural fat in most processed foods.

The Calorie Control Council states that 151 million Americans now consume low-calorie, low-fat foods and beverages, compared with 109 million in 1993.

The real-life results clearly show we have become fatter by eating more of these highly processed low-fat, low-calorie foods.

According to *Chemical Week's* Specialties section (another section of the magazine), *sales of artificial sweeteners are increasing at 7% per year.* They are currently at $1.5 billion dollars. Here are some of this article's high points:[60]

- The artificial sweetener market is dominated by *aspartame*, but there are opportunities for other manufacturers to supply the baked goods market, partly because *aspartame* can't be heated without decomposition.
- A new artificial sweetener, *Acesulfame K*, is currently used in the U.S. Hoechst, the company that makes it, is seeking FDA approval to expand its use. In 1996 the Center for Science in the Public Interest (CSPI) in Washington asked

60 "New and Established Products Vie for Share in a Growing Market," Bruce Gain, *Chemical Week*, June 11, 1997, Specialties: page 32.

the FDA to ban *Acesulfame K's* use in all foods. Ten scientists, including Arthur Upton, former director of the National Cancer Institute, found flaws in Hoechst's testing of the substance. However, the FDA said that, regardless of the protests, approval was all but assured.

- *Acesulfame K* will soon be released and will probably be adapted by "all the majors, such as Coke and Pepsi, in the U.S.," says John Simplicio, Hoechst's director of scientific and regulatory affairs. It will go into carbonated, non-carbonated, and fruit-based beverages.
- Monsanto has seen "double-digit" growth over the past 10 years for its lines of artificial sweeteners and food additives. Granola bars, pet foods, ice cream, and baked goods are targeted growth areas for the company.

Acesulfame K stimulates insulin secretion. Do you become hypoglycemic (low blood sugar) after drinking "diet" sodas or other artificially sweetened drinks? This will make it worse!

Given this increased trend in artificial food additives and fat replacers, will we be able to get real, unprocessed food in the future? How safe are these chemical additives? Little human testing is required for approval, so we will become the company's human test subjects.

Attention Deficit Disorder (ADD or ADHD) Takes a Hike

In the 1960s special education teachers were begging classroom teachers to place students into their special education classes. They didn't have enough students to fill those classes.

Times have certainly changed since then. Back then, there were, perhaps, one or two students who disrupted the classroom. Nowadays, often the majority of the students are disruptive, and at least four students are sent for their daily doses of drugs.

My mother was a school teacher for more than 30 years, before retiring in 1994. It was only during the late 1980s and early 1990s that this massive increase in "attention deficit disorders" emerged. According to her, it hit quickly. In only a few years, instead of the typical one disruptive child per class there were four or five disruptive ones.

I can attest to this, myself. I would typically visit her classroom of second-graders once a year and discuss science with them. This practice went on for several years, until 1992. What happened? For the first time in more than five years, students were either jumping around in their seats and disturbing each other so much that they weren't interested in what I had to say, or they had no science questions to ask. It wasn't until I threatened the class with leaving, unless someone asked a question pertaining to science, that one young student asked, "How does electricity work?"

After this ordeal, I vowed I'd never speak to her young class again. I couldn't take their lack of attention. My mother retired early because she couldn't take it anymore, either.

Later on, discussions with my mother confirmed that this phenomenon was something new. It was named Attention Deficit Disorder or Attention-Deficit Hyperactivity Disorder. I recall that three of her students were considered "hyperactive" and couldn't sit still. Too many of the remainder simply had no focus whatsoever. It wasn't that they were bored, because this very opportunity – a visiting scientist from out of town – was anything but typical.

There are now more than two million children taking the drug Ritalin, to manage their Attention Deficit Disorder.[61]

Ritalin is the most commonly prescribed drug for children. **In a pharmacy, it is classified as a "Schedule II" narcotic**. Ritalin reacts with the same brain receptors as cocaine.[62,63]

What can possibly explain the rapid rise of this disorder? Can it be a genetic problem? No, it can't be. As with obesity, a genetic disorder would take many generations to develop and transmit. This disorder has exploded much too quickly.

We must ask ourselves what has significantly changed over the past few years. The divorce rate has risen alarmingly, so family life for those involved has been impacted. Children also exercise less. Children eat much more processed food – in particular, more processed carbohydrates (sugar) – than ever before. Children eat more frequently at fast-food restaurants than ever before. The amount of sugar in their diet has risen, and the amount of EFAs and minerals has decreased to record lows.

---

61 *Energy Times*, January 1997, page 53.

62 "Imaging Cocaine in Action," Dr. Ricki Lewis, *Photonics Spectra*, May 1996.

63 Two further references are: *Brain Research*, 520(1-2): 303-9, 1990 and *Archives of General Psychiatry*, 52(6): 456-63, 1995.

From a *Life-Systems* Engineering analysis, EFA and mineral deficiency plus frequent fast-food meals and eating more processed carbohydrates, would be expected to cause a noticeable problem in a developing child. Could ADD and ADHD be symptoms of these nutrition changes? We should expect results of these deficiencies to be magnified in a child because their rapid rate of growth demands all the nutrients the body requires – in abundant supply.

Scientific research confirms this. Purdue University conducted a study which was published in the *American Journal of Clinical Nutrition*. At least 40 percent of children with ADD had deficiencies of EFAs as measured in their blood.[64] Did they count an adulterated EFA as an active one? The real numbers could be much worse!

EFA-deficient, carbohydrate-induced sugar "highs" stimulate the body to remove this excess sugar, then serotonin release makes you want to sleep. This can explain why the child's attention is so low. The corresponding sugar "lows" make you crave carbohydrates again and again.

In addition, all the chemical additives in processed food play havoc with growing bodies. Eliminating sodas and highly processed foods from children's diets has been shown, many times, to make a major difference. While this makes for an important start, the EFA deficiency must still be eliminated, and the buildup of toxins reduced, for the most effective results. Once again, the Foundation of Radiant Health comes to the rescue.

More real life results:

In 1996, 58-percent of all adult hospital admissions at The Methodist Hospital, in Houston, Texas, were diagnosed to be diabetic, as a secondary condition.

This statistic is based on more than 25,000 patients.

Source: Carolyn Moore, Ph.D, R.D., L.D., C.N.S.D., Manager, Clinical Nutrition Services, The Methodist Hospital, Houston, Texas, 1998.

64 "Attention Please," Rafael Avila, *Energy Times*, December 1996, pages 52-58

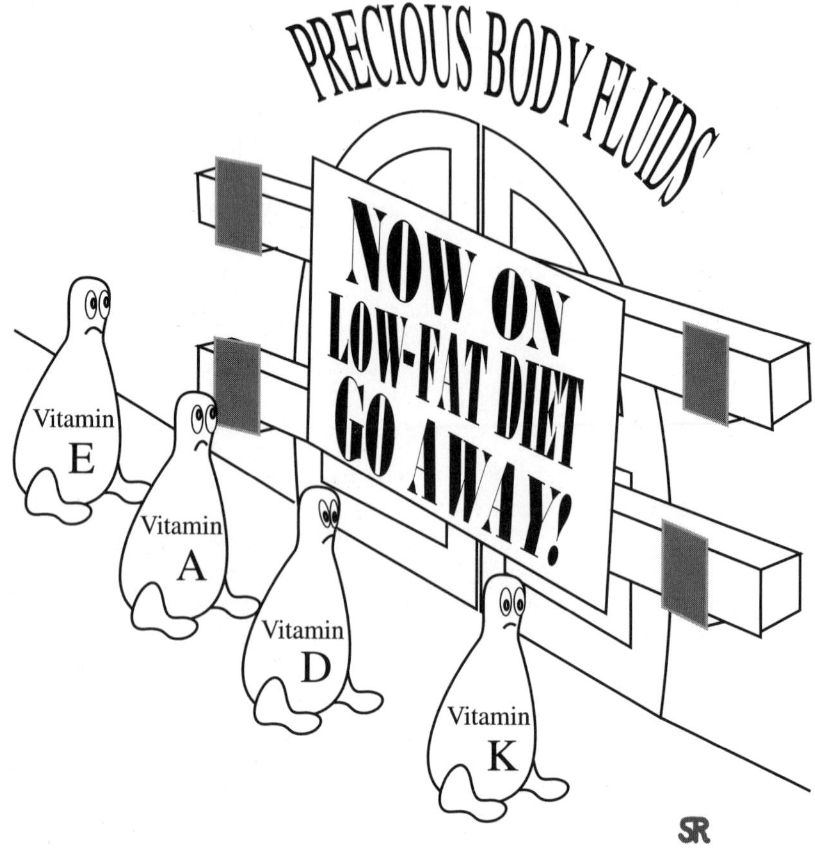

Vitamins A, D, E and K are fat- and oil-soluble vitamins. They don't dissolve in water. When you have a shortage of fats and oils in your diet, could your body's use of these important oil-soluble vitamins be reduced?

Milk: Does It Really Do A Body Good?

> *"Fundamentally, things never change."*
>
> Murray Gell-Mann – Nobel Prize-winner

Why? ... It bothered me for years. If dietary cholesterol is the cause of arterial blockage, why does this blockage take so long to develop? *Any theory that makes sense would have to account for the initial cause of arterial buildup.* Deficiency of EFAs, the body's natural lubricant, is one factor. Yet, there is another interesting possibility as well.

Our livers manufacture lots of cholesterol each day. We have plenty of cholesterol circulating in the bloodstream all the time. What would cause this cholesterol to suddenly collect in one place, much less cause a blockage? The only way such a buildup could even begin would be if an irregularity, something like a "cut" or crack, occurred on the inside of the arterial wall. The body's natural defense mechanism might create a cholesterol patch similar to a scab which forms when you cut your hand. If this type of wound happens often, a buildup of cholesterol-containing material could continue until a significant problem develops.

From my experience with magneto-hydrostatics, I learned that one could temporarily alter the electrical charges on minerals in water. Utilizing special magnets, I had designed specialized high-pressure (3,000 psi) systems to remain free of rust and buildup. A thin, protective substance resembling mud was deposited on the inside walls of the piping. No rust or buildup could attach to the inside of the metal pipes. It was amazing – almost unbelievable. In a similar fashion, the Slippery Elm in Essiac-concept tonic could coat and protect our arteries.

I thought that EFAs would naturally rebuild and heal the damaged arterial area with new healthy cells, but trying to figure out what caused the damage in the first place troubled me for years.

A colleague gave me a photocopy of an article called, "Homogenized Milk Could Kill You," by Tom Valentine. This article said that **cholesterol isn't the culprit in arterial clogging**. This was surprising, because almost everyone has blamed cholesterol. According to the article, Kurt Oster, M.D., a former chief of cardiology at Park City Hospital in Bridgeport, Connecticut, *blamed homogenization of milk as the culprit.*

N. Sampsidis' 1981 booklet, *Homogenized Milk and Atherosclerosis*, is based on Dr. Oster's research.[1] This booklet cites evidence from the Food and Nutrition Board of the National Research Council that clearly confirmed there is no link between cholesterol in the diet and cholesterol in the blood. The Board advocated against restricting fat or cholesterol intake. Their recommendations are still largely ignored. Fat and cholesterol intake still continues to be blamed improperly for arterial problems.

For decades now, our milk has been homogenized. Homogenization whips up fat globules at very high speed, breaking them into tiny droplets. Instead of coagulating together (cream naturally floats to the top in a bottle of unhomogenized milk), the fat globules are pulverized into many micro-globules so they don't float to the top – they stay in suspension. No nutritional value is added. In fact, it's just the reverse, as we shall soon see. The liquid mixture is then passed under enormous pressure through fine filters. These filters control the amount of fat that gets through in a certain volume of liquid. In this fashion, it's easy for the milk processors to obtain 1/2% milk fat, 2% milk fat, or whatever degree of fat they wish. Extending shelf-life and skimming off the expensive cream (which they use for other products) are their main motivations for doing this.

Dr. Oster's thesis proposes that these micro-globules of fat aren't well digested – in fact, they are so tiny, they enter the bloodstream directly without being broken down by the digestive process.[2] This can be a problem. The authors of *Fats That Can Save Your Life* state that undigested food entering the cell from the bloodstream triggers an inflammatory allergic response.[3] One thing that could help repair the damage from the inflammation would be a substantial quantity of EFAs in the cell wall. Whether or not this alone would protect you is unknown. What is known, however, is that Slippery Elm Bark can help protect the artery wall by preventing buildup in the first place.

---

1 Homogenized milk as a cause of clogged arteries was first proposed in 1973 by Dr. Oster.

2 Because it is water-soluble, and a natural food, butter can directly enter the bloodstream safely, but this is different.

3 *Fats That Can Save Your Life*, page 15.

Xanthine oxidase, commonly called "XO," in milk fat attacks the arterial wall.[4] When XO attacks the artery, lesions (tiny cuts or cracks) result. **Then the body's protective mechanisms come into play and normal cellular repair takes place.** According to Dr. Oster, this is how and where the arterial plaque starts. Normal blood cholesterol and other blood-components, as part of the natural healing process, adhere to this lesion. Over several years, as this process continues, the excess builds scar tissue like a scab. Mother Nature did not foresee this kind of continuous attack.

Is it just Dr. Oster who thinks this? No. Abbott Laboratories showed that xanthine oxidase is one of many substances which cause damage to the DNA in the cells. Any damage to the cell initiates the body's natural repair mechanism.

> We found that hydroxyl radicals generated by stimulated leucocytes (white blood cells) and iron caused eight different types of modified DNA base damage ... We found that stimulated leukocytes, cigarette smoke, and purine and <u>xanthine oxidase</u> were each capable of activating the K-ras proto-oncogenes into transforming oncogenes....[5]

XO is clearly specified as one of four possible causes of damage.

I must admit, this theory surprised me, yet it makes sense. It's also **the most realistic theory we've seen, addressing the initial cause of arterial plaque buildup**. This may not be the exclusive cause of atherosclerosis, because it would mean that everyone developing this disease must be consuming homogenized milk products – however, it could be a contributing factor.

In the meantime, we can ask ourselves: are there many people with arterial blockages who don't consume any dairy products, including: milk, yogurt, processed cheese, or ice cream?

Arterial degeneration is a *cumulative disorder* – it grows worse over time. This means it takes years to see the effects. Just as the effects of X-rays (radiation) add up each time you get them, so does the damage by XO.

---

4 Plasmalogen in the arterial wall acts like a glue that holds cells together. Homogenization assists XO's attack on plasmalogen by surrounding XO with a thin layer of fat. This also lets the XO into the lymph system — the center of the body's defense and immune system. Thus, the XO does other damage, too.

5 "Oxidative Processes and Antioxidants: Their Relation to Nutrition and Health Outcomes." Ross Products Division, Abbott Laboratories, Columbus, OH, 1994.

That little bit of homogenized milk in the coffee each morning, over the past 20 years, could be significant to arterial damage. But, while a little milk in coffee is one thing; drinking three cups or more of milk a day could be much more serious. Nature never anticipated us doing such a thing. How much homogenized milk and milk products do we consume? On average, **Americans consumed approximately 25 gallons a year of milk and milk products in 1996.**[6]

Recall how cholesterol has been inaccurately blamed as a cause of arterial blockage. More recently, the medical establishment has agreed that it might be the *oxidation of cholesterol,* not the cholesterol itself, that causes problems. Guess what the best solution still may be: a constant supply of fresh EFAs to combat oxidation of cholesterol.

Dr. Oster says that, with continued milk consumption, the XO literally eats plasmalogen[7] away over time, *leaving the artery wall damaged and weakened.* More and more plaque builds up as the body tries to respond. Can it be proven when XO is present in the blood? Yes. The body produces unmistakable XO antibodies (the body's natural defense against an intruder). They are easily detected in the bloodstream, and they only come from the body's response to XO. These antibodies are consistently found in the blood of homogenized milk drinkers but not in those who don't drink homogenized milk.

Homogenized milk is a processed food. No animal whips and tightly strains its milk before drinking it. Nor were humans meant to do this. Worse yet, we humans are so ignorant that we drink other animals' milk. *Milk is designed for one purpose only – to meet the needs of a newborn baby of the mother's species.*

To further add to our problems, cows are given a wide variety of drugs. Residues from many of them pass into the milk. The drugs detrimentally affect humans. They include antibiotics, growth hormones, and other chemical "enhancements." If you drink and eat organically-produced, unhomogenized milk products, at least your body won't have to deal with these chemicals. It may be difficult to obtain unhomogenized milk products in many places,

6 *Information Please Almanac*, 1997, page 73.
7 The cellular glue holding arterial cells together.

but look for them.[8] Most *real cheeses* use unhomogenized milk. Beware of "processed cheese foods," though: these products may be homogenized. Read the label or call the product's manufacturer to find out what process their milk undergoes.

Lactose intolerance is considered a problem. From a Life-Systems Engineering analysis, Mother Nature is simply working to protect these individuals. We weren't designed to drink lots of milk.

We are sometimes led to believe that only inactive people develop arterial blockage. Paavo Nurmi, a former Olympic gold medalist, who set an incredible 13 world records for Finland in distance running, died from heart disease. We frequently hear how running is exceptional protection against heart disease. He was from a country which consumes an enormous amount of dairy products. Interesting, isn't it?

Cutting back on the amount of *homogenized* milk (including *processed* cheese) should prevent a lot of arterial scarring. Skim milk or non-fat milk doesn't eliminate the problem. There is still XO in it.

Because of the way it is made, butter has no XO-associated problem. Butter doesn't involve homogenization.

Needless to say, the dairy industry wouldn't want this information publicized.

There is no need for manufacturers to homogenize milk used for real cheese. Look on the package to see if the milk has been homogenized. Organically produced cheeses don't have the additives or the processing.

Is this XO theory valid? I can't prove it conclusively. However, it does fit the data very convincingly. It makes more sense than those arterial-blockage theories that ignore obvious facts and direct causes. Without homogenized milk products you have one less health issue to worry about. *The Foundation of Radiant Health minimizes XO's cell-damaging effects.*

Nobel Prize-winner, Professor Richard Feynman, stated that, "Details that could throw doubt on your interpretation must be given, if you know them. If you make a theory, for example, and advertise it, or put it out, then you must also put down all the facts that disagree with it."

---

8 The Whole Foods Market chain in Texas recently started carrying a line of non-homogenized milk.

Here's a possible inconsistency with the XO theory:

Atherosclerosis or arteriosclerosis never occurs in veins. These conditions only occur in arteries. When a blood cholesterol test is performed, your blood is drawn from the vein. The vein is where cholesterol is measured. Why doesn't the vein have the buildup? Differences between arteries and veins may be very important.

1. *Actual stress in veins is less.* There is less muscle surrounding the vein to squeeze or deform it.
2. *There is much lower pressure in veins.* They are the low pressure return lines and blood reservoir for the circulation system.
3. *A vein is much more flexible.* It can withstand much more stress, as it can easily expand as much as six times more than an artery.
4. *There is very little oxygen left in the blood* by the time the it reaches the veins. The oxygen has been replaced by carbon dioxide, which is far less reactive than the oxygen it replaces.
5. *Is the amount of XO much lower* once the blood moves from the arteries into the veins?

Could we deduce from these facts why veins don't develop internal tears the way the arteries do? It's quite possible that the XO from the homogenized milk can't damage the inside of the vein because of the lower pressure, lack of oxygen and the expansive capability of the vein compared with the artery.

Possible arterial damage caused by homogenized milk provides a very plausible causal mechanism for triggering arterial buildup. If so, once again, food processing could be the culprit.

> One out of five Americans* - 20% - (and over half the world's adults) experience indigestion from eating or drinking lactose-based products like milk (*real* cheese is no longer lactose-based). Yet, virtually no infants or children are lactose intolerant.** Therefore, a *Life-Systems* Engineering analysis suggests that *cow's milk isn't a proper food for a human being*, especially adults. Mother's milk contains an EFA derivative, lacking in cow's milk, which is important in brain development.***

* *Basic Medical Biochemistry*, page 403.

** *Biochemistry,* page 472.

*** *Basic Medical Biochemistry*, page 498.

Something About Supplements

> *"Nutrition is the fuel of peak performance."*
>
> Marcus Conyers — Peak Performance Consultant

Health stores can be a help because they can be a good source of products. On the other hand, one wonders why there are typically so many products in a health store. Sales help may only know what manufacturers have told them – right or wrong. We can be easily misled.

Do you have any idea how many individual health store products there are? According to store managers, there are thousands. How could anyone know everything about so many products?

Health store personnel don't have an easy time. Customers aren't always reasonable. I've heard many customers ask one question after another without even listening to the answers. This can be very frustrating. Let's use a little courtesy: let's do some homework before asking salespeople a lot of questions about the products.

For best results, avoid general questions, like which vitamin is better than the others. Rather, ask very specific questions, like what methods does the manufacturer use to make the product.

For example, *some mineral formulations are much more effective and are more metabolically active* (or bioavailable) *than others.* This is important. If we want to fulfill our nutritional iron requirements, swallowing iron filings won't help – and may even be harmful.

Most health stores have book sections. Buy and read a few books on the topic of interest to become more knowledgeable. Then ask for the salesperson's suggestions. This way, you get better information, and the salesperson's comments will be more useful to you.

I am frequently asked, "What can I expect from health store personnel? Should I take their advice?"

These are good questions. As in any other field, some health store personnel are more helpful than others. There are good nutritionists and not-so-good ones, good plumbers and those you don't want to call. Unfortunately, you can't always tell the good ones from the not-so-good ones just by looking at them. **You need to educate yourself first.**

Clients sometimes tell me about wonderful results or terrible results from a particular product. I then ask them if they varied anything else at the same time they started taking it. For example, did they start a new exercise program or change their eating habits in any way? If so, how can they be sure this particular product was responsible for the results? We need to see how effective a particular nutritional supplement is alone. In order to see what works and what doesn't work for us, we have to perform personal trials on ourselves .

With multiple changes at the same time, we can't tell which factors or products caused the result.

This multiple-change factor is often used by exercise equipment companies to their advantage. They recommend that you use their equipment and *also change your eating habits* (diet). The diet portion of their "plan" is usually not mentioned in the advertising – it comes with the equipment. When the equipment doesn't give the advertised results (perhaps because the buyer ignored the diet plan), most people still don't send it back. It's a lot of trouble, and the equipment companies know this. *When exercise equipment appears to work, it is most often a combination of several changes that caused the improvement.*

To find a true cause-effect relationship, we must change only one thing at a time.

I can attest that taking basic essence, and changing nothing else in my diet or lifestyle, gave me noticeable and significant results. Drinking Essiac-concept tonic gives the same high level of definitive results. Together, the results are even more powerful. Add the nine minerals we don't get enough of from the soil, and we have the Foundation of Radiant Health.

Nutritional supplement manufacturers seldom provide information based on human "clinical studies." Information provided only by the product manufacturers, particularly when based solely on animal studies, is often not the best source.

A comprehensive collection of customer testimonials is the most useful measure of a product's effectiveness. Word-of-mouth product referral may also be a good indication. Most times, though, customers don't tell the salespeople whether they like a product. They simply repurchase it if they are satisfied. One might think a high repurchase rate alone would be enough to demonstrate that the product is good and effective, but is it enough? *The ultimate test is your own personal results.*

Lets examine some basic nutritional components:

Vitamins

"An estimated 100 million Americans are spending $6.5 billion a year on vitamins and minerals."[1] More than 10 billion multivitamin capsules and tablets are consumed each year, at a cost of nearly $700 million dollars.[2] Yet, Americans have never been as sick, exhausted, or overweight. Clearly, vitamins alone can't be the solution. Nevertheless, we need to look at what vitamins really do.

> Vitamins either enable biochemical reactions in the body to take place more efficiently, or they prevent specific substances from interfering with biochemical reactions. Vitamins are chemically organic: they only come from living things, either plants or animals. Vitamins A, E, D, and K are oil-soluble. If your diet is short on natural fats and healthy essential oils, these four vitamins can't get fully utilized. All other vitamins are water-soluble. The only vitamin the human body manufactures is "vitamin D." "Vitamin D" should not be called a "vitamin." It should be considered a powerful hormone because it has the chemical structure of a hormone.[3]

Vitamin D is critical for calcium absorption. Vitamin D is produced when sunlight interacts with the cholesterol and EFAs in your skin. With this understanding, it becomes clear that a shortage of EFAs compromises your body's use of calcium.

1 *New York Times*, October 26, 1997, page 21.
2 "Multivitamins," David Sharp, *Health*, March 1997, page 106.
3 *Sunlight*, page 144.

Many processed foods are supplemented with vitamins, so few people have vitamin deficiencies. Virtually no one suffers from the vitamin deficiency diseases scurvy or rickets anymore.

An article in *Forbes* magazine, November 1996, quotes Dr. Gary E. Goodman of the Fred Hutchinson Cancer Research Center in Seattle:

> **"I started taking vitamin A supplements around 1980. Later, I added beta-carotene, vitamin C, and vitamin E. I gave them all up in January 1996, when our study's results came out."**[4]

Dr. Goodman was referring to the Seattle study which looked at 18,000 smokers, former smokers, and workers exposed to asbestos.

> Note: they used a highly non-typical group for the sample, so we must be careful not to overgeneralize this particular study's results.

Vitamin A and beta-carotene were given to half of this group for six years.[5] The study was designed to measure the death rate of this group from lung cancer. After six years, the total death rate among the vitamin-supplemented group was reported to be 17 percent higher and their death rate from lung cancer was 47 percent higher – compared with the non-vitamin group. The subtitle of the *Forbes* article is: "How could so many scientists have been so wrong?"

The article goes on to state that, many months after the subjects were taken off the vitamins, they still had elevated beta-carotene levels. The same article describes two other studies, published in the *New England Journal of Medicine*, which monitored vitamin intake and death rate. **The death rate did not decrease for the vitamin users in these studies.**

The Forbes article suggests there might be a correlation between better health and people who eat an abundance of fruit and

---

4 "Spinach in a Pill: The idea that antioxidant vitamins prevent illness is biting the dust," Phillip E. Ross, *Forbes*, November 4, 1996.

5 Beta-carotene is converted by the body into vitamin A. Large doses of this combination don't make sense. One or the other should have been given, or two separate groups should have been used: one taking only vitamin A, and the other taking only beta-carotene.

vegetables, but then goes on to state that this isn't necessarily the reason for their better health. The people referred to may be doing many things differently, including exercise, meat consumption, carbohydrate (sugar) consumption, drinking, smoking, and so on. Hurrahs for Mr. Ross. This is one of the very few articles where the author addresses the possibility of multiple cause-effect relationships.

This study produced a startling and unanticipated result. Most people would have expected the vitamins to have helped at least a little. *No one expected these subjects to be more at risk with the vitamins.* Was there an unforeseen bias or mistake somewhere? This is an example of *what happens when everyone simply parrots what they think is supposed to work instead of verifying what really works. Life-Systems* Engineering was developed to solve this type of problem.

In the STAT-SMART chapter, we learn how to question whether there were any other conditions in the group experiencing the increased death rate which were not found in the other group. This questioning typically goes unanswered in many studies. How many of the 18,000 were given the vitamins and how many weren't? What were the dosage levels? What other ingredients were in the vitamins? Were all the 18,000 given the vitamins and were their results compared to other groups somewhere else? The report didn't answer these questions. Who funded this study? What results did they want to see?

Based on the article, we would have to say there are too many uncontrolled variables in a study such as this. Cause-effect conclusions cannot be deduced from the limited information available to us. But, it does *raise new questions about the benefits from vitamin supplements.*

> We aren't told the dosages of the vitamins administered to the subjects. *Vitamin A is oil-soluble.* Excessive amounts can build up in the body over time. Too much can be harmful.

Did the study overdose its participants?

This raises the possibility that the subjects were given excessive doses. So what good is this study? You can overdose on aspirin. One aspirin a day may be beneficial for some specialized groups, yet five aspirin a day can cause your stomach to bleed. There isn't room in the article to list all the study's details.

One might make the case that the participants in this study were predisposed to problems from their smoking or asbestos exposure, and the vitamin effect was compromised. That is, if these people had taken the vitamins years before they started smoking or were exposed to asbestos, then maybe the vitamins could have helped prevent health problems. Our *Life-Systems* Engineering team agrees, unless irreparable damage has occurred.

Have we been misled into thinking that massive doses (called "megadoses") of vitamins are beneficial? The basic truth is that, once we meet the body's requirements of vitamins, or most nutritional substances, additional amounts can't improve *Life-Systems* efficiency and may even be harmful.

Are we really meant to consume twenty to thirty oranges a day to obtain enough vitamin C in our diet? Fruits are major sources of sugar, and *an excess causes system imbalance*. Recall the insulin-carbohydrate connection. **The "megadose" theory doesn't make sense when it requires large amounts of any food in order to obtain suggested amounts of the vitamin or nutrient naturally.** Modern man developed the physiology (bodies) we have today long before supplements became available.

Victor Herbert, M.D., Professor of Medicine at Mount Sinai School of Medicine, may feel the same way. In his article called "America's Very Dangerous Vitamin Craze,"[6] he writes,

> **In amounts far in excess of the Reference Daily Intake (RDI), vitamins become drugs – with toxic side effects....**Excess amounts of fat-soluble vitamins are not excreted in the urine. Consuming high doses of these vitamins [A, D, E & K] on a regular basis can lead to toxic buildups. (emphasis added)

He suggests only 30 IU of vitamin E, and recommends getting a minimum of the daily recommended amounts of vitamins and minerals from non-food supplements.

If you take a nutritional product, it should be effective, no matter when it is started, and it should lead to noticeable improvements within a few months. We shouldn't have to be in good health already to benefit from nutritional supplements. If a product

6 "America's Very Dangerous Vitamin Craze", Victor Herbert, M.D., J.D., *Bottom Line-Health*, January 1998, pages 1-3.

doesn't work for us after a reasonable time, we should abandon it and try something else. However, if there has been severe tissue damage prior to a supplement's use, it might not be fair to always expect regeneration.

Any effective nutritional product should give results you can both see and feel – regardless of your initial condition.

Is a change in death rate over a short period of time a valid measure of nutritional effectiveness? Not necessarily. In the months and years before we die, we can be very sick or not sick at all. Most aged animals die quickly, experiencing no prolonged illness. Shouldn't humans? Too many of us are experiencing a drawn-out deterioration for years before we die. So, *our condition of health **before we die** is of significant interest.* A study's reported results may omit a lot of important details.

A Personal Test:

Start taking the Foundation of Radiant Health every day. Observe the difference in how your body reacts over the next 90 days.

This is the way to start personally verifying what works and what doesn't.

Antioxidants

The idea behind antioxidant theory is that an antioxidant substance will become the sacrificial lamb and be destroyed instead of allowing the EFA to become functionally altered. Antioxidant vitamins receiving the most press coverage are vitamin C, vitamin E, and beta carotene.

What happens if there are too many antioxidants in the body? Can they be harmful? This is a very good question. A *Life-Systems* Engineering analysis suggests that the balances may be seriously altered because oxidation reactions are required throughout the body all the time. If you take too many antioxidants, then hormone and eicosanoid (prostaglandin) production could be impaired.

Wouldn't it be unfortunate if critical reactions in the body were stopped because the antioxidants worked in the "wrong places!" For example, *oxidized* iodine is *required* for proper thyroid function.* We have no way to control *where* antioxidants are used or even *if* they are used. It often doesn't pay to attempt to control a system that was designed to work automatically. We don't get the desired results. Our body will work automatically when it is given the proper fuel.

The antioxidant theory was offered as a *guess* that antioxidants might be "the answer" to our health problems, because, vegetable and fruit eaters often *appear* healthy.

Just as the low-fat and high-carbohydrate diet was generalized and improperly recommended as ideal for everyone, the belief in eating excessive amounts of fruits and vegetables arose. From a *Life-Systems* Engineering perspective, the nutritional fields frequently tend to paint too simplistic a picture.

Many biochemists agree that, too often, the antioxidant aspects of certain vitamins are overrated.

This view is becoming more accepted, as negative effects from excessive amounts of antioxidants are surfacing. For example, it has been shown that antioxidants vitamin C and vitamin E, when taken in frequent megadose amounts, depress sperm motility, and therefore, decrease fertility. February 1997's issue of *Health Gazette*[7] published the following in big, bold letters: "**... it might be safer, if you eat reasonably well, not to take even an ordinary multivitamin pill everyday.**"[8] A *Life-Systems* Engineering analysis doesn't go that far, but *Life-Systems* Engineers certainly don't recommend "megadoses."

Of special interest to WOMEN:

> "Dr. Larry Norton, medical director of the Lauder Breast Center at the Memorial Sloan-Kettering Cancer Center, said research at his institution showed that **megadoses of vitamin C blunt the beneficial effects of chemotherapy treatment** for breast cancer. Their research shows the **cancer cells have**

---

* *Essential Histology*, page 346.

7 Volume 36, No. 2.

8 *Medical Tribune* (36#22:13, 1995).

numerous receptors for vitamin C, making the vitamin C act as a 'growth tonic for cancer cells.'"[9]

Here again, this really makes us re-think the megadose theory. A *Life-Systems* Engineering analysis never did recommend it.

Antioxidants are supposed to slow down natural deterioration of the body, by reducing the number of free radicals. They may work well in some laboratory experiments outside the body, but there is no indication that they work effectively in the body. More often than not, *laboratory "miracles" turn out to be real-life failures.* But "test tube" testing continues, in large part, because it's cheap. A product's effectiveness in the body can be extremely difficult – even impossible – to measure. Substances inside a cell can't be measured directly. So, an attempt is made to correlate with a component in the blood, which can be measured, with the substance we wish to measure in the cell. How accurate is this method? Often it is grossly inaccurate.

The method of *indirect* measurement can't be relied upon, but is, nevertheless, frequently used.

This may largely account for the ineffectiveness of many highly advertised nutritional products.

Free-radicals

A free-radical is simply an atom or molecule with a missing electron. This doesn't sound like such a big deal, but it can be.[10]

In one respect, a person's body works much like a furnace. We constantly burn fuel in our bodies by oxidation. **"All cells, regardless of their specialized function, oxidize fuels."*** Oxidation produces free-radicals as by-products. What many of us do not seem to understand is that the majority of free-radicals are formed by natural processes within the body.

Furthermore, **free-radicals are critical to life itself**. Free-radicals are among the most important components in our immune system – they help keep us from getting sick! Free-radicals are also required for important hormone production. The media rarely tell us that:

9 *New York Times*, October 26, 1997, page 21.

10 There are an estimated 10^{28} (1 followed by 28 zeros) electrons in our body.

* *Essentials of Biochemistry*, page 7.

"The life-producing effect of oxygen is only possible if oxygen is converted into free-radicals."[11]

Antioxidants are reputed to reduce the number of free-radicals, but there is little research showing how effectively antioxidant supplements actually work in the body. Many times the intended "solution" generates unexpected problems as well. Yet, great marketing has persuaded people in droves to purchase various antioxidant-based products. Just because something works in a test tube (scientifically called "in vitro" testing) *is no indication that it will work inside the body,* (called "in vivo"). We can be misled again.

Deepak Chopra's *Ageless Body, Timeless Mind* has this to say about antioxidants, particularly vitamin C and vitamin E:

> The eminent Japanese medical investigator, Dr. Yukie Niwa, has demonstrated that *dosing a culture of cells with antioxidants usually does little to decrease free-radical production.* Dr. Niwa found both vitamin C and vitamin E particularly unsuccessful when applied to test-tube cells. **It is even less effective to swallow these capsules, because the process of digestion nullifies them before they get into the cells they were meant to protect.**[12] (emphasis added)

Compared to basic essence, antioxidant supplements can't be very significant for bodily processes. Here's why. Many people take vitamins – loaded with antioxidants. They still get sick from a host of diseases. For many years I, too, tried megadoses of vitamins. I was still sick at least three times a year, and at least half of my airline trips resulted in a bad sore throat lasting many days. My allergies weren't helped, either. Megadoses of antioxidants and other vitamins simply didn't help enough. Many of my clients haven't observed any difference when taking megadoses of them, either. If they were "the answer," then most diseases would be cured simply by taking megadoses of vitamin C, E, A, or any other antioxidant. It simply doesn't work. Our team suggests a moderate approach to vitamin supplements.

---

11 *Enter the Zone*, page 107.

12 *Ageless Body, Timeless Mind*, Deepak Chopra, M.D., Crown Publishers, NY 10022, 1993, page 122.

Here's why megadoses of antioxidants may not be "the full solution":

When an antioxidant is used to neutralize an oxidant (free-radical) molecule, it becomes oxidized in the process, making it no better than the original molecule.[13]

If we start with a clean cloth to clean a dirty oven, the cloth then becomes dirty in the process. It can't clean the dirty oven anymore, and becomes an agent of "dirtiness" itself!

From a *Life-Systems* analysis, free-radicals are not a significant issue or a problem. A much more critical issue is to keep the supply of basic essence coming in – as nature designed.

If we are using a fire for heating our home, we don't want to smother it so that it goes out, or to provide the fire with too much oxygen, so that it burns too rapidly. A controlled balance is needed.

To keep the fire going, we must continue to feed it fuel. To allow the body to function, we must keep feeding it EFAs (fuel) – instead of attempting to manipulate its natural automatic control systems with excessive antioxidants.

A fundamental two-part principle in *Life-Systems* Engineering analysis is to operate at the optimum balance point, while avoiding an overload.

Attempting to protect an inadequate supply of EFAs doesn't work. Replenishing the supply does.

According to Doris E. Billek, a prominent cosmetic chemistry consultant, there are 10^{15} free-radicals inhaled *in each puff of cigarette smoke*. A large number is predictable. We are burning (oxidizing) tobacco. If free-radicals were as harmful as claimed, smokers should ***all*** *quickly become diseased and die*. This doesn't happen! The more permanent negative effects of smoking take a long time to manifest. I'm not saying that smoking is good for us. Of course, it isn't! But we need to make certain we understand the

13 *Rats, Drugs, and Assumptions*, page 299. Vitamin C (ascorbic acid) becomes oxidized into hydroxyascorbic acid — an oxidizer, itself!

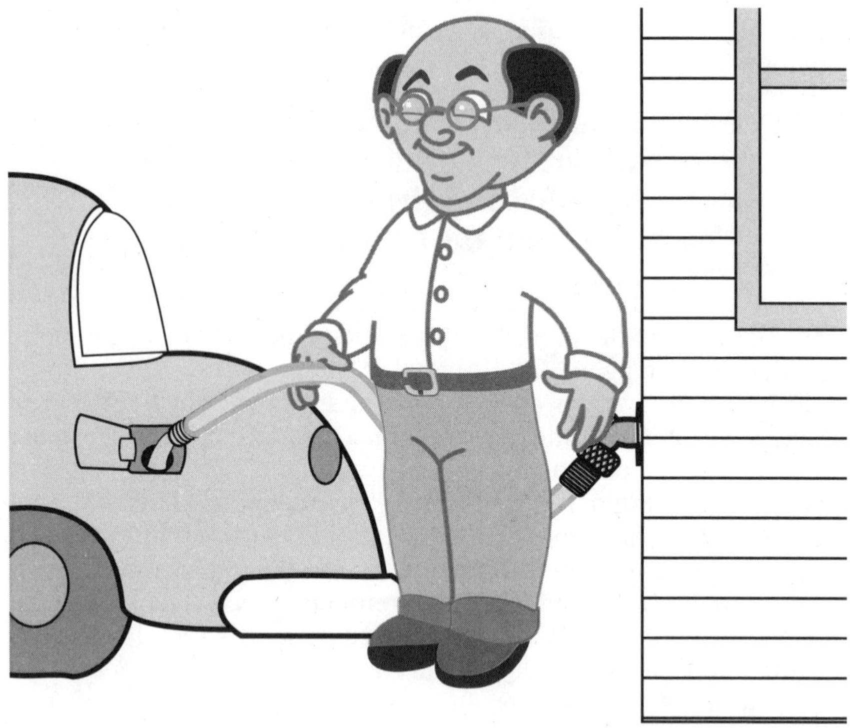

Excessive antioxidants are a lot like putting water in your gas tank – oxidation is what makes the engine run. Antioxidants, by definition, slow it down or stop it.

complexity of biological reactions in the body, and we must not jump to incorrect conclusions. Regarding damage from cigarettes, there may be even more of a concern about the chemicals in the paper, glue, and synthetic additives than with the tobacco, itself!

The body has built-in safeguards against damage caused by free-radicals.

Enzymes help keep free-radical reactions contained.

If enzyme activity is deficient, then free-radicals could become a significant problem. *All enzymes are made from proteins.* Even taking the Foundation of Radiant Health with its EFAs can't solve a protein deficiency.

Metals such as aluminum (from aluminum containers and cookware),[14] lead, nickel (used in margarine production), and mercury (from dental fillings) can be toxic to the body and can interfere with its operations. It is extremely useful to counteract these negative influences. An Essiac-concept tonic is the best detoxifying product our team has encountered.

Taking an Essiac-concept tonic is an excellent way to get rid of accumulated toxins from processed food sources and environmental pollutants.

Chemical reactions take place in cell membranes all the time. Many *Life-Systems* reactions use oxygen. That's why oxidation is so prevalent in the body. It is designed to be so. That's why we need basic essence on a daily basis – to replace the EFAs that get used and oxidized. There is no way around this. Vitamin C and vitamin E may help protect a little against damage, but *free-radical formation and disposal is a natural process and must continue.*

Also, free-radicals react quickly. They don't hang around for long, or travel far from where they originated. To do any real damage, free-radicals must be constantly generated and not disposed of, because they perish so quickly.

Taking the Foundation of Radiant Health daily is the best insurance to replace naturally oxidized EFAs.

When cell membranes are distorted from lack of new EFAs, enzymatic activity is also impaired. Then we are left unprotected.

The LDL (low-density lipoproteins) carry cholesterol and basic essence EFAs to the cells.[15] Without cholesterol, we'd die. Without basic essence EFAs in our cells, we'd die.

14 All carbonated soft-drinks are acidic, and they dissolve minute amounts of aluminum from the can, which can build up in your body over the years.

15 *Enter the Zone*, page 121.

Because of misunderstanding by the nutritional community and misinformation circulated by certain food industries, LDL-based cholesterol is still widely labeled "bad."

Have we fallen on the same misdirected path with free-radicals? Normal levels of free-radicals don't cause problems. Problems can result when we make too many of them or can't naturally dispose of them because of nutritional deficiencies. EFAs are easily attacked by free-radicals because of their easy-to-steal electrons. Once the EFA becomes oxidized (when an electron is stolen from it), the structure no longer works properly. Nature's solution is to replace this spent EFA with a new one. *Life-Systems* Engineering strongly suggests that megadoses of antioxidants are not the answer. Instead, bring in the Foundation of Radiant Health – with moderate amounts of vitamins.

What about vitamin E?

We are frequently told to take "megadose" amounts.

The frequently recommended daily amount of vitamin E is often 20-40 times above what occurs naturally in food.

Vitamin E is believed by many people to be an important nutritional substance. Vitamin E is an antioxidant which occurs naturally in foods before processing. *Vitamin E's role is to prevent oxidation of unsaturated essential healthy oils and natural fats, including EFAs.** You'll find naturally occurring vitamin E, called alpha-tocopherol, in foods containing unprocessed EFAs such as raw nuts and seeds.

Vitamin E protects the oil's natural ingredients before the body uses them. Only small quantities of vitamin E naturally occur in the oils, but a little vitamin E is all that is needed to protect them. When the body digests the food we eat, it takes what it needs and discards the remainder. Neither vitamin E nor other antioxidants affect this process. Once your body gets what it needs, it can't make good use of excesses. In fact, excesses may even be harmful. Consume an adequate amount of unadulterated EFAs, and you'll get vitamin E automatically with the EFAs. When we take nutrients in dosages many times higher than what naturally occurs, could this be another attempt to compensate for a shortage of EFAs? *Life-Systems* Engineering says YES!

---

* *Essentials of Biochemistry*, page 345.

You are better off taking basic essence with a more reasonable amount of vitamin E, because vitamin E's main job is to protect EFAs.

If you are EFA-deficient, then megadoses of vitamin E have little to protect.

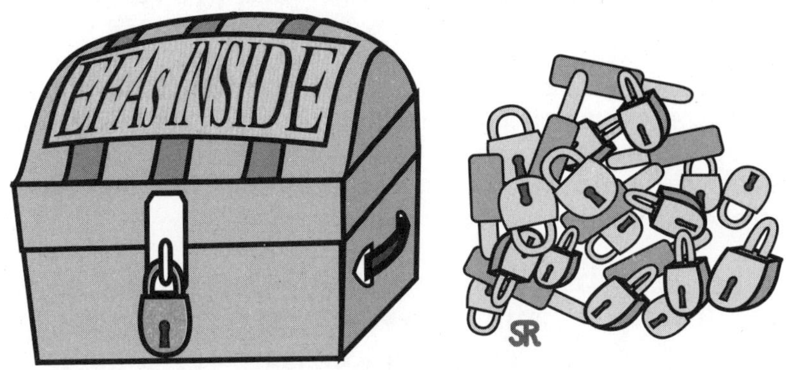

Vitamin E protects EFAs much like a lock protects a treasure chest. What good is a pile [megadose] of protectors with nothing to protect?

Basic essence includes naturally occurring vitamin E. Mother Nature designed it that way.

The analogy between vitamin E and EFAs and between calcium and osteoporosis is as follows: Without EFAs, vitamin E has little to protect. Without a strong underlying collagen-matrix structure, extra calcium can't prevent osteoporosis.

Here's a possible problem with taking vitamin E. Some chemical manufacturers use highly processed oils to make it. They may use the same oil full of *trans*fatty acids you want to avoid. You may be getting vitamin E in a "Killer Carrier." Do you really want this?

Vitamins aren't enough

Here's what a presenter at the *10th International Conference of Prostaglandins and Related Compounds* stated:

"... **We have very little information on the dose-response relationships of comparative potencies of antioxidant vitamins....** Despite this, consumption of vitamins for their antioxidant properties is widespread amongst the 'worried well' in Western societies, and support for phase three clinical trials of these compounds has generated confusion rather than enlightenment."[16] (emphasis added)

Without adequate basic essence and minerals, vitamins don't work properly.

Many biochemists and physical chemists will tell you that antioxidant supplements are overrated. However, Linus Pauling, who was one of the country's greatest physical chemists, fell into the trap of overgeneralizing, advocating massive dosages of vitamin C. He died of cancer – the very thing the vitamin was supposed to protect against!

The broad leap suggesting that megadoses of vitamins prevent everything from the common cold to cancer is unwarranted.

Am I saying that vitamins are worthless? No, not at all! I am simply suggesting that, if you aren't deficient in them, taking more (vitamin megadoses) won't help. Consider taking a more moderate amount of vitamins. A *Life-Systems* Engineering analysis says that megadoses of vitamins or any other nutritional substance must be carefully monitored. Nor are vitamins a cure-all. If they were, we wouldn't keep seeing such massive illness rates. The obesity problem keeps on growing, too. With record numbers of people taking vitamin megadoses, record numbers of us also have weight problems, suffer from low energy levels, and experience poor health.

From a *Life-Systems* Engineering analysis, the megadose vitamin theory doesn't make sense. Active vitamins are available in many foods. To obtain vitamin amounts from your food ranging from five to one hundred times the RDA[17] (minimum recommended doses) you would have to consume immense volumes of food. To obtain

16 "Novel indices of oxidant stress in cardiovascular disease: specific analysis of F2-isoprostanes," Domenico Pratico, Murdeach Reilly, John Lawson and Garret FitzGerald, Vienna, September 24, 1996.

17 RDAs (Recommended Daily Allowances) for vitamins were established by the government as the minimum levels needed so that diseases like scurvy and rickets didn't develop from lack of them.

40 times the RDA for B vitamins, you'd need to consume 40 times the amount of protein you normally eat. Could you eat 10 to 20 pounds of meat every day? The claim that eating indigestible fruit rinds "releases the inner nutrients," is just as unscientific. If you grind up apricot, peach, or cherry pits to "release the inner nutrients" you could die of cyanide poisoning!

(Basic Medical Biochemistry, page 316.)

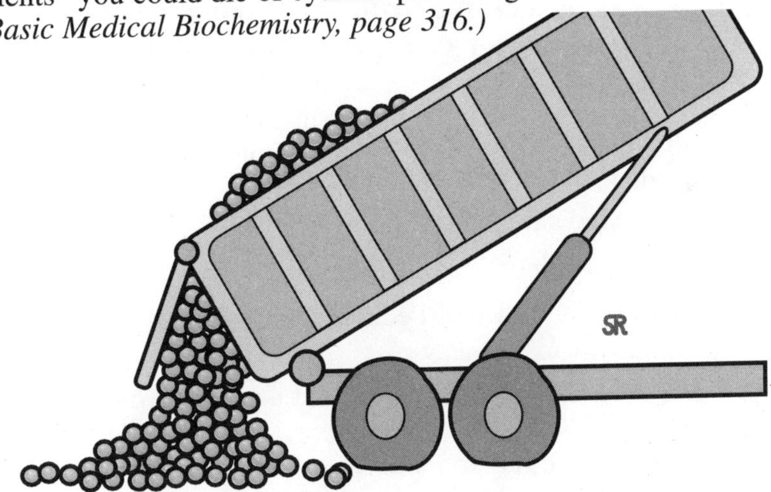

How many oranges would you have to eat each day to get a typical "megadose" of vitamin C?*

*Megadoses of vitamin C can be hazardous. Urine becomes too acidic and promotes kidney stone formation. *Essentials of Biochemistry*, page 347.

Here's a case of vitamin-overdosing insanity. Vitamin D is added to dairy products, cereal, bread, baby foods, macaroni, noodles, flour, beverages, and a host of other products, even though excessive amounts are known to cause magnesium deficiencies which can cause heart attacks. It has been known since 1975 that vitamin D *irritates the lining of blood vessels*.[18] It is also known that *excessive vitamin D causes atherosclerosis* (arterial blockage).[19]

How much is too much? Zane Kime, M.D., author of the book, *Sunlight*, calculates the average person consumes 2,500 IUs, or

18 "How Much Vitamin D Is Too Much?", *Medical World*, January 13, 1975, pages 100-103.

19 "Nutrition Imbalance and Angiotoxins as Dietary Risk Factors in Coronary Heart Disease," F.A. Kummerow, *American Journal of Clinical Nutrition* 32:58, 1979.

more than six times the recommended 400 IUs. If you get any reasonable amount of sunlight and have a diet supplying enough basic essence EFAs and minerals, *you don't need any supplemented vitamin D, because your body makes all that it requires*! So excessive supplements overload us with it.

Excessive vitamin D causes atherosclerosis (arterial blockage).

Why is this excessive vitamin D supplementation allowed, you ask? Good question. Here's a listing of some medical groups that recommended against it:

- British Medical Association in 1950.
- Canadian Bulletin on Nutrition in 1953.
- American Academy of Pediatrics in 1963 and again in 1965.
- Committee on Nutrition of the American Academy of Pediatrics has recommended that non-supplemented milk be available.

If you've never thought about what is done to the food you eat, you had better start or you could end up as another statistic, dying of cancer and heart disease.

Minerals, the rocks we eat

There are 3 major roles of essential minerals:

- support the energy conversion process*
- aid in growth and maintenance of the body tissues
- assist in the regulation of bodily processes.[20]

Chromium enables insulin (many other unfounded claims for chromium supplements have been widely promoted), and phosphorus is involved in the ATP molecule – which extracts energy from cells. Minerals contribute to the rigidity of bones and teeth, and are an important part of the lipid (fat and oil) metabolism and protein metabolism. As regulators of bodily processes, minerals preserve cellular integrity by osmotic pressure and are a component of many enzyme systems which catalyze metabolic reactions in biological systems.

Biochemistry, page 109.

20 *Introductory Nutrition*, H. Guthrie, C.V. Mosby Company, 1975, page 11.

* Minerals are non-protein co-factors that enable enzymes to work. *Basic Medical Biochemistry*, page 109.

Many minerals function in more than one role in the body. Calcium is critical for your heart and bones, too. Phosphorous contributes structurally, and also is a key element in energy production. Cobalt has a regulatory role (through vitamin B-12). Its effect on growth is as dramatic as calcium! Minerals' activities are highly interrelated with each other.[21]

If you are short on one essential mineral, or there is an overload (megadose), the others can't work properly.

For example, if both iron and copper salts in the diet are excessively increased (i.e., through a heavy intake of unbalanced mineral supplements), iron absorption is inhibited by the copper because of a greater affinity of copper for transferrin.[22] In this case, the animal displays symptoms of iron deficiency. This result may sound surprising. A proper *Life-Systems* analysis must always take into account how the body actually works. Theories may sound plausible but are frequently incorrect and may actually cause us great personal damage.

Chemically speaking, minerals are inorganic.[23] They come from rocks. Examples of minerals are: calcium, magnesium, chromium, and iron. Minerals are co-enzymes and need to be replenished frequently.* Some mineral producers may claim they have "plant-based" minerals. They are misleading you. Their source is typically clay (which is powdered rock).

Our bodies can't make use of raw minerals. When we take minerals in their inorganic form, they are not digested or used. Plants transform minerals from the soil into an organic form that animals and humans use. Animals eat plants and further transform the minerals into forms our bodies can readily absorb. We eat animals which ate the plants, as *meat and fish are excellent sources of minerals.*

21 *The Roles of Amino Acid Chelates in Animal Nutrition*, H. DeWayne Ashmead, Noyce Publications, Park Ridge, NJ, 1993, pages 2-3. Although somewhat technical, this is an outstanding book and gives the results of numerous studies.

22 "Binding of copper to mucosal transferrin and inhibition of intestinal iron absorption in rats," F. El-Shobaki and W. Rummer, *Res. Exp. Med.*, 174:187, 1979.

23 "Organic" means that a particular chemical contains carbon. All living systems on earth are carbon-based.

* *Enzymes*, D.A. Lopez, M.D., R.M. Williams, M.D., Ph.D., K. Miehlke, M.D., published by The Neville Press, Munich, Germany, 1994, page 67.

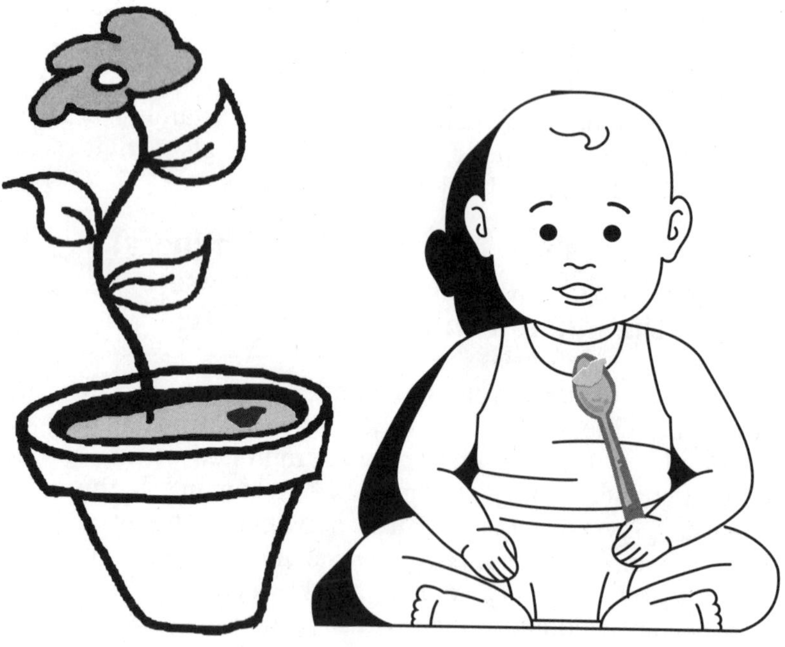

Do you regularly eat dirt to get your minerals?

Fruits and vegetables still contain active vitamins. But most of the plants we now eat are grown in mineral-deficient soil, so we are more prone to mineral deficiency than to vitamin deficiency.

Without a proper balance of minerals, the vitamins cannot be fully utilized, no matter how many may be consumed.

We need to learn more about minerals. Like basic essence, they are more difficult to obtain than other nutrients.

Mineral-deficient soil results in mineral-deficient plants — further resulting in mineral-deficient animals and people.

The Minerals We Need

We care about minerals which are known to optimize certain bodily functions in humans. Our bodies don't make minerals. Minerals must come from the food we eat. There are seventeen (17) minerals which have a demonstrated, important nutritional value in humans.

As with most nutritional substances, we need to understand how much of a particular mineral is required for optimum function and we need an awareness of other factors which influence mineral activity.

As with vitamins, once you have enough of a particular mineral, taking more of it isn't beneficial. In fact, it may be harmful, because excessive amounts upset the system-balance among all the other minerals.

Proportions Are As Important As Amounts

Making bread requires a balance between flour and water. Too much water or too little flour, and we end up with watery goop! With too little water or too much flour, we end up with lumpy paste!

Correct temperature and baking time are also required – we can "bake" the mixture all day long at 70 degrees and we still won't get bread.

We must understand the entire process and not just concentrate on one aspect to the exclusion of everything else.

Our *Life-Systems* Engineering research shows that, because of nutrient-deficient soil, the foods we eat no longer readily supply nine (9) of the seventeen (17) minerals we need.

We can benefit by balanced supplements of: boron, chromium, copper, iron, magnesium, manganese, potassium, selenium, and zinc.

The Calcium Connection

Contrary to the advertising blitz touting the benefits of calcium, our *Life-Systems* Engineering team analysis suggests that calcium supplements are highly overrated. The key to proper calcium levels isn't just taking more calcium, but rather increasing the absorption of what we already have. Our food supplies calcium – the problem is not how much – but what the body does with it!

What increases absorption of calcium? Vitamin D. Where does vitamin D come from? Sunlight reacting with the cholesterol and EFAs in your skin. Most people are surprised to find out about this. Here again, we see the profound system-wide impact of basic essence EFAs.

To ensure you don't develop osteoporosis (bone density loss) in later years, the Number One thing you can do outside of nutrition is is to work out with weights or isometrics. As the *Textbook of Medical Physiology* states, "Bone is deposited in proportion to the compression load that the bone must carry. Therefore, continual physical stress stimulates osteoblastic deposition and calcification of bone."

If you work out with weights and subject your skeletal structure to intense loads above normal, your bone density significantly increases.

Most of us aren't aware that, in adults, new bone grows and old bone is absorbed by the body in equal amounts. The problem is that, the older we become, the longer this dualistic process takes, so our older bone stays around longer. Older bone simply isn't as strong as newer bone. This is the main reason for bone problems in the elderly.

The Textbook of Medical Physiology states:

> "Osteoporosis is the most common of all bone diseases in adults, especially in old age.
>
> It is a different disease from osteomalacia and rickets because it results from diminished organic bone matrix rather than from poor bone calcium."[24] (emphasis added)

ARE YOU SURPRISED?

It's often **not a lack of calcium that causes bone problems**! Intensive advertising has misled us.

24 *Textbook of Medical Physiology*, page 991.

Causes of osteoporosis:

1. Lack of physical stress on the bone – from inactivity.
2. Shortage of protein – so the bone matrix can't be formed.
3. Lack of vitamin C.
4. Postmenopausal lack of estrogen.
   [Note: Estrogen is made from basic essence]
5. Old age – decreased growth hormone and other hormones inhibiting bone matrix.
   [Note: hormones are made from proteins and basic essence]
6. Cushing's disease (adrenal tumor).[25]

What's *noticeably lacking* on the list? Calcium! Lack of vitamin D isn't mentioned for the same reason – **osteoporosis has nothing to do with a shortage of dietary calcium**. Even rickets (which can cause bone problems) in younger persons, ordinarily results from *phosphate deficiency* in the extracellular fluid – not lack of calcium. Fluid calcium decreases (in the blood) are usually caused by lack of vitamin D – not lack of calcium in the diet![26]

If we're on a low-protein, low-fat diet, then factor No. 2, lack of protein, can easily apply to us. Vitamin C, factor No. 3, is vital to strong bones because it helps the collagen in bones to ossify, that is, to form the matrix.

Could factor No. 5 be based not on old age at all but on the year-after-year cumulative effect of basic essence-and-mineral deficiency? A *Life-Systems* Engineering analysis suggests this could be true, because EFAs are raw material for many hormones and critical prostaglandins.

Epidemiologist Dr. Bonnie Specker, of the University of Cincinnati, reviewed 17 calcium studies and noted a pattern.

Only when women exercised did a calcium supplement of 1,000 mg a day produce stronger bones.[27]

---

* **A new study of 32,000 women showed those who ate the most meat were 68% less likely to break a hip! (*Journal of Clinical Nutrition, 1999;69:147-152*). Protein Helps Bones Heal Quicker (50% faster) and Stronger Too. (*Prevention,* October 1998, pg. 143).**

25 *Textbook of Medical Physiology*, page 998.

26 *Textbook of Medical Physiology*, page 998.

27 *Your Health*, March 4, 1997, page 4.

From a *Life-Systems* Engineering perspective, the additional calcium did little, if anything at all. The increased bone density was entirely due to the increased stress on the bone – just like the previous chart indicated.

Although bones are made with large amounts of calcium phosphate, virtually everyone must obtain enough calcium. **Otherwise we would see significant numbers of children and adolescents with bone malformation and other obvious signs of a calcium shortage**. This doesn't occur,[28] because we obtain plenty of calcium from lots of foods, including: cheese, milk, yogurt, egg yolk, peas and beans, dark-green leafy vegetables, such as spinach and broccoli, and so on.

Symptoms of calcium deficiency include:

- Tetany (spontaneous muscle twitching) in the hands.
- Heart palpitations.
- Poor blood clotting.

Virtually everyone has calcium concentrations above the level needed to calcify bone.[29]

Years ago, when there weren't any "Drink milk" advertisements plastered all over magazines and billboards, we consumed less milk and milk-based products. Did many children develop osteoporosis? No. If they had, one might make a case for calcium lacking in our food. Because children grow quickly, their calcium requirements far surpass mature adults' calcium requirements. They don't have a problem, because lack of calcium is not the cause of osteoporosis, as the *Textbook of Medical Physiology* clearly states.

Do you take calcium supplements or eat processed foods with added calcium?

Virtually all non-chelated mineral forms of calcium are converted in the body to calcium chloride, which irritates your intestinal tract.

---

28 Pure reason and deduction leads to this conclusion. Look closely at the source saying otherwise.

29 *Textbook of Medical Physiology,* pages 988-989.

Since kidney stones and gallstones contain lots of calcium, could their formation be aggravated by this irritation from excess calcium supplements? Could arthritis be caused, in part, by excess calcium depositing in the joints?

Some physicians aren't aware of this yet, but calcium carbonate (a common antacid ingredient) also causes acid rebound – a system imbalance – three to five hours later. An even greater danger: the possibility of milk-alkali syndrome, a very serious disorder.

The Milk Council has produced several brilliant advertising campaigns. For those of you who think that drinking large amounts of milk will prevent osteoporosis, consider the following. A clinical study gave a group of patients 1,000 mg of calcium per day and gave a second group 1,000 mg of calcium per day along with trace minerals.[30] The first group, taking just the calcium, still had bone density loss over time, although the rate of bone density loss was slowed down. The article didn't say by how much. But in the second group, taking calcium and minerals, the bone loss stopped.[31] Wouldn't you like to know what would happen if a third group was given trace minerals without calcium? Would the bone loss stop? This question wasn't addressed.

Too many of us are wasting money on products which the body can't utilize effectively. Calcium is a perfect example. Swallow a big 2,000 mg pill and less than 14 percent may be used. Take a 500 mg pill and almost 30 percent (more than twice the proportion) may get used.[32] The calcium absorption rate for milk is less than 30 percent. In other words, we use less than one-third of the calcium in milk.

How effectively a nutritional supplement is absorbed is far more important than how much is taken.

30 Calcium is, of course, a mineral. "Trace" minerals are those that the body needs, but in lesser amounts. Chromium is a trace mineral and magnesium is a mineral needed in much larger amounts.

31 "Spinal Bone Loss in Post-menopausal Women Supplemented with Calcium and Trace Minerals," Straise, L. et al., *Journal of Nutrition* 124(7): 1060-1064, July 1994.

32 14% of 2,000 = 280 mg utilized for a 2,000 mg tablet, and 30% of 500 = 150 mg utilized for a 500 mg tablet. If you still insist on taking calcium supplements, save yourself some money and take two 500 mg tablets twice a day.

The vast majority of calcium supplements and additives are in the form of calcium carbonate – ground limestone (rock). As you may imagine, the body can't make efficient use of this form of calcium.

To raise money for research, some foundations will "license" their name on products.[33] Physicians may be misled, just like the rest of us into thinking such a connection is an endorsement.

Physicians are so busy treating the symptoms of nutritional deficiency, that they don't often have time to keep current on the hundreds of monthly medical publications relevant to their speciality.

A natural calcium regulator?

After all the advertising about how great calcium is, you may be surprised to know that the most common drugs prescribed to decrease blood pressure (anti-hypertensives) also block calcium utilization. Each of your body's cells has an automatic mechanism for controlling its calcium levels. These drugs actually interfere with this mechanism.

Is there a natural calcium regulator that might work in place of the drugs? Yes, magnesium, and it works slowly without the adverse effects. A fundamental postulate of *Life-Systems* Engineering is that the body always has natural automatic control mechanisms – when and where they are needed. We only have to take the time and effort to look for them.

Calcium and Alzheimer's?

In an Internet article, "National Institute on Aging, National Institutes of Health," tech net, July 18, 1997, there is an interesting comment on Alzheimer's disease and calcium. The article states, "Too much calcium can kill a cell, and some neuroscientists suspect that in the end, a rise in calcium levels may be precisely what is killing neurons in Alzheimer's disease." A *Life-Systems* analysis poses the question – could a mineral imbalance be at the root of this problem and other ailments?

Calcium and arteriosclerosis?

Arteriosclerosis, commonly called "hardening of the arteries," is a condition where the arteries become like rigid tubes. What isn't

33 It's not necessarily an endorsement.

commonly published is that **calcium is deposited on top of the plaque buildup**. That's what makes the plaque mass so hard and bonelike.[34] Once the calcium is deposited onto the plaque, the calcified mass won't go away! With all the "megadoses" of calcium we are often told to take, are we are helping cause excessive calcification of plaque?

EFAs and Alzheimer's?

An Internet article referenced a study that reported women who underwent estrogen replacement therapy (ERT) have about a 45% lower rate of Alzheimer's than those who don't.[35] EFAs are building blocks for hormones and critical prostaglandins.

An even better solution may be to increase the quantity of EFAs, too, so the body can naturally produce the hormones it requires!

Chelation

Minerals, in their raw form, have no nutritional value to humans. To chelate means to bind. The body is designed to assimilate minerals in natural food form. For minerals, that means attachment to specific amino acids – the building blocks of proteins. This is a natural form of chelation that we *Life-Systems* Engineers call *bioavailable*. (Compatible with and readily available to our bodies.) By contrast, most mineral supplements commonly described as "chelated" have an organic molecule, like a citrate or a gluconate, chemically tied to the mineral. This is only *partially compatible* with the needs of the body. The most effective chelation process combines specific amino acids with the mineral through a controlled chemical process called "amino acid chelation." This is not just a mixture. An amino acid chelate supplies minerals in the form the body needs for maximum absorption.

Here's what Darrel J. Graff, Ph.D., Weber State University, Ogden, Utah, has to say about chelated minerals:

> "From 25 controlled studies by 42 different authors in five different countries, a diverse array of data is presented. These data validate the effectiveness of mineral nutrients presented

34 *Textbook of Medical Physiology*, page 873.
35 *Ask NOAH About:* Alzheimer's Disease (Well Connected).

as amino acid chelates when compared with the ionic forms derived from inorganic salts."

H. DeWayne Ashmead, the world's leading mineral expert, provides a little background:

> The term "chelate" was used by Morgan and Drew, in 1920, to describe the molecular structure discovered by Werner.
>
> ...The word [chelate] is derived from the Greek word "chele", meaning lobster's claw. Because the claw, or ligand [attached to the mineral], held the cation, the metal [mineral] was no longer free to enter into other chemical reactions. Thus it quickly became evident that when a metal was chelated, the chemical and physical characteristics of the constituent metal ion [mineral] and ligands were changed. **This had far-reaching consequences in the realms of chemistry and general biology.** It was not until the early 1960's that anyone thought seriously about using this molecule for nutritional purposes.
>
> ...Two schools of thought quickly developed. At that point in time these amino acids were called "metal proteinates" instead of chelates. Concurrently, with the development of amino acid chelates, a second school of thought approached animal nutrition with synthetic chelates based on *ethylenediaminetetraacetic acid* (EDTA). These synthetic chelates were heavily promoted in the decade of the 60's and the early part of the 70's. When they could not deliver the enhanced mineral nutrition promised by the chelation concept, all nutritional products using the word "chelation" lost favor with the animal nutritionists. The "c" word became a word to avoid if one wished to amicably discuss animal nutrition.[36] (emphasis added)

It turned out that the EDTA method worked too well – the body had too hard a time getting to the mineral. We find, time-and-time-again, that the nutritional communities sometimes suffer from a deficiency in conducting a proper analysis.

As time went on, it became clear that, for optimum use by the body, even more was required than the proper mineral-carrier chelation technique. One problem was that the chelate could be too

---

36 *The Roles of Amino Acid Chelates in Animal Nutrition*. Although somewhat technical, this is an outstanding book and gives the results of numerous studies.

large to be absorbed. This is one of the problems with the widely promoted "*colloidal minerals.*"

EDTA has been successfully used to hasten elimination of toxic metals in the body. However, concerning mineral nutrition, EDTA chelates are ineffective.

The chelate is a ring structure and has both an ionic and a covalent bond. Dr. Ashmead continues, "It is important to note that as part of the chelate molecule *the amino acids do not function biologically as individual amino acids* [you can't use them to satisfy a protein requirement], *but as unique transfer molecules.*" (emphasis added)

For ideal mineral absorption,
four important criteria MUST be met:

- The ratio of minerals to amino acid bonding must be in the ratio between 1 unit of mineral to 3 units of amino acid.
- The weight of the amino acids in the mineral chelate must be very small (150 daltons).
- The total molecular weight must be less than 800 daltons.
- The chelate must not ionize in the digestive system.

Do many mineral suppliers meet this specification?

Proteins are readily absorbed by the intestinal wall. Cells welcome them. The cell accepts the protein, getting the mineral with it. This is how minerals are naturally transferred from our food.

A truly biocompatible mineral form duplicates organic mineral structures in the food that Mother Nature designed.

Most beneficial nutritional substances must be coupled with a protein or amino acid to enter our body's cells.[37] There are many so-called "organic chelating agents" that are not protein-based. They are of little use to the body. These include: citrates, sulfates, gluconates, phosphates, and so on.

37 *The Physiology Coloring Book*, plate 75.

Most mineral formulators claim they have "chelated" minerals, but they really don't.

Instead of natural amino acid-bonding, they use mineral salts and other so-called "chelating" complexes. Also, simply mixing in processed protein with the minerals does not increase mineral assimilation.

One of the critical factors for optimizing mineral absorption is to make the mineral-protein combination stay together during digestion. **We don't want it to separate or break down.** If it does, the minerals will recombine haphazardly. This is why we are told not to take calcium and magnesium together. One mineral can block another mineral's absorption into the cell – especially when large concentrations are taken.

Minerals that are properly chelated don't suffer from this problem. It doesn't matter how many of these minerals are taken together, because, if they are in the biocompatible protein-chelated form, they don't interact with each other.

By understanding how the stomach and the small intestine work, we can design the mineral-protein combination so that the cells will use it effectively. *Life-Systems* Engineering always directs its course of action in accordance with how Mother Nature designed us – not just what may sound good.

Does this discussion lead you to believe that eating meat (protein), eggs (protein), and fish (protein) would be a great way to ensure against mineral deficiency? It's true. Eating animals (who ate vegetation) ensures that you will assimilate whatever minerals are in the meat or egg. However, when the animals feed on plants grown in mineral-deficient soil, the minerals we need simply are not available.

Could a mineral deficiency result in the pale and less healthy (gaunt) look of many vegetarians?

Our *Life-Systems* Engineering team thinks so. If you are short on proteins and minerals, you get a double whammy. This reasoning is further supported by the fact that people are designed as omnivores – needing both plants and animals for a complete diet.

Organically raised eggs are an ideal protein source for vegetarians. Our *Life-Systems* Engineering team finds that eggs are Mother Nature's "perfect food."

Digestion quickly separates the commonly used "chelating" mineral salts or complexes from any mixed-in protein. This is the purpose of digestion. We want the mineral-protein combination to remain free of positive or negative ions (charges). Otherwise, the mineral will bond with something else and may never get used. With proper chelation – if the molecules are very small and stable – the digestive process doesn't break them apart. You won't get an upset stomach from taking properly formulated bioavailable minerals, either.

RDAs for minerals are often inflated to allow for poor absorption.

The U.S. Food & Drug Administration recently replaced the Recommended Daily Allowance (RDA) with Reference Daily Intake (RDI). Most mineral RDIs are likely deliberately set high to allow for general low bioavailabilities. For example, two-thirds of the calcium from milk never gets used. That's one reason why the dairy industry tells you to drink several glasses of milk every day. Remember the less-than-30% calcium absorption rate?

When it comes to mineral absorption efficiency, the key is to raise the bioavailability (assimilation). When we increase the bioavailability, we need less. Remember, too, that *these RDAs, as with most "normal" standards, are based on studies with EFA- and mineral-deficient people*.

When you take mineral supplements you can actually lose more of those minerals than you are taking! It may sound strange, but it can be true. What you don't know *can hurt you.*

Here's what scientists at Albion Laboratories – the world's foremost mineral specialists – have to say about minerals in an article titled, "A Healthy Start":

> To get his day off to the right start, Joe has a healthy breakfast of his favorite high-fiber cereal,with low fat milk, a side of fresh papaya, a little high-fiber toast, and a glass of fresh-squeezed orange juice. Joe's days are hectic, so to be sure that he is properly fueled, Joe takes his multivitamin/mineral supplement along with some good antioxidant....

It appears that Joe has done all the right things. However, on a closer review, we find that Joe's stomach has become a combat zone....

Non-chelated minerals ionize in the gastrointestinal tract. Once these types of minerals ionize, the fiber that was consumed during breakfast latches onto them to form complexes that are nonabsorbable and effectively decreases the bioavailability of the minerals from the multiple supplement.

But wait!! Some of the ionized minerals have evaded the fiber, and they are trying to head for their absorption sites and the carrier proteins that await them at the mucosa of the small intestine. Now these ionized minerals start to fight amongst themselves for absorption sites – a form of intra-intestinal mineral revolution! Calcium and zinc fighting against iron. Iron fighting back against zinc. Copper joins the fight against zinc.

The researchers found that **the fractional absorption of these minerals from the fiber-rich diet was not enough to overcome intestinal and urinary losses of these elements**. *All the subjects were found to be in negative mineral balance for the supplemental minerals.*

Natural sources of fiber, such as cereals and fruits, generally have a depressing effect on absorption of minerals such as calcium, iron, zinc, and copper. *Imagine taking mineral supplements and still going into a negative balance for the very minerals that are being supplemented!*[38] (emphasis added)

The highly promoted fiber we keep hearing about actually depletes our minerals! Truly chelated, bioavailable minerals easily solve this problem – they don't ionize, so the fiber can't grab them.

For a personal test, instead of your usual mineral supplement, try, for at least 90 days, a truly amino acid chelated blend of the nine minerals lacking in our diets. You can even take them on an empty stomach, because they are real food for your body. You'll feel the difference!

---

38 *Albion Research Notes* — A Compilation of Vital Research Updates On Human Nutrition, Albion Laboratories, Clearfield, UT, Volume 6, No. 2, June 1997.

We now know how to efficiently turn raw minerals into small organic molecules which the body uses, with no more upset stomachs. The key is the process called "amino acid chelation."

"Miracle" minerals?

Let's take a look at *chromium picolinate*, one of the so-called "miracle" minerals. It is claimed that chromium picolinate burns fat and increases muscle. Product after product now contains this chemical – all claiming its wondrous effects. Chromium may be an important trace mineral for overall health, but it hardly seems to measure up as "miraculous."

Our *Life-Systems* Engineering team never has believed the chromium picolinate hype; nor do many others. In 1992, R.G. Lefavi stated that studies suggesting it burns fat and increases muscle were flawed.[39] Few paid him notice, though. With consumer purchasing being driven by immense advertising campaigns, manufacturers often overplay a single study's results prematurely. You now know better than to take these conclusions at face value; especially when they are supplied only by the manufacturer.

Less than one percent of the chromium from food is even used![40] The amount of chromium actually used by the body is about one-millionth of a gram a day – it's virtually insignificant. Understand, this doesn't mean that we need more chromium to make up for its low absorption rate. It means the body simply doesn't want much of it.

An article in *Prevention* magazine states: "One by one, studies are failing to find that chromium supplements help you lose weight or build muscle." The author cites three studies from: the *Official Journal of the American College of Sports Medicine*, January 1996, the *Journal of Sports Medicine and Physical Fitness*, December 1995, and the *American Journal of Clinical Nutrition*, June 1996.[41] **Each study showed insignificant results of chromium picolinate adding muscle and dumping fat** – so don't feel bad if it didn't work for you. It did nothing for me, either, during my bodybuilding days.

39 Lefavi, R.G. et al., *International Journal of Sports Nutrition* 2(2):111-122, 1992.
40 *Nutrition For Fitness & Sport*, page 229.
41 "Why chromium isn't shining," Holly McCord, RD, *Prevention*, November 1996.

Chromium is most frequently sold in the picolinic acid form. Why – because it's more effective? No, it's cheap to make. Unfortunately, this particular structure often causes more health problems than it helps. Picolinic acid is known to deplete your body of other minerals in exchange for the mineral the picolinate is attached to. This means that, when your body does receive some chromium, *iron and other minerals are removed.*

It is interesting and distressing to note that picolinic acid is another name for nicotinic acid (niacin) – it could be that any noticeable effects from this compound are more from the nicotine residue remaining when chemically synthesizing the nicotinic acid than from the chromium!

Does chromium picolinate still have the same appeal when we call it "nicotine chromate"?

When chromium picolinate came out as the latest "miracle mineral," there were numerous studies purportedly proving its usefulness in weight control.

Colloidal mineral products: what are they really?

There has been a lot of publicity about the "miracle" of colloidal mineral supplements. With all the enthusiastic claims, it is important to separate facts from fiction.

The *Random House Dictionary of the English Language* gives this definition of a colloid: "... a substance that when suspended in a liquid will not diffuse easily through vegetable or animal membrane."

Because colloidal minerals are often claimed to have huge absorption rates (98 percent, according to a widely distributed audio tape), this presents a contradiction. Can the dictionary definition be wrong? Let's look at another reference book.

Dorland's Illustrated Medical Dictionary, 24th Edition, says a colloidal is: "A state of matter in which the matter is dispersed in or distributed throughout some medium called the dispersion medium. The matter thus dispersed is called the disperse phase of the colloid system. The particles of the disperse phase are larger than the ordinary crystalloid molecule, but not large enough to settle out under the influence of gravity."

to the bottom. The bottle never has to be shaken.

Don't let this technical jargon cloud the concept:
Colloidal minerals are not readily absorbed.

"Nor can colloidal solutions pass through a semi-permeable membrane. Since colloids **do not pass** through a semi-permeable membrane, they are retained in the vascular system."*

Homogenized milk is a good example of a "colloidal substance" — so is whole blood. In milk, the fat, carbohydrates, and proteins are suspended in water. Homogenization is a mechanical process that rips the fat globules (cream) into extremely fine particles so they can be dispersed rather than rising naturally to the top.

Some people think colloidal minerals are so small they bypass the digestive process and are directly absorbed by the cells. This simply is not true.

Digestion can be bypassed,

a. if the substance is small enough,

b. if it remains pH-stable in the stomach's highly acidic environment, and

c. if it is in a form compatible with how your body assimilates food.

*But this is **not** the case with colloidal minerals.*

The colloidal structure is too big to be absorbed by the cell. If the minerals were dissolved in a solution, they might be a little more useful – the mineral would be in a smaller form – but the **colloidal minerals are not dissolved** – they are merely in suspension.

What is in liquid colloidal minerals? "Colloidal" refers to the structure, not the content (the specific minerals and amounts) in the liquid. The formulations of various brands of minerals vary greatly.

Our team reviewed an analysis of one colloidal formulation and found five toxic minerals in it – aluminum, arsenic, cadmium, lead, and mercury. There was a tremendous amount of aluminum: 1,857 parts per million (ppm). The arsenic level was nine ppm, lead levels were three ppm, and the mercury level was one ppm. *No level is considered safe for these toxic metals.*

Levels of valuable minerals in this sample were found to be 10 to

* *Body Fluids And Electrolytes*, pages 62-63.

Levels of valuable minerals in this sample were found to be 10 to 100 times too low in concentration to be significant.[42] This is in marked contrast to marketers' claims of their products being highly concentrated. For example, five milligrams (mg) of zinc is considered to be a minimum daily requirement. A tablespoon of this colloidal mixture contained only two-tenths of a milligram. The magnesium RDA levels should be about 100 mg. A tablespoon of the colloidal mixture contained only 10 mg of magnesium.

The specific amounts of each colloidal mineral aren't usually labeled – perhaps because most have insignificant concentrations. The manufacturers certainly don't want you to know the levels of toxic minerals, either.

Some people believe that very low doses of medicines stimulate the body's natural defense mechanisms. The field is called "homeopathy."

Could this same rationale apply to extremely low amounts of minerals? A *Life-Systems* Engineering analysis says NO. The body uses minerals in a completely different way. Drugs stimulate, inhibit or regulate natural processes; minerals are raw materials for those processes – when the raw materials run out, the process stops!

Numerous tests are available to determine bioavailability of minerals. Some of these tests are: X-Ray Diffraction, Infrared Spectrometry, and Nuclear Magnetic Resonance Spectroscopy.

Our *Life-Systems* Engineering team has never seen any such tests, analyses or results showing bodily absorption rates of colloidal minerals. *We have seen analyses showing absorption rates of other mineral forms.* When evidence doesn't exist to the contrary, promoters can say anything they wish – and some promoters of colloidal minerals certainly do!

Alexander G. Schauss, Ph.D., Senior Director of Research, Southwest College of Naturopathic Medicine and Health Sciences, delivered a 12-page report to the National Nutritional Foods Association:

> In an effort to locate scientific support for many of the claims made for colloidal minerals, databases incorporating nearly **30 million papers** published over the last 40 years were

42 These products are food supplements and not intended to supply all of the nutrients in food. However, certain minerals are no longer found in food, in significant quantities; we need most of these minerals from the supplement.

utilized, including the well-known Medline. **Not a single reference could be located that could support the many claims being made for these products**.

They [clays] are essentially hydrous aluminum silicates, and are usually formed from the alteration of aluminum silicates. This explains why some "colloidal minerals" contain 2,000 to 3,000 parts per million (ppm) of aluminum. By comparison, foodstuffs may contain up to 100 ppm as bound complexes that are often very difficult to absorb.

To date the only element among minerals that seems to protect the brain from excess levels of aluminum is magnesium. Yet characterizations (analyses) of numerous colloidal minerals rich in aluminum often reveal low levels of this important element relative to the aluminum content. [At present, **aluminum is considered a "toxic" element.**]

Or, take the claim that colloidal minerals are "negatively charged, hence increase intestinal tract absorption." *This is news to gastroenterologists and physiologists* since the walls of the lumen of the small intestine where many minerals are absorbed, when at a neutral pH of seven, are negatively charged. The wall is composed of mucopolysaccharides which negatively ionize at a pH of seven. For this reason, the intestinal walls would repel negatively charged colloidal clay particles, since similar charges oppose each other, as any child who has ever held two magnets knows.

Another claim some purveyors of colloidal minerals have made is that the minerals in their product are 95-percent absorbed. Again, cite one study that demonstrates this is true. **None can be found in the scientific literature**.

Colloids have the capacity to scatter light, allowing them to appear opaque or milky in appearance. This is important to know, since some products claiming to be colloidal minerals do not scatter light or appear opaque, hence lack the qualities to be truly colloidal, and are mainly plain water.

Do Colloidal Minerals Contain '65,' '74,' or '92' Elements as Claimed?"... Again, **proof is lacking**. Of the 92 elements that comprise the inorganic portion of the soil on this planet,

> **all but ten usually occur at concentrations of less than 0.1%** (i.e., 1,000 micrograms/gram, milligrams/kilogram or parts per million (ppm)) and are referred to as "trace elements.
>
> Some purveyors of colloidal minerals might claim that they have all the elements in their product at the parts-per-billion or -trillion level, but one would have to ask how such an infinitesimal amount could benefit trillions of cells in the human body.
>
> Analyses of many of the colloidal products reveal bizarre ratios of elements not found in human cells, or reflective of ratios found in fluids, organs, or tissue. (emphasis added)

In his landmark book on amino acid chelates,[43] here's an interesting comment by the world's leading mineral expert, Dr. H. DeWayne Ashmead: "[Bioavailable] Chelation also prevents the strong adsorption [non-absorption] of the mineral onto insoluble colloids in the intestine." In his book, Dr. Ashmead makes it clear that he is referring to genuine chelation with amino acids, not with chemical salts. "Adsorption" (not absorption) means sticking to the surface. Insoluble colloids are not easily digested or absorbed. Dr. Ashmead is offering another, independent argument that proper amino acid chelation protects us from ineffective colloidal minerals.

By the way, Dr. Ashmead's book costs $65 and it's only available by special order.

Minerals must be in the right form in order to be absorbed.

Like ground-up rocks, many mineral supplements offer very little benefit.

If you feel different when taking colloidal minerals, then possibly,

1. you are so extremely deficient in a particular mineral that any tiny amount may be noticeable (although probably not enough),
2. you are taking very large doses,

43 *The Roles of Amino Acid Chelates in Animal Nutrition.*

3. your body is responding to the toxic ingredients (colloidal minerals can be highly acidic too), or
4. the psychological "placebo effect" is at work.

Depending on the specific circumstances, the placebo effect (expecting results) can account for sizable nutritional and medical success rates. As a result of reviewing 275 scientific articles, placebo-based effectiveness was found to be significant (at least temporarily) in many cases of so-called "miraculous results."

This finding was published in the *Journal of the American Medical Association.*[44]

Hormones and prostaglandins (cellular counterparts)

Hormones are controllers in a big way. A little input from them causes a big result. We could compare a hormone to a transistor. A tiny bit of current going into a transistor causes a large output current.

Insulin, estrogen, and progesterone are all well-known hormones. Others include DHEA and melatonin. If a diabetic takes too much insulin, it can produce such a decrease in blood glucose that a coma results. When attempting to manipulate *Life-Systems* artificially with hormone supplements, one must be very careful.

Especially for WOMEN

"Insulin causes the adrenal glands to produce androgens such as testosterone, which can prevent ovulation and wreak havoc with women's natural hormone cycle."[45]

Overloading on carbohydrates can make women more aggressive, and negates their feminine qualities.

P*lus, it piles on unwanted fat and cellulite.*

Add carbohydrate overloading to the EFA/mineral deficiency epidemic, and the avalanche of recent health and appearance problems becomes predictable.

44 "The Importance of the Placebo Effect on Pain Treatment and Research," Turner, et.al. *Journal of the American Medical Association*, May 1994, 271:1609.

45 *Beyond Pritikin*, page 7.

DHEA and melatonin have been proclaimed as "solutions" to health problems more often than many scientists would presume to do. Here's why our *Life-Systems* Engineering team does not advocate the use of any hormone, unless it has been prescribed, for a specific deficiency, by a physician – no matter how popular it may be.

1. **A tiny bit of hormone causes drastic changes in the body**. Some hormones can now be legally purchased by anyone. Dosage is unregulated. Does this lack of regulated use make sense? No. Hormones are much weaker when administered orally than when injected into the bloodstream, but that doesn't guarantee safety in using them. This decrease in effect, when hormones are taken orally, shows us that the body alters hormones during digestion. The body doesn't want them that way! From a *Life-Systems* Engineering view, taking hormones, without being under a physician's direction, is not a prudent path to radiant health.

2. **All hormone production typically decreases with age.** By mentioning only the hormone they sell, manufacturers often imply through their ads that only certain levels decrease as you age. Thus, they encourage you to increase the levels of the hormone found in their particular product.

   Here's what you aren't being told: Overall reduction in hormone production is a typical occurrence with adult maturity. If you just take more of one or two hormones, you upset the overall balance by not taking more of all hormones. There is a multi-faceted automatic control-system at work which must be respected.

3. **Many hormones (and all prostaglandins) are made from EFAs.**

Could a reduction in hormone production be another symptom of long-term EFA deficiency?

Hormone promoters haven't addressed the long-term deficiency of basic essence. With an EFA deficiency, we shouldn't expect a fully functional hormone system.

Judging by the droves of people purchasing hormone supplements, we see one more probable effect of basic essence deficiency.

4. **Taking hormone supplements may not correct the underlying problems**, even though they may affect a symptom. Nutritional supplements should address the underlying problem – not just attempt to compensate for symptoms of a critical deficiency by overriding the body's automatic control systems.

5. **DHEA, a heavily promoted hormone supplement, is converted in the body to androgens and other steroid hormones.** Excessive steroids are known to suppress the immune system. *DHEA used to be a controlled substance available only by prescription from a physician*, and it was only available from a pharmacy. **Steroids are regulated because they can be dangerous.**. Be cautious of self-medicating with DHEA supplements. Pharmacists and physicians are.

6. **There are risks with indiscriminate use of any hormones**. Some of melatonin's and DHEA's unpublicized, yet reported, common side-effects are: mental impairment, drowsiness, morning-after headaches, and excessive dream-disruptive sleep. Many people experience insomnia and nightmares instead of restful sleep. Clinical depression can occur, and there are also possible harmful effects to the thyroid and reproductive systems. You'll soon see new cautions about melatonin supplements. Canada and Great Britain have banned nonprescription sales of melatonin. Use of DHEA supplements gave two members of our *Life-Systems* Engineering team sleep-disrupting dreams.

Melatonin's recommended daily three-milligram dose is *at least ten times greater than what the body naturally produces*. This higher dosage is intended to compensate for digestive degradation. The *Pharmacist's Letter* warns that caution should be used, because, contrary to the frequent "safe at any dosage" claims, no one has yet studied its long-term effects at any dosage.[46]

---

46 *Pharmacist's Letter,* Vol. 12, No. 10, Oct. 1996. "FDA Reports Nonprescription Pharmacy," 4(34):13, 1996, *Lancet* 348:551, 1996. *Pharmacy Times* 1996, Aug. 1997, page 67.

> **If you have arterial blockage, retinal disease, or if you are taking estrogen, you are strongly advised to avoid melatonin entirely.** [We are further advised that] melatonin should only be used temporarily, a few days at a time, for example, to lessen the effects of jet lag or workshift changes.[47]

If you are already depressed, *melatonin typically increases depression.* Depression makes sleeping more difficult, so if you take melatonin with this condition, you will make the condition worse. *Melatonin also constricts arteries.* This provides more resistance to blood flow, increasing your blood pressure (and stress on your heart). Safe at any dosage? Our *Life-Systems* Engineering team says NO.

More "miracle" products?

Nutritional manufacturers sometimes mislead the public. What's a ceramic pot made from? Clay. What's that? – dirt. We have observed "detoxification" products containing "*bentonite*" and water. Bentonite is a fancy-sounding word for *clay* (purified dirt). That's right – dirt. The pharmaceutical industry has used it for years as a pharmaceutical binder. For that purpose, it is fine. But for a nutritional product to imply that it will act as a detoxifier in the body is another thing. Still, it doesn't stop their marketing campaigns. How much dirt would you choose to eat?

Another product, made from ground crustacean shells, is called "chitosan." Supposedly it's a "fat-blocker." But we've already seen that blocking the body's natural life-systems is detrimental and doesn't cause us to lose excess bodyfat or slow the rate of adding new bodyfat. What do we do with the shells of a shrimp or oyster? Most of us would either throw them away or use them as plant food, because they are nutritionally worthless for humans. Imagine, taking a waste product and marketing it to hordes of unsuspecting customers desperate to lose excess bodyfat!

"Beriberi *continues* to be a serious disease in the Far East because rice, the major food, has low thiamine content."*

47 *Dr. Alexander Grant's Health Gazette*, Indianapolis, IN, Volume 19, Number 10. Source: *Journal of the American Medical Association* (276:1011,1996).

* *Biochemistry*, page 518.

Basic fuel – the raw materials

After considering vitamins, minerals and hormones, we are now concerned with two types of basic fuel, or raw material. They are

essential healthy oils (lipid building blocks) and

essential amino acids (protein building blocks).

These two substances interact with the vitamins, minerals, and any other nutritional supplements you may be taking.

We must consume enough protein each day to provide our body with all the essential amino acids. We get lots of these amino acids from eggs, poultry, fish, cheese, meat, and seafood. Other sources typically have less bioavailability. Proteins are used by the body to make your enzymes, which are necessary for effective digestion and a host of other critical functions.

Many people in the U.S. don't eat enough protein because we have been misled into thinking that too much protein is bad. Vegetarians often have a difficult time obtaining all the essential amino acids through their selected foods — vitamin B_{12} *must come from animal protein!*[48]

Note: Virtually none of these essential building blocks are found in any processed carbohydrate!

Without basic essence, many people don't have enough healthy essential oils for their system to work properly.

No matter how many vitamins, minerals, and other supplements you take, they do very little good if the raw material isn't there for them to work with.

Surprise: Not all cells divide and renew. Once they are damaged, heart muscle cells form scar tissue. Most nerve cells can't be rejuvenated, either. What you are born with is all that you have for life.[49] **You had better know how to protect these limited resources!**

48 *Essentials of Biochemistry*, page 348.
49 *Essential Histology*, page 47.

Why haven't you been told this?

As reported by Reuters Health (May 24, 1999), omega 3 (an EFA) fights colon cancer in laboratory studies. "The growth inhibitory effect was most prominent in rapidly proliferating [cancer] cells," according to graduate student Abgela Jordan and colleagues at J.W. Goethe University, in Frankfort, Germany. "They seemed especially effective against COLO-320, the most aggrressive of the two cancer cell lines, ***halting all growth within 72 hours of exposure.*** *This inhibitory effect appeared to stem from 'both growth arrest and apoptosis [death of cells].'"*

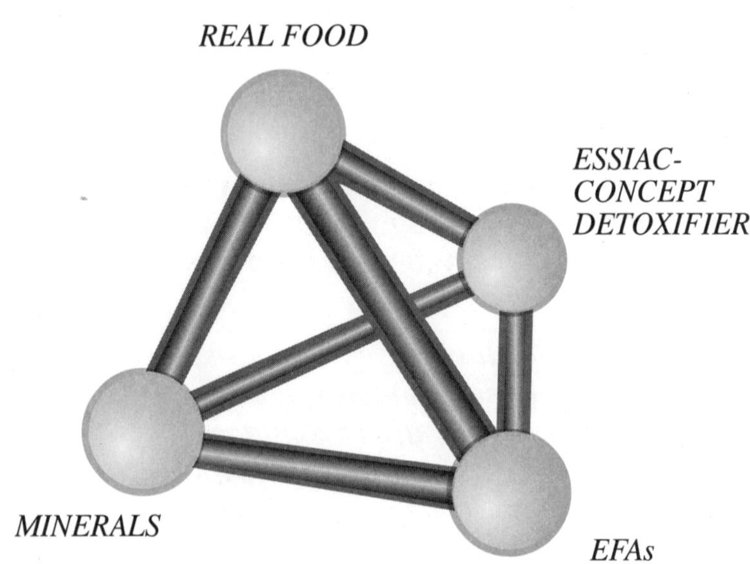

Radiant Health

Cellulite Takes A Hike

> *"Everything should be as simple as possible, but not simpler."*
> Albert Einstein – Nobel Prize-winner

(Men – show your wife or girlfriend this section)

Every cell of your body requires basic essence in its structure to function at its best. One of the wonderful ways in which this is demonstrated is through its visible effects on personal appearance. With basic essence, most people are amazed at how their skin and nails take on a whole new dimension. For many women, "skin conditioners" are no longer necessary.

Skin conditioning happens from the "inside-out," as it should. External moisturizers only give the illusion of softer skin. Basic essence gives you the real thing – naturally. Most women are amazed at the decrease in their cellulite too.[1] Basic essence is so effective it actually gets rid of cellulite. Finally you can eliminate and prevent the ugly plague of cellulite.

I am extremely excited to present this discovery to America's women!

Your skin will feel as smooth as butter.

and

Your nails will feel like fine crystal.

What's even more exciting, better skin and nails are noticed by virtually everyone within 90 days, once you start taking EFAs.

A while back, some women friends, who knew my scientific background, asked me how to get rid of their cellulite. They said they had tried everything and *nothing* worked. I told them, at the time, that I didn't know how to get rid of it.

---

1 For most women, major reduction occurs within 90 days. It virtually disappears within a year.

Before I could intelligently discuss the topic, I needed to understand cellulite's structure. After a week of constant thinking about it, I happened to fold a piece of paper into an accordion shape. I looked at it from the edge, and – low and behold – there was the same hill-and-valley structure that cellulite exhibits.

The "valley" is a direct response to the "peak." They are directly connected, not two separate things. Both structures must be caused by the same effect. For those of you with a physics or engineering background, cellulite ripples resemble the field-structure of the gravitational field around a black hole in outer space – an appropriate description, isn't it?

Now that the apparent nature of the underlying structure was clear to me, the next issue was to determine why the body would wish to support such a strange structure. It turns out that our bodies don't favor this effect, but have been stuck with it.

There were a few more issues to consider:

- From years of watching runners, I observed that even thin women often have significant amounts of cellulite. Cellulite is not directly related to the amount of excess body fat. This was interesting.
- At the gym, I observed women body-builders with cellulite, even though these women had more muscles than I did!
- After seeing many women in swimsuits over the years, I saw that cellulite appears mainly on women's rear upper thighs. You don't find much cellulite on the stomach or other areas. There are fat deposits in other areas, yet little or no cellulite. Why?

Let's not be sexist about it ...

Do men have cellulite, too? Men have hair to "cover it up." Without the hair, would men's cellulite be more visible? While watching runners in the park, I finally did notice several men with cellulite, as predicted.

Still, men seldom appear to have cellulite. Part of the explanation may be that men's skin is thicker than women's, and women have a higher percentage of bodyfat than men, by nature's design.

These two facts led me to suspect that cellulite would be magnified in women if it is related to the types of fat we eat.

Generally speaking, women have about 50 percent more bodyfat than men and 20-percent thinner skin. Thus, cellulite on a woman should be much more visible than cellulite on a man.

Women have a different hormonal makeup than men. This could have an influence on cellulite, too. If the hormones influence cellulite, and the hormonal system was impaired, we should see an effect of this impairment manifesting as increased cellulite.

Once my study of EFAs was in full swing, I learned that EFAs were critical to estrogen and all other hormone production.

Women's PMS problems often decrease with basic essence.

I knew that food processing destroys or deactivates EFAs. Because every cell needs EFAs, I also knew that muscle and fat cell structure could be altered by our diets. Could this alteration explain the hill-and-valley effect?

I had to explain the fact that even many thin women had cellulite, and some slightly overweight women didn't. It could go either way. Many diet foods are low in total fat, but high in adulterated EFAs. Furthermore, extremely thin women often exist on a diet severely lacking in all fats, so this could explain the apparent paradox.

Cellulite's main cause is lack of pure EFAs!

Cellulite's annoying structure is tied to the molecular bonding between the fat and collagen in your skin. With cellulite, these two substances unnaturally attract one another. Try to picture the cellulite as two magnetic silicone implants (one positive and one negative). When they are close, a strong attraction field will hold the two pieces together as one unit. This is precisely what happens with cellulite. Like fluid silicone, instead of two hard magnets, our tissues are flexible. Otherwise, the bonding is essentially the same. I wondered why this bonding happens.

*Trans*fatty acids from processed oils and fats are not as flexible as the EFAs they replace in the cell membranes. Their rigidity interferes with natural cell flexibility. Lack of cell flexibility further magnifies cellulite's hill-and-valley effect.

With the
Foundation of Radiant Health
I can do my job.

Functional Cell

NUTRIENTS
GET USED

DISEASE
KEPT OUT

SR

DISEASE
GETS IN

Dysfunctional Cell

NUTRIENTS
NOT USED

HELP!

I can't do my job without the
Foundation of Radiant Health.

Food processing destroys nutrients and alters the chemical structure of fat. In your body, EFAs are building blocks for each cell's membrane. If a significant number of them are altered, we should expect some observable effect. Cellulite is a result of this effect.

When EFA intake is increased, the cells resume the type of structure you had as a young child. When this happens, those "magnetic bonds" are broken, and the cells are flexible again – cellulite takes a hike!

How long will it be before you notice a difference? That depends on how much cell integrity has been lost. Typically, noticeable improvements are seen within 90 days. It could take as long as one year, but you will lose the cellulite over time, and it doesn't take any effort.

The more basic essence you assimilate, the less cellulite you will have.

Another important cellulite factor is eating too many processed carbohydrates. AGEs (advanced glycosylation end-products) cross-link with proteins and act like little magnets in the wrong places, too. Processed carbohydrates end up full of AGEs, which cross-link with proteins. AGEs are also known to build up, causing problems with arteries and DNA. Could they be part of cellulite? Yes. So once again,

EFAs come to the rescue: Less processed carbohydrates = Less cross-linking.

When you eat less carbohydrates, you'll have less insulin output. It is known that both the size and weight of fat cells shrink with decreased insulin levels. This reduces the surface area for adulterated EFAs to attach to your skin, so the cellulite effect will decrease further.

Over the years a lot of incorrect information has been published regarding cellulite. Let's sort through the myths, so that we may gather further insight into the true nature of cellulite:

- Some say cellulite is caused by "fluid trapped in the tissues." It is true that there is extra cellular fluid throughout the body, but there is no "trapping." This fluid (mainly water) is uniformly distributed throughout the body. This fluid can't be the cause of cellulite, because the fluid is everywhere and cellulite isn't. Furthermore, many runners still have cellulite. The amount of shock and stress a runner subjects her body to would force this "fluid" out of the problem areas. Plus, with all the running, she gets as close to dehydrated as anyone can, and the cellulite stays "behind." So this theory can't be true.
- Others say it's just "uneven deposits of ordinary fat." If you look closely at the dimple structure of cellulite, this doesn't make sense, either. There is nothing irregular or stringy and fibrous at all. While not pretty, it is a visibly regular structure. Nor does this theory explain why cellulite occurs preferentially in one location – the rear upper thighs.
- "Aerobics burns cellulite" is another myth. Have you taken a good look at the women in aerobics classes? They may be a little thinner, but their cellulite is just as bad as everyone else's. Do you know anyone who lost their cellulite from doing aerobics?
- "Massage eliminates the problem." Supposedly, massage breaks up fat cells or untraps the fluid between cells. This doesn't work for the same reason running doesn't. You can't undo strong magnetic attraction with a little movement. You have to demagnetize the area at the molecular level. Only basic essence can do this.
- Last but not least, high-fiber, vegetarian foods with whole grains are suggested, along with diuretic foods (cucumbers, celery, grapefruit, etc.). Translation: "We don't know, but this sounds great, so it has to work." No, it doesn't. You've probably already tried that method.

The reason why cellulite appears predominantly on women's upper back thighs, from a Life-Systems viewpoint, is because this is the least problematic area for the body to deposit adulterated EFAs which don't function properly.

Because there are so many vital areas that need EFAs – the brain is the most important – our bodies distribute EFAs with a priority agenda. Adulterated EFAs may fit in the cell membrane, but the cell can't make good use of them, and the cells know the difference.

The amount of cellulite is a good indicator of your EFA deficiency. The only effective way to eliminate this deficiency is to consume *basic essence*.

Many clients have told me that their cellulite appeared soon after they had their first child. This is because the female body gives every advantage to the child. This includes good EFAs. Where does it get them from? The body can't make EFAs. If your dietary intake isn't adequate, your baby gets YOURS, and it has nine months to take them from you – even longer when you breast-feed.

A pregnant woman really needs basic essence throughout her pregnancy for both her own and her child's benefit. Also be aware that **a woman's immune system is at its lowest during pregnancy**.[2] So the fetus isn't rejected, nature makes a compromise – temporarily lowering a woman's immunity. Doesn't it make sense to have the highest degree of natural immunity possible during this critical time? Only basic essence naturally ensures this.

Additional benefit:
Basic essence gives you more elastic skin = less stretch marks.

Cellulite articles disregard most of these facts and attempt to push the approach that "exercise and low-fat eating cures all." We've seen that the low-fat method has disastrous results. More vigorous exercise may be beneficial, but won't help decrease your cellulite – it can't.

I don't like to see people wasting their time, and I don't want you wasting yours, either. **Low-fat eating actually increases the cellulite**, because you'll never get the EFAs you need!

Now, with basic essence, stop cellulite cold!

2 "Pregnancy-Associated Immune Suppression: Risks and Mechanisms" by Eugene D. Weinberg, *Microbial Pathogenesis* (3:393-397, 1987).

"I don't care if test results proved our product doesn't work. Just write the description so **people will assume** it works. The placebo effect will take care of the rest."*
PLACEBO, INC.

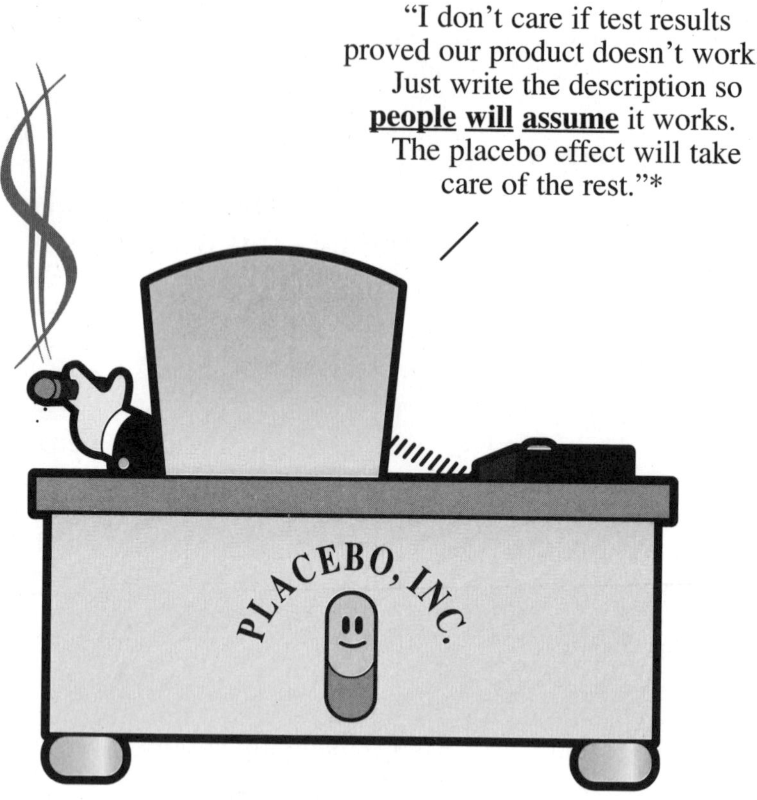

If you don't believe that we are routinely misled, then read this:

We get misled all of the time – *especially women...*

*The rationale for estrogen replacement therapy relies mainly on **two** types of evidence, **both of which are flawed** ... This is indeed a strong **assumption.**"

Source: *Therapie* (French), 1999 May/June;54(3):387-392

Your Thoughts Can Eat Your Lunch

> *"A new scientific truth does not triumph by convincing its opponents and making them see the light, but, rather, because its opponents die and a new generation grows up that is familiar with it."*
>
> Max Plank — Nobel Prize-winner

We have discussed the biochemical basis of food. Consider the psychological basis of hunger and eating. We know by observing real-life results that diets don't work. Over 80 million Americans are way too fat.

97 percent of people who go on a diet regain all the weight (or more) back within just 2 years.[1]

A recent study at the University of Toronto confirmed that: **"The more worried you are about how much you've been eating, the more you eat."**[2] (emphasis added)

Intuitively, *we know that there should be a simple solution to our problem with hunger* and our continued drive to overeat. From the previous chapters we can see why the fundamental EFA-nutrition link has been overlooked for so long. Attempting to alter the body's automatic control system is clearly not the answer. Instead, what works is feeding the body the fuel it was designed to run on: basic essence – essential healthy oils, – proteins and minerals. Once the body's physical needs begin to be met, there are emotional aspects that can still impede your efforts to achieve radiant health.

Maximize the Mind-Body Connection

We are greatly influenced by advertising and often don't realize it.

---

1 *Beyond Pritikin*, page 45.

2 "The Dieter's Paradox," Mary Roach, *Health*, November/December 1997, pages 96-99.

Here are six things that most of us have heard repeated many times, and would swear are true beyond a shadow of a doubt:

1. **What is the most important meal of the day?** If you didn't read this book, you would have bet your last dollar that a full breakfast is required, even if you aren't hungry, to "fuel the metabolism" for the day. You now know that essential nutrients are critical – not so much the rest of the food, or when the food is eaten.

2. **What causes osteoporosis?** Before you read this book you may have felt certain that it was lack of calcium. Why? Because most of the advertisements say, or imply, that lack of calcium is the primary cause and that taking more calcium is a "cure." You now know it's not the calcium.

3. **What does the body do with the fat you eat?** Until you read this book, you would probably have bet your last dollar that "eating fat makes you fat." and clogs arteries. You now know that fat does not go to fat.

4. **What is important about cholesterol levels?** In the past, you may have wagered that LDL is "bad," HDL is "good" and that you need to avoid eating cholesterol. You now know that cholesterol in the food you eat has little to do, if anything, with cholesterol in the body or plugging the arteries. It is also critical for the proper functioning of virtually every part of your body.

5. **How can we get the minerals we need?** You may have heard that "colloidal" minerals are a good answer. Could the nationwide distribution of millions of audio tapes bearing a carefully crafted advertising message have had any effect on your answer?

6. **Is a bagel a great food?** That it has no fat and no cholesterol is only a small part of the whole picture. Now you know a bagel is the metabolic nutritional equivalent of six teaspoons of sugar and little else. Far from being a good food, it is almost nutritionally worthless "baked paste" – mainly flour and water.

Food Psychology

Appetite is the *desire* for food, and hunger is the *need* for food. Because I eat so rapidly, my wife says I "eat like a dog!" I take this as a compliment, because a dog is a very noble creature. But she says I can't possibly appreciate my food this way. I'll tell you why she may not be correct on that point.

Contrary to popular belief, digestion doesn't rely on salivary enzymes to break down the food. Those of us who eat fast let the stomach do its full job. As we age, our salivary enzymes become weaker, and if we "chew" our food extensively, we rely too much on something which may hurt us later on. This is similar to the way people develop insulin resistance, which I spoke about earlier.

When you eat your food, can you really tell whether you are consuming meat, vegetable, or fruit? We should be able to, but typically we have lost or dulled a lot of our taste awareness.

With adequate EFAs, your sense of taste dramatically increases.

You will soon be able to really savor the flavor of food. Lack of EFAs has made your sense of taste less sensitive – only you aren't aware of it. Wait until after a few months of taking EFAs. Real food becomes delicious, and your desire for highly processed food ("junk food") will get smaller and smaller. Contrary to what you may assume, this increased sense of taste won't encourage you to eat more. You can eat less, because you now get so much enjoyment out of the food.

Like good sex, once you are satisfied, you don't need more for awhile. Food shouldn't be any different. But only if EFA and mineral intake is adequate will this satisfaction occur. Otherwise your stomach's "EFA switch" stays on and you are never satisfied.

A system-imbalance can lead to obesity. The system imbalance can be either physical or mental. Once EFA intake is increased, many physiological imbalances will stabilize themselves. Oftentimes, bodily problems strongly influence the mind.

This is true for many of our clients. Each of us wants to enjoy the foods we eat. In the natural order of things, we are obviously designed to enjoy what we eat. But Mother Nature couldn't foresee the explosion in nutrient-destroying commercial food processing.

There is no need to feel guilty about eating for pleasure.

When you get hungry, does a big bowl of salad come to mind? I doubt it. Sure, a small salad with hardboiled eggs, maybe some feta cheese, tomatoes, cucumber, and lettuce with creamy ranch dressing is tasty, but it doesn't come to mind first with most people.

You might try to make the case that it should come to mind, and that our taste is "screwed up" for all the reasons previously mentioned. That could well be true, except even after 12 months of the Foundation of Radiant Health, the desire for salad doesn't increase much. That is because Mother Nature didn't design us to live on salad – it is mostly water and indigestible cellulose. Mother Nature designed us as omnivores. The desire to eat less processed foods is very significant, though. So don't feel like anything is wrong if you don't desire more "rabbit food." You probably won't.

With adequate EFAs, your desire for sweets and other processed carbohydrates (sugar) diminishes to virtually nothing. So does the amount you desire. I now eat half the food I used to eat.

What if this doesn't happen to you when basic essence is added to your diet? Good question. Give yourself 90 days, though, to see results. If you still don't get the expected results, then the problem is very likely to have psychological aspects that need to be addressed.

For 30 years, I bit my fingernails. After just one session with a hypnotherapist, I didn't bite them anymore. True, I had wanted to stop, just as you want to change your eating habits, but I hadn't been able to do it on my own. Will power wasn't the solution. Biting fingernails is totally psychological (mind). While overeating is mostly physiological (body), there are also many possible psychological components as well.

Most of us salivate, like a conditioned dog, at the sight of chocolate. We are conditioned to think of chocolate as mouth-watering. A particular kind of candy bar is my favorite. Before the Foundation of Radiant Health I would eat one of them daily. Now, I seldom have a desire for one. It really is amazing.

The "Air Force diet" of restricted carbohydrates was instituted many years ago because air crews were getting fat on processed carbohydrates (doughnuts, soft drinks, candy, and other snacks).

When you realize that the taste for sweets is really an illusion, this conscious knowledge will put the "icing on the cake" in altering your desire to consume them. Basic essence provides the *physical basis for the reduction of your body's desire for processed carbohydrates.*

Many of our clients (including myself) used to eat processed snack foods all the time and thought they tasted great. Not anymore! The first time your body signals its dislike of them, make a mental note of how that feels. The next time you see a pack of processed snack foods, you probably won't want it as much as before. For most people, the desire really decreases dramatically. With the Foundation of Radiant Health, even most of the psychological barriers go away, in time, because the body is finally able to send the correct signals, naturally.

Emotional forces are real. If you find out that an illness or unhealthy condition is primarily "in your head," the most powerful solution is to understand what's happening.

A baby enjoys a finger or pacifier in his mouth. Psychologists call this "oral gratification." A *Life-Systems* Engineering analysis predicts that less breast-feeding is tied to increased smoking, nail biting and excessive eating. *As we grow older, eating continues to be associated with feeling better.* When an overweight person is upset, hungry or not, he usually heads for the kitchen. Instead of blindly reaching for food when difficulty occurs, ask yourself, "Am I really hungry?" If the answer is "no," then you are empowered to do something else.

Restaurant Dining

Restaurant dining should remain a great experience. You can eat anything you desire – your desires change as your body finally gets the EFAs it needs, within a matter of months. The main point to remember in a restaurant is to minimize the carbohydrates (sugar), especially the processed ones, like bread, potatoes and pasta. You may have to challenge some previous assumptions – like these foods were assumed to be good for you.

Who wants much bread anyway? There's much better food to eat. Go ahead and enjoy the delicious meat: steak, veal, duck, chicken, plus eggs, cheese, vegetables and fruits. Skip the rolls. They are primarily there to give you something to do while you wait for the food, and to make you feel full at the end of the meal, so you think you got your money's worth.

When dessert time comes, you probably won't want much of it, because your appetite will be satisfied. Remember that your appetite goes down compared with the amount of food you "needed" (craved) before basic essence. When you are consciously aware of this change in your system, it makes the process work more quickly and effectively. Instead of fighting the satisfied feeling because of your ingrained habit of eating more, you can relax and enjoy your new-found freedom from cravings.

If you are just starting with the Foundation of Radiant Health, split a dessert with someone else. Let them have the bigger portion while you enjoy yours. Eat whatever you want. Within 90 days you should rarely desire more than a few bites of dessert.

In the drink category, beer has lots of carbohydrates, yet the light beers generally have a little more than half as many carbohydrates as regular beer. Dark beers and nonalcoholic malt beverages typically have at least a third more carbohydrates than regular beer.

Distilled liquors are mostly free of carbohydrates. Avoid the sugary or processed drinks like soda and juice. Margaritas are fine if made fresh with real lime juice, without added sugar. Prepared drink mixes and any sweet drinks will rack up the carbohydrates, along with adding to your "bottom line." So, minimize beer and sweet drinks.

Why do you drink what you do, when you do and as much as you do? Is it for taste, something to do, being sociable, or because you are actually thirsty? For quenching thirst, nothing beats cool, clear water. When you choose to drink, be aware of what you are drinking, and its effects on your system.

A few nuts make a good snack, but the potato chips, pretzels, and sugar-coated nuts can make you fat.

With sandwiches, eat only half the bread. The main purpose of the bread is the convenience of an edible wrapper. Many plain breads are virtually devoid of taste as well as nutrients, but they still have lots of carbohydrates.

Most commercial fried food has lots of hidden calories from carbohydrates in the batter, plus health-threatening transfats, so be careful of them. Skip the french fries, unless they are really good. If they are, just a few of them should satisfy you.

One of the more challenging habits to overcome for many of us is the "clean plate" syndrome. We were taught as children to eat everything on our plates, no matter how full we might feel. While it is inappropriate to waste food, putting it around your waist is not a useful alternative.

As you become more in touch with your body and carry a conscious awareness of how it feels, it becomes much easier to save some of the food for later. When eating in a restaurant, you can ask for a carry-out container for leftovers. Just because the food is there in front of you, doesn't mean you have to eat it all right then.

Consider eating only half of the potato at restaurants after starting the Foundation. Our clients often tell me that they don't miss them one bit. You'll get the same taste and enjoyment with less food. With EFAs in your system, your sense of taste significantly increases, so there is never any need to "deny yourself." Bottom line: If you really crave it, eat some of it, then pay attention to your body's response. The next time, you'll want to eat less, as you learn to pay more attention to your body's signals.

What is that hungry feeling?

Your stomach is connected to your brain via what we call the "appestat." When our body needs nutrition, the appestat signals the stomach. Unless we are eating all the time, the stomach responds with a message to the brain that it needs food. This triggers the appestat to send a message stimulating the rest of the digestive system to be alert for food. We call this "hunger."

As time passes, and the need for nutrients goes unfilled, the hunger message automatically grows stronger. If it were a buzzer, we would hear it growing louder. The longer the body's nutrition needs go unmet, the stronger these feelings become. If we ignore hunger long enough, it becomes strong enough to cause physical pain. It can also drive us to extreme and nonsensible behavior. *When we feel really hungry, we will eat almost any type of foods and in quantities well above normal.*

The hunger response is not just "on" or "off." It has variable intensity: when it is on high, look out! Years ago, my wife decided we both needed to go on a diet. So, for two weeks, I went along with it. When mealtime came, I'd be extremely hungry.

The feelings of hunger completely dominated my thoughts all day long. If any food had been available during the day, I would have devoured it. I was ravenous all the time, and pity anyone who came between me and my food when mealtime arrived. The small amount of food I was "allowed" to eat only slightly took the edge off my hunger. I constantly maintained a conscious degree of hunger – it never went away. At the end of the two weeks, I was informed that there was a mistake in the calculations, and that I had been eating 400 calories a day less than the diet had called for.

It was a good lesson on how powerful hunger and the mind can be. *I was ready to do almost anything for food.*

The appestat senses nutrition – not volume.

Since we have not been getting the nutrients we require, our hunger switch is always "on." When we eat, it reduces the degree of hunger's intensity, but it only shuts off when the nutrient need is filled, or temporarily, when we stuff ourselves – until the appestat senses there is little nutrient value. When the appestat stays on for extended periods of time (virtually all of the time, with a deficiency of EFAs) even at lower intensities, the message can become garbled and turn into periodic cravings – intense appetite for specific foods. It can stimulate "feeding frenzies" when we do eat. It can also drive us into eating all the time.

When the mind is preoccupied with things other than food, like working and recreation, this sets up a conflict between the body and the mind. With a continuous deficiency of needed nutrients, we experience a constant inner conflict.

Which is stronger? The body or the mind? The real answer is that neither is always stronger. When hunger is strong enough, the body wins the battle. Do you know anyone who would choose to live only on water for 30 days? Even if they desperately wanted to lose weight? When the mind is determined enough, it can win – but only short-term. The mind cannot overrule the body for long. Even if you consciously cut back on eating, you will probably become irritable and physically and mentally inefficient. The forced restriction will show up as problems elsewhere. We are not designed to be internally at war with ourselves.

Many of us have developed ways to cope with a constant low- to mid-level of hunger. The most common way is to ignore it as much as possible. Likewise, if we hear a sound all the time, we tend to tune it out most of the time. If we do some hard work with our hands, the skin thickens (a callus develops) in response, to protect us. The human body has an amazing array of coping skills for survival, and the awesome power of the mind is one of them. When misused or overused, this power can backfire and bring about unforeseen and unwanted results.

When we ignore our hunger, it really hasn't gone away – we have just pushed it out of our conscious awareness. Keeping it in check requires a lot of mental energy. We may not even be conscious of the hunger any longer, but to control it, we must keep expending valuable energy – energy that could be put to much better use. The denied hunger keeps building until we binge out, often becoming nauseated afterwards, and we are so stuffed that our poor stomach has to call a halt.

We then suffer the consequences of this overload: discomfort, reduced energy, and often self-disgust. While the metabolism works the same for all of us, our perceptions as well as survival skills and methods are often quite different. We have developed quite a variety of dysfunctional ways to deal with food.

As we continue these survival behavior patterns over the course of many years, they become powerful habits – automatic, ingrained behavior that no longer requires conscious thought. We become automatic eating machines!

When we begin to rebuild our bodies with the Foundation of Radiant Health, it is important to understand how radiant health can affect these long-term habits. As the body's nutrient needs finally become met, a whole new perspective on food and eating opens up. If the mind is still stuck in the old patterns, we will have trouble recognizing all of the wonderful benefits.

Let's address a few key issues:

• **The worse our condition, the longer it takes to see results.** When our body has an extensive amount of rebuilding to do, it channels most of the new energy into areas that need help the most. Remember, every cell needs these nutrients – we are rebuilding the entire body. This takes time. It's a lot like boiling water. You put it on the burner and keep adding heat, yet it doesn't boil for some time – until enough energy is put into the water – then suddenly it is all boiling. Be aware that the results from the Foundation of Radiant Health can be very subtle to many of us, and the changes are gradual – not at all like the "big bang" we have learned to expect from drugs and stimulants. It is more difficult for us to recognize gradual changes. *We need to become more aware of ourselves and our individual condition – before and after – to fully appreciate the benefits we receive.*

• **Most people are not fully aware of their body or their personal energy levels**. They have been intent on ignoring how they look because they are unhappy with their appearance. They may not even recognize themselves in a photo – except perhaps a shot of just the face. When you ignore any part of your body, you cannot be aware of subtle changes there. For most of us, it's enough of a struggle to get through the day – let alone frequently monitoring our energy levels, too. Besides, that would only serve to remind us how poor we usually feel at the end of each day. As we start on the path to radiant health, this can be emotionally painful when we realize how far we have fallen from that path. As we progress on the new road to radiant health, we must become more aware of ourselves in order to see the benefits as they occur.

• **Does overloading on carbohydrates induce a fight or flight response**? The body uses stored sugar for either emergency responses (adrenaline) or strenuous muscular activity. By overloading on carbohydrates, we could be stressing our physical emergency response system and backing up the signals into the nervous system, triggering stress response. The adrenal hormone *cortisol* raises blood-sugar levels.[3]

Nobel Prize-winner Dr. Walter R. Hess demonstrated that the "fight or flight" response could be evoked by stimulation of a portion of the brain.

• **Can your mind make you fat?** Yes and no. The mind does not directly make us fat. It does not order the digestive system to pile on fat. Yet, it can set up conditions so that the body has little choice. Some of these conditions have larger physical components than others, but they can still be very powerful. The only way to deal effectively with the power of our mind is to bring a situation or behavior into full conscious awareness. We then have three choices: keep the dysfunctional behavior or judgment, modify it, or eliminate it. Until we consciously become aware of a particular pattern or habit and acknowledge it as ours, we are at its mercy.

3 *Essential Histology*, page 350.

Let's look at some examples of these behavior patterns:

- How often do I eat? Is my schedule fixed and rigid, or flexible? Do I respond more to my body, or more to influences like time of day and other people's schedules?
- Do I know a carbohydrate (sugar) when I meet one? If it's not protein, fat, oil, or water, it's carbohydrate.
- What is the "emotional content" of my meals? For example, do I associate eating apple pie (almost 100% processed carbohydrate) with mom's love and approval?
- What are my eating habits? Do I know precisely what I eat and when? Try making a list.
- Does my mind override my body with food desires or vice versa?
- Do I eat for taste and stop when I'm satisfied?
- Do I want more food even when I'm physically full?
- Do I subconsciously want to avoid intimacy? Overeating will develop the ultimate body armor – a thick layer of bodyfat.
- Am I simply eating out of boredom? Eating has become our nation's No. 1 form of recreation. Get a real hobby.
- Am I overeating to be sociable? That is, I don't want to offend anyone.
- Am I bending my elbow too much? How many processed carbohydrates (sugar) do I drink? Beer, juice, milk shakes, soft drinks, and so on, are all chock-full of carbohydrates.
- Do I eat because I'm blindly following some "eating program?"
- Do I misguidedly think that I need or should enjoy the so-called sugar "highs" throughout the day? And am I fully aware that there is always a corresponding low?
- Have I been misled into believing that I can eat all I want, as long as the food is called "low-fat"? I didn't realize that the only stretch exercise here is expanding my stomach and fat deposits.
- Do I eat a lot of snacks just to keep my hands busy while watching TV? Find an activity or craft to do.

We eat – even when we're not hungry.

Years before television and food processing, this problem would not even have been worth mentioning. Back then, few people ate after they were full. Today, with extensive time spent immersed in the television set, most of us want something to do with our hands while we are couch potatoes. So, we eat too often. The Foundation of Radiant Health will take away the physiological cravings, but TV bombards us with food and drink ads. Basic essence may not so quickly and easily take away years of learned and reinforced eating habits without some extra, conscious awareness.

Fortunately for most of us, eating when we aren't hungry isn't as common as eating when we really are hungry. Most people are hungry when they eat. Actually, they never stop being hungry except for a short while after stuffing themselves to become physically full. Chronic hunger can be stopped with basic essence. We have seen our clients' desire to eat even when they aren't hungry significantly decrease – once the Foundation of Radiant Health Program is implemented. You gradually, but naturally, stop "needing" to eat as often. My wife grew up eating multiple dinners and snacking all evening while watching television. I was amazed when even she stopped doing it – without conscious effort – over the course of 12 months.

Are we better off eating less – to "shrink the stomach?"

The stomach signals when food is needed for nourishment. It also is accustomed to taking in a certain quantity of food. We eat to satisfy our taste and to obtain the accustomed sensation of pressure which the stomach experiences when it contains this quantity of food. With basic essence, the quantity of food your stomach considers "normal" is gradually reduced.

"Wander nerves" branch out across the walls of the stomach. These nerves give rise to the sensation we call "hunger" when they don't sense the accustomed pressure. Thus, the stomach can become accustomed to lower quantities of food as well as higher quantities. But how capable are you of intentionally reducing your food intake for the necessary time to adapt to a lower volume and pressure?

Fortunately, basic essence naturally decreases the volume of food required to reach nutritional contentment. This leads to satisfaction of quantitative fullness (less volume), too. Over a few short months, you become adapted to eating less food each day. The stomach slowly and naturally becomes used to a smaller volume, and a new balance point is reached naturally.

Overeating: genetic or environmental?

There is no genetic relationship to obesity, and experiment-after-experiment, such as the leptin receptor theory, keeps confirming it. The main reason why obesity tends to run in families is primarily because of learned behavior. A family tends to have consistent types of meals and repeated eating patterns. In some families, frequent trips to fast-food restaurants may have taken the place of home-cooked dinners.

> A preliminary 1996 study of identical twins showed that after they left the household (and split up), their new bodyfat level was based on new living conditions.

If we are still not ready to take full responsibility for our choices, we may feel comfortable with the convenient "genetic" excuse.

Bodyfat comes from what we eat and drink – not our genetics.

If we examine what a family eats and the weight of the individuals, it isn't too difficult to see the correlation and deduce the culprit. Our clients have often demonstrated the connection – excessive carbohydrate (sugar) consumption coupled with EFA- and mineral-deficiency. The high carbohydrate consumption was reinforced by the incorrect idea that carbohydrates are good for us. Many of us unknowingly consume many more processed carbohydrates (sugar) than we think. So that you can be aware of foods that are high in carbohydrates, a listing of carbohydrate content for many common foods is located in Chapter 13.

Does calling something a "food" make it one?

Do you deliberately eat sand or sawdust so you will feel full? A lot of people do, although, of course, they don't always know it. These are two very common additives in processed food. Of course, they are purified and made into a very fine powder. Sometimes you will even find them on the label of products found in health stores and supermarkets. They will be called silica (sand) and cellulose (sawdust). If you don't willingly eat sand or sawdust with your food, what about other indigestible stuff like psyllium husks? Some people actually pay to add this by-product fiber to their diet so they will feel more full. From a Life-Systems Engineering analysis, this method is detrimental. The purpose behind this method of eating indigestible bulk is that: 1. you physically expand your stomach to short-circuit the hunger sensation, and 2. you improve water absorption so that your bowels work more efficiently.

Once again, you are attempting to trick your natural automatic control system. Your stomach works to process this "material" not knowing there is nothing to be processed, because, for humans, it isn't food. For a human being, psyllium husks are nutritionally worthless. From high-fiber fruits and vegetables, we obtain vitamins and minerals. No one would naturally choose to eat husks on their own without the misguided suggestion that they may be useful for weight loss. Biologically and nutritionally, they are the same as sawdust.

For the length of time the fiber stays in your stomach, you'll have a sensation of physical fullness. Remember, the appestat senses nutrients, so you'll still feel hungry. The other downside is that the fullness effect is temporary, and you'll be starving yourself nutritionally, plus upsetting your body's natural digestive rhythm.

It's nice to know that, with the basic essence discovery, such counterproductive "methods" as filling up on sand and sawdust are obsolete.

I'll eat less if I chew more, won't I?

There are two reasons that I learned to eat rapidly. First, I grew up with two brothers. When dinner was served, if I didn't eat quickly, the food was gone. Second, when I was sixteen, I worked at a fast-food restaurant. Breaks were short, so I had to eat quickly. When I became a manager there, I didn't have time for a formal break, so I ate even quicker. With me, eating patterns are a learned behavior.

Is that terrible? If I learned to chew thoroughly, would I enjoy my food more because I'd appreciate the taste? Would I eat less because I would get more benefit and nutrition from the food, since it gets partially digested before it enters my stomach?

I can tell you that chewing a lot and eating slowly doesn't help you to eat less or help you lose weight. Both methods are ineffective. I have many clients who tried this approach and still remained overweight. Experience clearly shows that you don't lose bodyfat by eating slowly or by chewing your food more.

Understanding affects perception!

As a young man, many years ago, I always tried to chew (masticate) thoroughly before swallowing. Once, I was on an expedition with a group. We had stopped to eat at a restaurant, and we met an old man. I later found out he was from Persia. When this old Persian saw the way I was chewing, he asked me why I chewed so thoroughly.

He said, "Tell me, young man, why do you eat like that?"

I was embarrassed at this question. I was ashamed for the man. Wasn't it obvious to any learned being that food must be chewed thoroughly?

Repeating verbatim what I had once read, I replied, "I chew thoroughly so that the food's value will be better assimilated in my intestines. Properly digested food gives all the food's value to the organism." I repeated everything I had learned out of various books on the subject.

Slowly shaking his head, the old Persian shared the following saying, which I'll never forget: "Let God strike him who does not know, and yet presumes to show others the way to the doors of His Kingdom."

When I heard this, *my opinion of the old man changed and I listened intently to the rest of his comments.*

"If you chew your food in this way as a means to health or for the sake of other attainments, then I shall have to say, if you would like to know my sincere opinion, that you have chosen the worst possible way.

By chewing your food so carefully, you reduce the work of your stomach. Now you are young and everything is all right, but you are accustoming your stomach to do nothing; and when you are older, owing to the lack of normal work, your muscles will be to a certain extent atrophied. And that is bound to occur if you continue this system of chewing. You know that our muscles and body get weaker in old age. Now, in addition to the natural weakness of old age, you will have another form of weakness brought on by yourself, because you are accustoming your stomach not to work. Can you imagine how it will be then?

On the contrary, it is not at all necessary to masticate carefully.[3,4] At your age, it is better not to chew at all, but to swallow whole pieces, to give work to your stomach. I can see that those who have advised you to practice this mastication, and also those who have written books about it, have, as is said, "heard a bell without knowing where the sound came from."

I was devastated. I had counted on the wisdom of the consultants in these matters. I decided to take advantage of the opportunity to ask this old man what he thought about controlled yoga-style breathing, because I had practiced this for years, too.

The old Persian explained that "yoga-style" breathing, which he termed "artificial inflation," would be very detrimental. Only if one knew every small screw and every small pin of our machine (the human body) could one know what to do. He said I risked a great deal because the machine is very complicated. He asked me: "Do you know yourself so well?"

He ended our conversation by saying, "I repeat, our body is a very complicated apparatus. It has many organs with processes of different tempos and with different needs. You must either change everything or change nothing. Otherwise, instead of doing good, you might do harm." The manner in which he spoke, and his depth of insight, gave me the impression that this Persian was a true specialist whose understanding of the human body was unquestionable. This old Persian may have been one of the first true Life-Systems Engineers!

I thought I was doing everything correctly — was I WRONG!

Most of what we were taught about nutrition is wrong.

---

3 This is true. *Life-Systems* science now knows that insignificant breakdown of carbohydrate occurs from chewing. Lipid (fat) digestion begins in the intestine. Protein digestion begins in the stomach. *Essential Histology*, pages 186, 217, 261.

4 In the human, salivary amylase (in the mouth) accounts for very little of the total amount of carbohydrate (starch) digested. *Basic Medical Biochemistry*, pages 405-406.

Advertiser's Motto:
"Money is the muscle that moves minds."

You can see how the advertisers use money to influence us. Incorrect information from advertisers can lead us to harmful and unnatural behavior. We have locked ourselves in a prison of our own delusions. The great news, though, is that you have the key in your hand. It is the *power of understanding* that can make you free.

Before we can escape from prison, we need to know that we are in prison.

Many articles have been published about how it is alright to be overweight. They promote denial that being overweight is a problem. These articles usually start with the premise that the person has had a constant battle with excess bodyfat for many years. Because they don't know how to eliminate the excess fat, they rationalize that it "must be" OK to be overweight; otherwise they wouldn't be overweight. It doesn't make rational sense, but it is an attempt at justification. Life-Systems Engineers understand these people's years of frustration – we all suffered through it, too, and we now have the solution. If you are overweight, or not as physically fit as you'd like to be, accept that fact, because now there is an easy solution.

We have come a long way in our new understanding of the body and its life-systems. Much of this information is not yet understood by health professionals. As we saw in the beginning of this book, it usually takes 25-50 years for new ideas to be implemented by the established "experts."

Most of us can't achieve ideal bodyweight by sheer "will power." Our bodies won't let us. Even if we did this by overriding our bodies' Life-Systems, to do this causes illness, exhaustion, and other system imbalances. We would be putting ourselves on the fast track to ill-health! Under those conditions, a woman will rapidly develop cellulite, too.

The first key to developing the ideal mind-body connection is to give the body what it requires – the Foundation of Radiant Health. With it, we no longer need someone else telling us what is best for us. Once our body has what it needs to work efficiently, we can train the mind to maximize the nutritional benefits.

Three basic principles will help guide you on your path to radiant health.

1. Even an ideal mindset will yield limited success as long as the body doesn't have its Foundation of Radiant Health requirements met.
2. Even with the body working at full capacity and unimpaired, the mind can still interfere with the body's functioning.
3. Setting a positive mental intent and taking the Foundation of Radiant Health at the same time yields up to a 1,000-percent (10 times the original) improvement.

It also helps to be aware of some of the more common mental and behavioral complications to attaining radiant health.

• **Depression**: This will sap energy out of us no matter how fast our body generates it. We weren't meant to be depressed. Our Life-Systems Engineering analysis blames EFA deficiency as a frequent factor contributing to depression, because many of our body's hormones and all of our prostaglandins are made from EFAs. One symptom of hormone deficiency is depression.

• **Habit**: We behave as though we are hungry, even when we aren't. Once we start with the Foundation of Radiant Health, we begin to develop a sensitivity – we can learn to avoid eating whenever we aren't actually hungry.

• **Emotional Escape**: Are we gaining excess weight (a form of armor) to avoid intimacy or social closeness? Most people aren't; but if we are, hypnotherapy may be a powerful way to help us gain conscious awareness and the release of emotional blocks.

• **Emotional Substitute**: Is food being used as an emotional substitute – for love or acceptance?

• **Escape from Boredom**: Snacking on virtually anything but processed carbohydrates is ok, but if we become an eating machine while watching television each night, even when we aren't hungry, we need to change our behavior.

• **Celebration**: We are trained from childhood to eat as a way of celebrating special events. Are we going overboard?

• **Recreation**: Are we eating just to have something to do? Do we get anxious when our hands or mouth are idle?

Heal the Body First...

" ... Eating disorders affect approximately 8.5 million people in the United States alone, and should not be taken lightly. Because of the many complex psychological/physiological issues that surround eating disorders, seeking professional help is often crucial to diagnosis and recovery. **One of the guiding principles from the American Psychiatric Association is that nutritional balance must be achieved <u>first</u> when treating people with severe eating disorders. ... Often, once nutritional rehabilitation occurs, many mood disorders and other <u>psychological</u> <u>symptoms</u> exhibited by eating disorder patients <u>improve</u>.** ... Heart problems, anemia and electrolyte imbalances are just a few of the serious health issues surrounding eating disorders.* **Consequently, heal the body <u>first</u> and the mind follows."**

Source: Nancy Locke, LSW, Licensed Psychotherapist
Excerpt from private publication.

The most common mental roadblocks to radiant health:

- Continuing unproductive or detrimental habits.
- Failing to recognize carbohydrates and thinking they are good for you.
- Lacking awareness of your body – the mind-body connection has been short-circuited from long-term nutritional deficiency.
- Irrationally expecting what hasn't worked in the past to start working in the future – "hoping for the best."

**American Psychiatric Association: Diagnostic and Statistical Manual of Mental Disorders*, 4th edition, 1994, pgs. 541-542.

Your nutritionist, diet center, or physician has failed you!

If your nutritionist's or physician's recommendations haven't helped, it's not your fault! They need to understand the insanity of the great 25-year carbohydrate eating *experiment*.

"Insanity: doing something that doesn't work, over and over, in spite of its obvious failure."

Anthony Robbins

"Saturated fat and cholesterol in the diet are not the cause of coronary heart disease. That myth is the greatest 'scientific' deception of the century, and perhaps any century."

George V. Mann, M.D. (1991)
Professor of Biochemistry and Medicine – Vanderbilt University

Better Than Free and Save Time Too

> *"It is easier to resist at the beginning than at the end."*
>
> Leonardo Da Vinci

The Foundation of Radiant Health puts money in your pocket.

1. Most people experience a 30%-50% reduction in food consumption with the Foundation of Radiant Health.
2. For the average American, that means *saving more than $100 per month in food costs* – after paying for the Foundation of Radiant Health.
3. Eating fewer meals gives you more time. *The average person will **save more than 300 hours each year*** (based on 18 hours daily awake time). That's adding more than 17 extra days of free personal time to your life each year.

How Much Do You Spend On Food?

One soft drink	**$0.75**
Breakfast	**2.00**
Lunch	**4.00**
Dinner	**5.00**
Snack	**1.50**
Packaged Drinks	**2.00**
Total daily cost	**$15.25**

($106.75 per week)

Add $14.00 more for two modest meals in a restaurant.

Weekly Total = $120.75

Foundation of Radiant Health
Saves You Money: You Eat Less Food

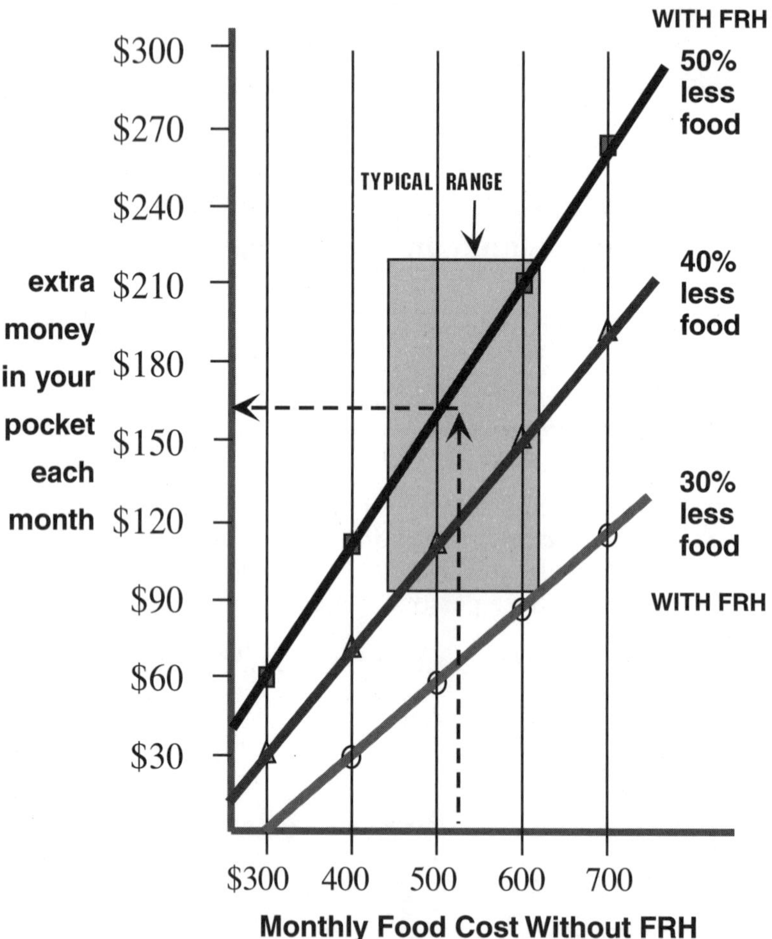

1 Across the bottom of the chart, find your monthly food cost.

2 Look up to the diagonal line representing the amount your appetite decreased since starting the FRH

3 Read across to the left to see how much money you save each month *after* purchasing the FRH.

Foundation of Radiant Health (FRH)

Eating Fewer Meals Gives You **More Time**

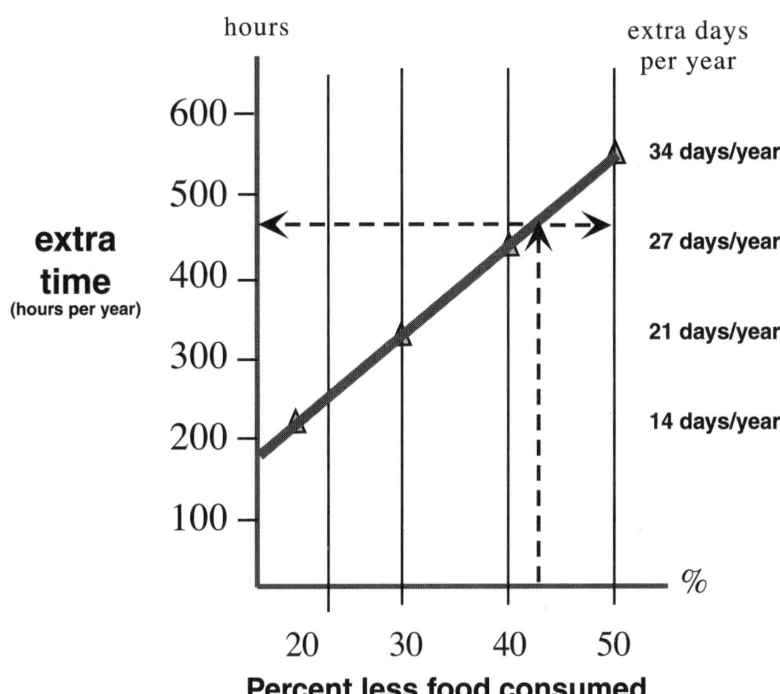

1 **Locate on bottom of chart how much less food you now eat since starting the FRH.**
2 **Look up to diagonal line on chart and read how many hours of extra time you will gain in the course of a year.**
(This is shown as hours on the left and days on the right side.)

The Only Menu You'll Ever Need

There is no Foundation of Radiant Health "plan" or "eating program." When appetite functions correctly, there is no longer a need to consciously control it. We don't count our breaths or "program" our hearts. We don't have to. Automatic life-systems take care of it for us.

If there is a basic program, this is it:

1. Give your body the Foundation of Radiant Health.

2. Eat what you desire.

Once EFA- and mineral-deficiencies are overcome, you'll be amazed how you feel, and how food cravings are no longer the controlling force in your life.

As promised, here's a list of carbohydrate-based foods. This listing is by no means a "do not eat" list. Rather, if you find yourself not losing excess bodyfat or eating more than you think you should, once you are *regularly* taking basic essence, then you may be unconsciously consuming too much of these foods. Just cut back on them. That's all there is to it. Cutting back will be much easier with the Foundation of Radiant Health.

Carbohydrates come in 2 varieties – "sweet" or "filling."

The sweet ones include:

desserts, cakes, candies, juices, processed snack foods (including potato chips and corn chips), and ice cream.

Sugar – in any form, including glucose, sucrose, fructose, maltodextrin, and honey – is almost pure carbohydrate.

The filling ones include:

bread, potatoes, rice, cereal, and milk.

A bowl of cereal (sweetened or not), milk, and some sugar give you as much as 160 calories, nearly 8 full teaspoons of sugar!

Look at the great American lunch: a sandwich, a piece of pie or cake, and a soda, maybe even some french fries or chips. With at least 350 calories of processed carbohydrate (17 teaspoons of sugar), the unfortunate news is that, *not only are you overloading your system with processed carbohydrates, but also you'll be starving and craving again just two-three hours later.*

Carbohydrate content of some popular foods
(in equivalent teaspoons of sugar)

Extra heavy sources:
pancakes and syrup, bread, pasta (spaghetti, macaroni, etc.), cereal, potato, rice, ice cream sundaes, milk shakes, juice, dried fruit, grits, oatmeal, baked beans

20 carbohydrate calories (five grams) = one teaspoon of sugar.

The Quick Carbohydrate Summary:

Very High carbohydrate: sugar, dried fruits, jams, jellies, canned fruits in syrup, fruit juice, fruit drinks, soda, cereals, rice, beans, lentils, peas, potato products, corn, pastries, pretzels, cakes, cookies, bread, crackers, flour, yams, pies, rolls, honey, (maple) syrup, beer, rice

Low carbohydrate: squash, string beans, cabbage, turnips, cauliflower, mushrooms, asparagus, spinach, lettuce, celery, onions and most other vegetables.

Very Low carbohydrate: eggs, real cheese, fish, beef, pork, ham, bacon, lamb, chicken, turkey, duck

Does this mean I shouldn't eat some of these foods? No. Simply *eat less of those in the very high category*. One generous piece of cake will give you more carbohydrate calories than you require for the day. So will four pieces of bread. When enjoying a hamburger, you may choose to not eat half of the bun. The point is just not to overindulge in high carbohydrate foods.

As your body readjusts itself to radiant health, your habits and eating patterns will change, too. Remember, with basic essence, you won't want very much of these high-carbohydrate foods. A little will now "go a long way"! If you truly desire any of these high-carbohydrate foods, by all means eat some, but be consciously aware of the effect on your body. With basic essence, your body's "feed-back" system will quickly send the signals to stop eating.

Sugar Content of Common Foods

Alcoholic drinks:

8 oz. beer 1.5 tsp.
brandy 0
bourbon & ginger 3 tsp.
8 oz screwdriver 3 tsp.
whiskey 0
brandy sour 1 tsp.
bourbon 0

Beverages:

black coffee 0
1 cup apple juice 6 tsp.
1 cup fruit punch 8 tsp.
1 cup fruit juice 4 tsp.
1 cup carrot juice 2 1/2 tsp.
12 oz. carbonated non-diet soda 5 -10 tsp.

Breads:

bagel 6 tsp.
English muffin 6 tsp.
bun, hot dog / hamburger 2 tsp.
2 slices white bread 4 1/2 tsp.

Cereals:

8 oz puffed rice 6 tsp.
8 oz oatmeal 4 tsp.
bowl of corn flakes 4 tsp.
(add more for milk, sugar, and fruit)

Cheeses: Only creamed cheese and cottage cheese have any carbohydrate to speak of, and even they are very little. Make sure you purchase real – not processed – cheese.

Cookies: Average 2 tsp. per cookie.

Pasta/flour:

8 oz. pasta 6 1/2 tsp.
4" diameter pancake 2 1/2 tsp.

Fruit:

apple 4 1/2 tsp.
1 banana 5 tsp.
1/2 cantaloupe 2 tsp.
4 oz. grapes 3 tsp.
peach 2 tsp.
8 oz. papaya 3 tsp.
1/2 cup raisins 10 tsp.
avocado 1 1/2 tsp.
1 cup blackberries 3 1/2 tsp.
4 oz. cherries 2 tsp.
1/2 grapefruit 3 tsp.
orange 4 1/2 tsp.
pear 4 1/2 tsp.
8 oz fresh pineapple 3 1/2 tsp.

Ice Cream:

banana split 20 tsp.
ice cream soda 7 1/2 tsp.
1 scoop any flavor 4 tsp.
milk shake 10 tsp.

Milk:

1 cup half & half 2 1/2 tsp.
1 cup heavy cream - neg.*
1 cup milk (all varieties) 5 tsp.
1 cup plain yogurt 2 1/2 tsp.
1 cup sour cream (not "lite")1 1/2 tsp.

Nuts:

1 cup almonds 1 1/2 tsp.
1 cup peanuts 4 1/2 tsp.
1 cup roasted cashews 7 tsp.
1 cup pecans 2 tsp.

Pie: 1 piece 7 1/2 - 10 tsp.

Puddings:

1/2 cup 1 1/2 tsp. (sugar-free) to 6 tsp. (sugared)
1/2 cup custard 2 1/2 tsp.

Salads:

3/4 cup fruit 4 1/2 tsp.
1/2 cup potato 2 1/2 tsp.
tossed greens neg.*
1/2 cup chicken salad 1/2 tsp.
egg salad (with real mayonnaise) 0
cup macaroni 10 tsp.
1/2 cup shrimp neg.*

Sandwich with 2 slices of bread: 6 - 10 tsp.

Sweet toppings:

1/4 cup caramel 12 tsp.
1/4 cup marshmallow 5 tsp.
1/4 cup fudge 14 tsp.

Soups (1 cup):

bean 5 tsp.
lentil 10 tsp.
potato 5 tsp.
corn chowder 3 1/2 tsp.
oyster stew 6 tsp.
most other 2 1/2 tsp. - 5 tsp.

Candy:

average candy bar 4 tsp. -10 tsp. (some bars are very high!)

---

* negligible (means insignificant amount)

Vegetables:
(even large servings of some vegetables have little carbohydrate)

6 stalks asparagus neg.*	1 onion 2 tsp.
stalk celery neg.*	1/2 cup squash 2 tsp.
1 cucumber neg.*	1/2 cup mashed potato 2 1/2 tsp.
med. tomato 1/2 tsp.	1 cup pumpkin 3 1/2 tsp.
1/2 cup mushroom 3/4 tsp.	med. baked potato 4 tsp.
1/2 cup zucchini 3/4 tsp.	20 potato chips 4 tsp.
1 cup cabbage 1 tsp.	15 french fries 5 tsp.
1 cup cauliflower 1 tsp.	1/2 cup lima beans 5 tsp.
1/2 cup green beans 1 tsp.	1 cup peas 5 tsp.
head lettuce 1 tsp.	1 cup tomato sauce 5 tsp.
1 cup spinach 1 tsp.	ear of corn 6 tsp.
1 cup broccoli 1 1/2 tsp.	8 oz. rice 9 tsp.
1 cup brussels sprouts 1 1/2 tsp.	1 sweet potato/yam 9 tsp.
cup beets 2 tsp.	serving baked beans 10 tsp.
1 cup carrots 2 tsp.	1 cup hash browns 12 tsp.

*neg. = negligible (insignificant)

Frozen/canned/ packaged foods:

Packaged foods come with labels describing the contents. Multiply the listed grams of carbohydrates by 4 to get calories, then divide by 20 to get equivalent teaspoons of sugar. That comes to one teaspoon equivalent of sugar for every five grams of carbohydrate.

A simple guideline: if one serving carries more than twenty grams of carbohydrate (four tsp. sugar), take this into consideration at your next meal.

NEVER FORGET:
"To stop **gaining** weight is as important as losing weight! Be patient. *Radiant Health* helps stop the weight gain."
Dr. Robert Nemer

Seven Rapid Recipes For Radiant Health:

I love to eat. We all should enjoy eating – that's why Mother Nature gave us a taste for so many delightful foods. During the multi-generation carbohydrate experiment, many of us had our taste buds dulled. Once you start enjoying **Beyond The Zone** meals, you'll soon awaken your taste buds.

I don't have much time to spend preparing food and cleaning up. You probably don't, either. I like a delicious meal in 15 minutes, and I don't like depriving myself. These recipes should satisfy you and ensure your peak performance throughout the day. I've included one of my favorites dishes from my favorite Houston restaurant – Aldo's Dining Con Amore´. I dine there often, and Master Chef Aldo was kind enough to let me include this recipe for your enjoyment. To me, there's no equal to a delicious filet mignon.

You will find that each of these recipes gives you energy instead of making you sluggish!

Three-egg omelet:

Heat about 2 tablespoons of real butter, or ghee, in a frying pan on medium heat (a true brass omelet pan is best because it makes anyone into a great cook – it's harder to burn anything).

While the butter is heating, crack 3 eggs and add a pinch of salt into a mixing bowl and beat. Let sit about 1 minute. The (scientific) reason for the salt is that salt "denatures" (relaxes) the protein in the eggs, so cooking fluffs them up. No milk, cream, or water is needed to make a great omelet.

While your omelet cooks, clean the bowl. When the omelet is close to finished, you can add a little fresh pepper to it, a little freshly grated Parmesan cheese (or Regiano Parmesano for the gourmets), or a pinch of Tarragon. You can add whatever "extra" you enjoy before you "flip it in half." A couple of sliced tomatoes make a tasty complement. If you want bread, you'll find a German black bread delicious, and doubly good with real butter.[1]

1 A slice has about 60 carbohydrate calories. It's very flavorful, and you won't get bloated from one slice. Soon, you may find that "white bread" doesn't taste good anymore. Mestemacher or Schinkenbrot brands (both from Germany) have little processing and can usually be ordered from your favorite grocery store. If they can't order it, try rye or pumpernickle.

Hamburger:[2]

A hamburger is one of my favorites and an American tradition. Mother Nature gave us a taste for beef, because it is good for us. The 80% fat grade chuck has great flavor. You don't need to waste your money on leaner beef.

If you don't already have one, you might consider getting a cast iron pan (hardware and gourmet stores have them). They are great for cooking because of the easy cleanup and great heat radiation.

Preheat the pan on medium high for 5 minutes. Add some ghee. Put in your hamburger patties. Turn when cooked enough. Put some real cheddar cheese on your burger for a real treat. Use 1 piece of bread if you like. My personal favorite is 2 'burgers and a salad with Sass brand "sesame-garlic" dressing. (It's made by Sisters & Company in Austin, Texas, and should be available at your local natural food market.)

Egg Salad:

Place a half- or full-dozen eggs in a pot, and cover with water.

Heat to boiling.

Simmer gently about 25 minutes. (You can tell that an egg is done when is spins smoothly like a top.[3])

Cool and shell the eggs.

Add *Spectrum* Natural brand Canola Mayonnaise – it's the best I've found (or use your favorite).

Mash the eggs. Add a dash of freshly ground pepper and salt to taste. For variety, add some chopped celery. It'll keep for days, when covered, in the refrigerator. It's ideal on half a slice of bread with some pickles.

---

2 You can easily buy inexpensive chuck roast and grind your own. It's delicious, and you have a better idea what's in it. If you choose to grind your own meat, it pays to purchase an electric meat grinder. Many cities have stores selling organically raised chuck roasts for a price competitive with other meats. For two people it's easy to grind about four pounds at a time, make the hamburger patties, and freeze them.

3 An uncooked egg has a lot of internal drag, so it spins slowly and wobbles on a flat hard surface like a table or countertop. Knowing physics makes cooking easier!

Tuna Salad:

Use your favorite brand of tuna fish.

Add mayonnaise to taste.

Add chopped celery. Like the egg salad, it'll keep for days, covered, in the refrigerator. It's great by itself or with a slice of bread.

Poached eggs:

Fill your skillet about halfway with water.

Bring to boil.

Add 2 tablespoons of vinegar (white or apple cider) to reduce the eggs' tendency to stick to the pan.

Shut off heat and drop eggs into water.

Cover. It only takes a few minutes for the eggs to cook.

Use a slotted spoon to scoop them up. They will either easily scrape off the bottom of the skillet or float to the top.

Put them on a buttered English muffin. They are great with bacon and a piece of cheddar cheese. A particular brand of bacon, called "Sunday Bacon," is delicious – any day of the week.

Filet Mignon:

Even though it looks complicated, this recipe isn't complicated. Master Chef Aldo cooks this dish in just 9 minutes! It's a great taste-treat.

Preheat your cast-iron pan on medium high for 5 minutes.

Add some ghee.

Sear an 8 oz. filet (for 2 people).

Turn heat down to medium.

Add:

1/2 tsp. chopped shallot
1 tsp. Gorganzola cheese
a pinch of sage
3 oz. meat or vegetable broth (ready-made)[4]
1 tsp. green peppercorns
2 oz heavy (whipping) cream
a pinch of thyme
salt and pepper to taste
add 2 oz of brandy and 1 oz of sherry – optional

4 Pacific Foods of Oregon makes terrific organic broths.

Cook on low until beef is cooked and sauce is how you like it. If you want a simpler dish, just sear the filet, then reduce the temperature to medium to finish cooking.

For a side-dish, I enjoy some mashed potatoes (half a cup) made with half-and-half, butter, and salt. It's easy to make them while you cook the steak.

Snacks:

A favorite snack is small pieces of real cheese, like Cheddar. A little cheese goes a long way to fulfilling your appetite without weighing you down. Freshly shelled nuts, especially almonds and pecans, are another good source of non-fattening energy. Try them.

One of the delightful things about being **Beyond The Zone** is that you can enjoy the pleasure of eating again. Meats and delicious sauces are guilt-free.

You'll find many more dining delights in our forthcoming book, *Rapid Recipes for Radiant Health.*

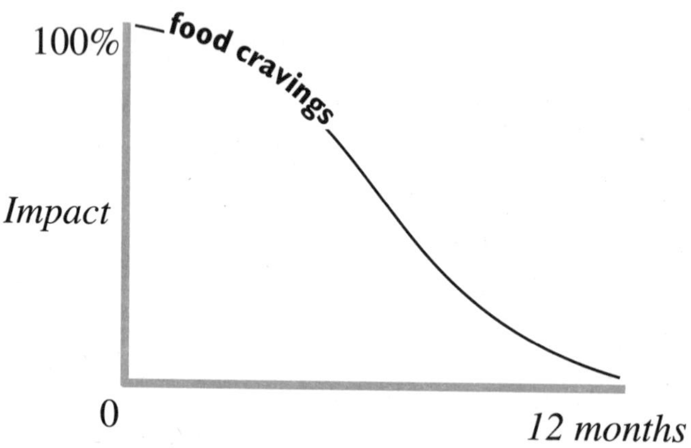

The Foundation of Radiant Health reduces food cravings.

Your Ultimate Detoxifier

WARNING! Detoxifier required: Pesticide impact fertility!
Methoxyclor, a widely used pesticide since 1972 can destroy testosterone production. "...this metabolite can adversely affect testosterone in men." The researcher's suggestion: "Protect yourself against exposure by eating organically grown fruits and vegetables."

Biology of Reproduction, 2000;62:571-578

Q: What does an Essiac® [1]-concept tonic actually do?

A: It is a highly effective, yet gentle, detoxifier.

Q: What is a detoxifier?

A: It systematically cleanses body systems and organs. In other words, it activates removal of impurities and toxins from our bodies.

Q: Why does toxicity occur?

A: It occurs because we are exposed to polluted air, impurities in our water, harmful pesticides, preservatives and synthetic chemicals in our processed foods, and other harmful exposure such as found in "sick building" syndrome. Also, it has clearly been shown that mercury used in virtually all dental amalgams (fillings) impedes the functioning of many of our organs. Mercury is considered toxic yet is still a standard component in many tooth fillings.[2] How many more questionable items which may be toxic are routinely used in food processing?

It is a tragedy that virtually all foods we eat and drink have been highly processed and adulterated. It matters little whether we dine at the finest of restaurants or prepare the food ourselves. Food additives and processing take away beneficial nutrients and in many cases cause harm by altering the food's molecular structure. Even popular terms such as "freshly made" or "homemade" are virtually meaningless given the vast number of food additives, preservatives, and processing of the raw ingredients used almost everywhere today.

It's not an easy job for our bodies to combat all these foreign "man-made" additives and processes. We need every possible advantage for an added "edge" in today's stressful world.

1 Essiac is a trademark of the Resperin Corporation, Ontario, Canada.

2 *International DAMS* (Dental Amalgam Mercury Syndrome) *Newsletter*, Albuquerque, NM, Summer 1992, page 7.

Q: What are the benefits of detoxification?

A: When all body-systems function properly, our body is a highly efficient machine. Detoxification rids the body of compromising impediments to ideal physiological functioning. Essiac®-concept tonics are the most effective (yet extremely safe) detoxifiers we have come across.

Q: Are any other characteristics associated with detoxification?

A: Some users gain a heightened intolerance for alcohol. One drink often makes them feel "wiped out." This reinforces the idea that the human body is a very fine-tuned machine when it is properly functioning. It doesn't respond well to being harmed and therefore provides immediate feedback in the presence of alcohol and other detrimental drinks and foods.

Q: Are any side-effects or negatives associated with detoxification?

A: Typically, very few with this tonic. There is usually none of the temporary sweating or decreased energy associated with most other detoxification formulas. This tonic works gradually to maximize system balance.

Initially, flushing the toxins may cause some temporary effects lasting two-three weeks. Detoxification influences all life-systems and shifts them to a new balance point.

For those with extreme system imbalances, some users find taking the tonic just in the morning ideal, for the first few weeks, so sleep won't be disrupted while the body begins to normalize itself.

Q: Is Essiac® helpful in dealing with cancer?

A: That was its original purpose, over 60 years ago. According to the many who have used the formula, it can be most beneficial. Essiac®-concept tonic has historically been used as a cancer preventative. So much has already been published on this subject, we will limit the remainder of our discussion to non-cancer related benefits of the formula. Your nutritional consultant or physician can guide you to publications, such as the *Townsend Letter For Doctors*, showing its effect on cancer-related conditions.

Q: Why should I believe that this formula is good for me?

A: You should maintain a healthy skepticism, but *this particular formula has been well-established for over 60 years with the same consistent results*. Few products have this long history of consistent results – and with no side-effects. There is no reason for anyone not to try the formula.

Q: How does this product compare to the "mushroom tea"?

A: There are several possible health concerns in using the mushroom tea (Kombucha). Before using the mushroom tea, read at least one of the books about it.

Q: I've noticed some brands have an acceptable taste and others taste horrible. Why the big taste difference between brands?

A: Taste depends on a multitude of factors. There need not be any unpleasant "medicine" taste. Although the original formula doesn't call for it, some manufacturers add a small amount of apple cider vinegar to increase product stability and decrease the formula's natural bitterness.

Q: Can yeast-sensitive users take this tonic?

A: There are no yeast related effects, if the formula is correctly bottled at over 180 degrees F. Yeast-sensitive users can safely take the formula.

Q: What is the closest comparable product to this formula?

A: Nothing else is comparable. Numerous vitamin and herb department managers reported this product is unique and "in a class by itself."

Q: What makes Essiac®-concept tonic so different from other supplements?

A: Its methods of formulation, assimilation, and action are completely different from those of vitamins, amino acids, or virtually any other product because *the process of digestion is bypassed – the formula is immediately utilized by the body*. It also helps purify the blood.

Q: Why does it work so well?

A: The special 12-hour brewing process for this combination of herbs, using distilled water, releases their full potency. The formula works in a way that no pill or tablet possibly could.This is the most effective way to utilize the formula we know of.

Q: Is 12-hour brewing really required?

A: Tests have verified it is. The TDS (total dissolved solids), which is a measure of ionic activity, peaks at 12 hours and doesn't increase further after 12 hours. Therefore, 12 hours is the optimal brewing time to release all the herbs' nutrients. This is an extremely long time for a manufacturer to tie up expensive brewing equipment. Most manufacturers won't even consider the idea.

Q: Why is water-based brewing so great?

A: Our bodies absorb water-based nutrients quickly and easily. With water-based formulas, the digestive process doesn't destroy potency as so often happens with capsules, pills, and most oil-based formulas. "You're not what you eat, you're what you absorb," says Jeff Bland, Ph.D.[3] No other medium is so readily utilized by the body without negative effects.

Q: Is this special herbal blend irritating like so many other herbal formulas? Many experts say to stop using a particular formulation after a while, to give the body a short "rest."

A: No. Each of these herbs (as used in this formula) is non-irritating. They "feed" the body – they don't irritate it into increased short-term performance which must be paid for later!

Q: Can children take the formula?

A: We know of no reason why not. None of the herbs are irritating. Simply give children a proportionately smaller amount based on their weight.

Q: I have high blood-pressure. Will the formula help lower it, and will taking it interfere with medication I am taking?

A: We know of no interference with any medications. If you are taking a blood thinner, you may need less of that medication. Consult with your physician.

Depending on the reasons for the increased blood-pressure, the formula's Slippery Elm Bark reduces resistance in the vascular system, and both Burdock Root and Sheep Sorrel increase circulation (blood flow to the extremities), so the formula often helps. If you can find the formula brewed with

3 *The Energy Times,* published by The Energy Times, Long Beach, CA, July/August 1995, page 20.

Cat's Claw, that is probably your best approach.

Q: I'm concerned about possible future heart problems. I've worked too hard in my business to suffer a heart attack at an early age. Will the formula help?

A: The original 4-herb Essiac® formulation can make a noticeable improvement, but for this purpose we *highly recommend the Essiac®-concept formula brewed with Cat's Claw.* Only one company we know of (Maximum Efficiency Products) produces this formula by adding a significant amount of Cat's Claw to the original formula. Our research shows it may be the ideal preventative. Cat's Claw bark has the ability to inhibit platelet aggregation and thrombosis, so it helps to naturally increase circulation, lower blood pressure, and inhibit the formation of plaque on the arterial walls. The heart works with less effort. Dangerous blood clot formation is also inhibited throughout the body. A useful analogy would be the difference between pumping thick cream through a pipe or pumping water. The water has lower viscosity, which translates to less drag and resistance; therefore, less work is required.

Q: Can I take the tonic for extended periods of time?

A: We have found no drawbacks to continued usage. In the literature we have come across, there was one instance of someone allergic to Sheep Sorrel (1 of the 4 herbs in Essiac®) reported. That user was also allergic to many other substances – the tonic wasn't the problem.

There are various Essiac®-concept tonics in the marketplace. Be sure to read the ingredient list on the label. Some products have been altered from the original formula to include stimulating or irritating herbs. Make sure you understand what you are taking. Because most of us keep eating processed foods, drinking water of marginal quality, breathing polluted air, and suffer from high stress, we virtually never stop abusing our bodies. Therefore, daily usage provides maximum benefits to combat these harmful effects. In this respect it's just like taking a daily vitamin supplement.

Q: What happens when I stop taking the formula? Are there withdrawal complications?

A: No. If you have been taking the formula consistently over a significant period of time, you will be significantly detoxified.

Depending on the level of harmful additives in your food, the quality of air you breathe, the level of water pollution, etc., over time you will simply revert to a similar condition you were in before taking the tonic. The first sign of stopping use is likely to be the skin's oils reverting back to the "pre-Essiac®" condition. There are no known physical or psychological addictions whatsoever, so there are no withdrawal symptoms.

Q: Can the tonic be used topically?

A: Yes. Although not the primary method of action (oral ingestion is the primary method), it has excellent results topically. Skin conditions are often improved. Healing of burns, cuts, and sores are aided with external application. One member of our team was painfully burned and applied just the tonic to the burn. A few days later, doctors were amazed how quick and complete the healing was! One of our editors found that twice-daily exposure directly to canker sores quickly reduced the pain and speeded their healing.

Q: I've read many testimonials speaking about Essiac® helping with fuller and thicker hair and decreased hair loss from brushing or shampooing. Will the formula bring color back to the hair? That is, will it eliminate the grey?

A: We have heard of a few cases where it has brought back color, although it hasn't done so for any of our team. However, it has decreased typical hair loss observed when brushing and shampooing as well as increasing its body.

Q: Does the formula assist in weight loss?

A: Although not directly, it appears to help significantly.

Q: How?

A: First, the formula is a natural diuretic, so excess water retention decreases. Second, if all body-systems work correctly, we are less likely to desire or crave "junk-foods."

Q: I'm on multiple medications. Will Essiac®-concept tonic interfere?

A: Our research did not uncover any reported drug interactions. It appears that the Essiac®-concept formula is uniquely compatible with any vitamins, nutritional supplements, or medications you may be taking. Check with your physician.

Q: Even when taking numerous vitamins and supplements, I still catch colds, flu, etc. – most discouraging. Will Essiac®-concept tonic help raise my immunity?

A: We spoke with numerous users and, yes, immunity appears to increase tremendously. White blood cells become much more efficient, hence the increased immunity to infection. Numerous users report insect bites don't become nearly as inflamed or itch as much. This is a clear example of an increase in immunity.

Q: How will I know what degree of detoxification has been accomplished, and how long does it take to become detoxified?

A: Many users gain a new, highly refined sense of taste. The flavors of every food really stand out, and for many users, the sense of smell is improved. Calmness abounds as nervousness decreases, and fatigue goes away. Users get tired when they are supposed to become tired – not before. Many users become aware of an incredible sense of general "well-being." This has to be personally experienced to be understood.

Maximum effect usually takes about 6-12 months of continuous use. Of course, depending on your physical condition (whether you smoke, etc.), this could take longer. Depending on your specific condition, the body will work in different personalized ways to enhance this detoxification. Stressful situations become easier to deal with, too.

Q: I observe a noticeable calmness when taking the formula. Could the formula help with hyperactive children? Diagnoses of Attention Deficit Disorders (ADD's) have become widespread. Is there anything that can help these kids besides Ritalin? I'd rather not risk possible drug-induced side-effects.

A: Extraordinary results have been reported with ADD's. This type of disorder is caused by an imbalance in the body's endocrine system. The formula can be impressively effective against this imbalance – the formula encourages a harmonizing effect throughout the body. Consult your physician.

Q: I've heard one's "regularity" will be altered when first starting the tonic. Is this true? If so, why?

A: It seems to be true for some people. The formula's strong detoxifying effect can cause a temporary "flushing action" (looser bowels). Typically, it will be most noticeable during the first weeks of taking the formula. For most users, constipation is eliminated after just a few day's use. The Slippery Elm Bark coats the entire intestinal tract, soothing it and allowing elimination to proceed with less effort. The formula also aids the regularity of those not suffering from constipation.

Q: What is blood purification?

A: Toxins in the blood and the lymph system are eliminated.

Q: Does the formula help do this?

A: Yes.

Q: I am taking antacid for acid indigestion. Will the tonic help?

A: If you read the article by Johnathan V. Wright, M.D.,[4] you may not take antacids so often. Dr. Wright says they may cause problems, such as interfering with mineral and amino-acid absorption, effectively causing malnutrition.

The Essiac®-concept formula actually aids digestion. It soothes the entire intestinal tract and allows healing of the inflamed areas which could cause this discomfort. A Cat's Claw brewed formula is even better. Cat's Claw is the best intestinal cleanser there is – and, as used in this formula, it is totally non-irritating!

Q: Does the tonic work in the manner of "chelation therapy"?

A: In the area of detoxification and blood purification, there is a similarity. Like magnets, components of the tonic "grab onto" metals and other impurities which don't belong in our body and help eliminate them through our excretory system.

Q: How much more energy can be expected?

A: Significantly more. When the body-systems are optimized, we don't have to waste energy to overcome deficiencies, and less energy is required to maintain normal activities. Also, the chlorophyll in the Sheep Sorrel appears to increase the oxygen carried by the bloodstream. This helps all body-systems to operate more efficiently. The mechanism used in an Essiac®-concept tonic to release energy is unique. There is no sudden

---

4 *Let's Live*, Hilltopper Publications, Inc., Los Angeles, CA, September 1995, pages 14 -16.

release of energy (no "blast") as with most "green" drinks. It's like having race car performance on demand – the energy is always available, yet you sleep sounder, too.

Virtually all who regularly use this tonic – business people, students, athletes – don't "crater" or become exhausted (either mentally or physically) as easily. This is another unique attribute of the formula! You will rarely become mentally tired – just physically tired, as we were meant to become when we need rest.

Q: Is this formulation useful for bodybuilders, powerlifters, and other athletes?

A: Outstanding. Increases in endurance and strength are reported along with decreased recuperation time. Many martial artists are now using the formula because it has significantly helped them to recover from the aches and pains of taking numerous falls and hits. Bodybuilders often find workout soreness and inflammation is significantly reduced. This tonic, brewed with Cat's Claw, is an excellent supplement for all athletes.

More sedentary people have reported noticeable increases in strength and stamina. In many cases, the pain and inconvenience of old injuries decrease. The formula seems to be compatible with any other supplements you may presently be taking.

Q: Does the formula shrink swollen ankles? I've tried everything, and nothing seems to work!

A: There have been excellent results on swollen ankles – typically starting during just 1-2 bottles' usage!

Q: Is the formula good for diabetics?

A: **Outstanding**. Type 2 diabetics can often reduce insulin requirements, and their glucose levels stay more consistent. The Burdock Root's *inulin* (not insulin) yields impressive results. The formula increases circulation, so many diabetic-related conditions have been reported to improve. Often, the elderly develop mild diabetes without their knowledge. This formula is excellent – it can minimize the effects of diabetes, including reduced circulation and cold extremities.

Q: Are any "female" problems relieved?

A: Frequently, severe headaches are minimized, and periodic

bloating decreases. Numerous users report urinary tract infections and yeast infections are often quickly eliminated with use of the formula.

Q: Are any "male" problems relieved?

A:Essiac® users have reported decreased prostate size and inflammation. Because overall energy increases, there are numerous "performance" benefits as well.

Q: Will the formula help hemorrhoids?

A: Yes. Numerous users have reported decreased inflammation.

Q: I noticed the tonic's nutritional label shows very little: no calories, very little vitamins, or other traditional nutrients. Why?

A: The Essiac® formula is not a vitamin, mineral, or enzyme supplement. It contains the natural nutrients from herbs and works in a different way. Traditional measurements don't tell us much about herbal formulas.

Q: The health benefits seem outstanding. Are there other benefits such as appearance related ones?

A: Many users say the formula is the **best skin moisturizer and conditioner they have ever used**. Women are raving about *their nails being much stronger and not splitting*. Even better, you just drink it – the formula works from the "inside-out."

Q: Are there additional health benefits I may not see or notice?

A: Yes. The majority of the formula's benefits won't be directly visible. For example, the antibiotic, anti-microbial Slippery Elm Bark coats virtually all the joints, digestive tract, and vascular (circulatory) system with a "protective" layer. Any internal inflammation is eased and healing is rapidly promoted before you may have been aware of a problem.

In this respect the formula could be described as an effective *preventative tonic*. Several of us have taken the formula for more than twelve months and still continue to see new improvements even though we would have been pleased just continuing to maintain our wonderful "optimized" state.

Q: How many of the benefits can I expect to experience?

A: An excellent question. Many of the formula's attributes work on "the inside," so you may not be directly aware of how much good is being done to their vascular, digestive, and endocrine systems. Also, the more ailments one has, the more noticeable the effects of the formula will be.

This is a very personal experience. Even if you don't notice specific changes for awhile, the formula is working. But the typical user will notice observable improvements in at least one area.

Q: Will changes in the formula decrease its efficiency?

A: Some modifications will ... others won't. A small amount of apple cider vinegar can be added to increase the formula's stability (resistance to spoilage), and decrease its bitterness. Apple cider vinegar has a multitude of trace minerals – especially potassium – which provide benefits in a form that is readily absorbed by the body. *Your Health* magazine calls apple cider vinegar "miraculous."[5] You can also combine the tonic with juice, tea or other beverages.

Q: I am interested in maximizing intestinal cleansing. If the intestinal wall is clean, it makes sense that food nutrient transfer will be more efficient. I've heard that eating lots of fiber is best for this. Are you saying Essiac®-concept formula is good and a Cat's Claw brewed version is even better?

A: We are, although what matters is that you experience the difference. Years ago, our team analyzed the "high-fiber" diet. *Life-Systems* Engineers predicted fiber's effect is *minimal*, at best. The regular Essiac®-concept formula improves the efficiency of cleansing, and the Cat's Claw brewed version is even better. Once you try it, you will see for yourself.

Q. What Might This Tonic Assist Me With?

A. Please remember that each of us has a different level of "healthiness." For example, a smoker will have a different accumulation of toxins than a non-smoker. The waiting time to see results will vary with each user. Depending on your personal condition, this could take as long as a year, although the majority of users report noticeable results within the first month. This is especially true of the enhanced feel and appearance of their skin (the skin's essential oils re-balance themselves).

---

5 *Your Health*, Boca Raton, FL, July 25, 1995.

In many cases, hair reportedly becomes much thicker and fuller with substantially decreased hair loss from shampooing and brushing – just as it did with our staff. The beauty-related effects are wonderful, but many of the tonic's users quickly experience other beneficial, yet more subtle, effects.

Be reasonably patient. Allow at least 90 days for a fair evaluation.

The Herbs

The original tonic formula utilizes a special blend of four herbs. Some manufacturers add other herbs which they claim increase the original formula's effectiveness. Added ingredients have included Kelp, Milk Thistle, Red Clover, and Cat's Claw – among others. We prefer the addition of Cat's Claw. The prestigious *Townsend Newsletter For Doctors* has described extensively many of the benefits of this special herb, and it is completely compatible with the formula.

All of the original four herbs, as well as Cat's Claw, have been used for hundreds, if not thousands, of years. Unlike some herbal formulations, *these herbs have no irritating effect as used in this formula and can be taken every day.* General properties of each herb are listed here along with some of their reported effects.

Burdock Root – This herb is best known for its beneficial effect on the skin. It increases circulation to the skin and helps to detoxify (cleanse) the epidermal tissues. Many users report exceptional smoothness and especially healthy appearance of their skin. "Some of the conditions which may benefit from this root are: psoriasis, eczema, acne, boils, sties, carbuncles, ulcers of the mouth or stomach ..."[6]

The root (in a way similar to garlic) has been reported to destroy bacteria and fungus cultures. Anti-tumor properties have also been noted. At Nagoya University in Japan, researchers found that the root helps reduce cell mutations.[7]

Another beneficial feature of this root is its action as a "blood purifier." This term means the formula helps eliminate toxins from

---

6 For detailed information, *Your Health*, Boca Raton, FL, December 27, 1994, page 56.
7 *The Essiac Report*, page 81.

the blood and lymphatic systems. Its action is also reported to work on the respiratory and urinary systems.

The liver, gall bladder, kidneys, and digestive system benefit from the properties of Burdock Root. It may also help with the elimination of excess fluids from the body.

Burdock Root is rich in Vitamins B-complex and E. Its trace minerals include potassium, phosphorus, chromium, cobalt, iron, magnesium, silicon, zinc and sodium.

Because of its diuretic action, conditions of arthritis, rheumatism, and sciatica may be improved. Many users report a rapid decrease in swollen ankles even if the condition hasn't responded well to other treatments.

Burdock Root contains *inulin* (not to be confused with insulin) which helps regulate sugar (glucose) in metabolism. Diabetics may be helped. Inulin has also been shown to possess exceptional restorative properties. It increases immunity by improving the efficiency of white blood cells.

Sheep Sorrel – Like Burdock Root, this ingredient has been reported to aid in healing a wide variety of skin disorders, as well as assisting in the destruction of tumors and easing some degenerative diseases.

Carotenoids, a component of Sheep Sorrel, are present at a concentration of approximately 8-12%. Beta carotene (a strong antioxidant member of the carotenoids) is converted to Vitamin A in the liver. Vitamin A has been shown to strengthen the immune system by aiding production of white blood cells. White blood cells are what attack many of the body's harmful intruders, including cancer.

Sheep Sorrel is rich in vitamins A, B complex, C, D, K, and E. Its minerals include significant levels of calcium, iron, magnesium, silicon, sulphur, zinc, manganese, iodine, and copper.

Sheep Sorrel is also rich in chlorophyll. Chlorophyll increases oxygen content in the blood. High blood oxygen content can increase the body's action against many invasive conditions. Research at the Linus Pauling Institute and at M.D. Anderson Cancer Hospital has shown chlorophyll to enhance the body's immunity against certain carcinogens (cancer-causing substances) and has been shown to strengthen the immune system. According to these studies, it appears to be effective against chromosome damage – which is considered to be a precursor to cancer.[8]

Sheep Sorrel is rich in potassium oxalate. It aids digestion, and has been reported to relieve stomach hemorrhage and jaundice.

Slippery Elm Bark – This herb's main constituent is mucilage. Mucilage is a gum dissolved in the bark's juices. This material has extraordinary cleansing properties. It has been reported to reduce the pain of ulcers – the mucilage coats any area it passes through.

Slippery Elm Bark has a lubricating property which helps protect membrane linings and joints. Relief of inflamed areas is commonly reported.

An antibiotic and anti-microbial effect has also been reported along with an ability to remove toxins from the body.

Turkish Rhubarb Root – This root has been used in China more than 2,000 years! It has impressive detoxifying properties, especially in the liver. This root also has antibiotic, anti-microbial, and anti-tumor properties. Although the original formula called for Indian Rhubarb Root, that particular variety typically can't be obtained in the USA without chemical contamination. Judging by our research, the Turkish variety works just fine.

The Essiac® formula is based on a tonic originally developed and used by Ojibwa Indians in Canada, who gave it to Rene Caisse, a nurse. This tonic is very special. Specific barks, roots, and leaves must be boiled, then **carefully simmered for at least 12 hours** in a special process. This is no simple "tea." No synthetic preservatives, flavorings, alcohol, glycerine, or other ingredients should be added.

Herbs grown in the United States are preferred because many imported herbs undergo fumigation (gassing) and "protective" radiation. These processes can virtually destroy the potency of the

8 *The Essiac Report*, page 80.

herbs. Be sure the brand you choose contains only organic herbs completely free of fumigation or irradiation.

The importance of growing methods

The most important point is to use no pesticides. Any of the following growing processes are acceptable*:*

1. "**Certified organic**" – These are cultivated crops grown without man-made chemicals. Many times, this certification is unavailable because certification is a complicated and costly governmental procedure and takes significant time for the approval process.
2. "**Organic**" – cultivated as above but without accreditation.
3. "**Wildcrafted**" – grown in the wild without man-made chemicals. Many feel this produces a heartier plant than a cultivated crop. We feel wildcrafted Sheep Sorrel is best – it is heartier and more nutrient-rich.
4. "**Commercially grown without pesticides.**"

Other important considerations

For maximum effectiveness, herbs should be natural and unadulterated – organically grown or wildcrafted – so the product's taste may vary slightly from batch to batch. For example, herbs grown in Washington state taste different from those grown in California. Sheep Sorrel's taste varies greatly from sweet to mellow depending on the growing area, and can even "deepen" and develop a smoother flavor after a few days in the refrigerator. Also, the amount and appearance of particulate may vary from bottle-to-bottle.

Herbs are light-sensitive, so amber-colored glass bottles should be used to retain maximum potency and value.

Distilled water is best for brewing this formula. Although it's more costly, distillation provides the purest water to maximize the power of the herbs. To adhere to any lower of a standard of purity would decrease effectiveness of this product. With today's high water-pollution levels, city tap water, bottled spring water, or even "purified" drinking water can often leave much to be desired for brewing Essiac®-concept tonic.

This tonic should be prepared with stainless steel vessels and instruments. Stainless steel, while much more costly than other metals, is the most sanitary and nonreactive. No harmful preservatives should be used. Preparation must be meticulous.

If you don't think a daily detoxifier is required, then read this:

Use of Antimicrobial Growth Promoters in Food Animals and *Enterococcus faecium* Resistance [Vancomycin resistance] to therapeutic Antimicrobial Drugs in Europe

"Supplemental animal feed with antimicrobial agents [added] to enhance growth has been common practice for more than 30 years. ... until recently, clear evidence of a health risk was not available. ... Finally, antimicrobial drugs should not be used for growth promotion if they are used in human therapeutoics."

Sources: *Emerging Infectious Diseases* 5(3), 1999.
Centers for Disease Control

***Life-Systems* Engineering Analysis:** Have you wondered why drug-resistant infections have become rampant? It isn't just because humans are taking antibiotics too frequently, it's because of antibiotics and growth hormones commonly used in animal feed. Radiant Health increases your immune system. Now you can understand why a *daily detoxifier* is so important.

In 1937, John Wolfer, M.D., director of the tumor clinic at Northwestern University Medical School, treated 30 terminal cancer patients at their clinic. At the end of a year of treatment, a panel of 5 physicians at Northwestern wrote, **"Essiac prolonged life, shrank tumors, and relieved pain."**[10]

Surprisingly, for all its possible positive benefits, we know of no negative side-effects reported over a 60-year period! Daily use apparently poses no known risks.

Many users have conducted their own personal tests – they stopped taking the tonic for a short time, only to find their physical condition returns to the "pre-tonic" state. The tonic functions as an optimizer and detoxifier – *it apparently has the unique ability to improve the efficiency of virtually all of the body's natural mechanisms.*

Remarkable skin smoothness and glow is reported by many of the formula's users. It works equally well on both men and women. The tonic works from the "inside-out" at the cellular level. This is in marked contrast to most creams, which may merely give the illusion of smoother skin. Just an ounce a day is all it takes to accomplish this result.

Warning: Unforseen damage to you and your environment.

"So many Europeans are using the cholesterol-lowering drug clofibrate and excreting it into domestic sewer lines, according to the Physicians Committee for Responsible Medicine (PCRM), that **detectable levels are being found throughout the entire North Sea,** which is awash in **50 to 100 TONS** of clofibrate annually. Clofibrate is a **cousin of the weed-killing herbicide** 2,4,D. PCRM. Researchers are similarly **concerned** about **estrogen supplements,** which are excreted in the urine and can change the sex characteristics of certain fish at **concentrations of just 20 parts per trillion – well below levels triggering governmental scrutiny."**[11]

10 *Recliaming Our Health*, John Robbins, H.J. Kramer, Inc., POB 1082, Triburon, CA, 1998, page 271.

11 *Natural Pharmacy*, Liebert Publishing, 2 Madison Avenue, Larchmont, NY, Vol. 3, No. 6, June 1999, page 4. (Ref: *Good Medicine,* Winter).

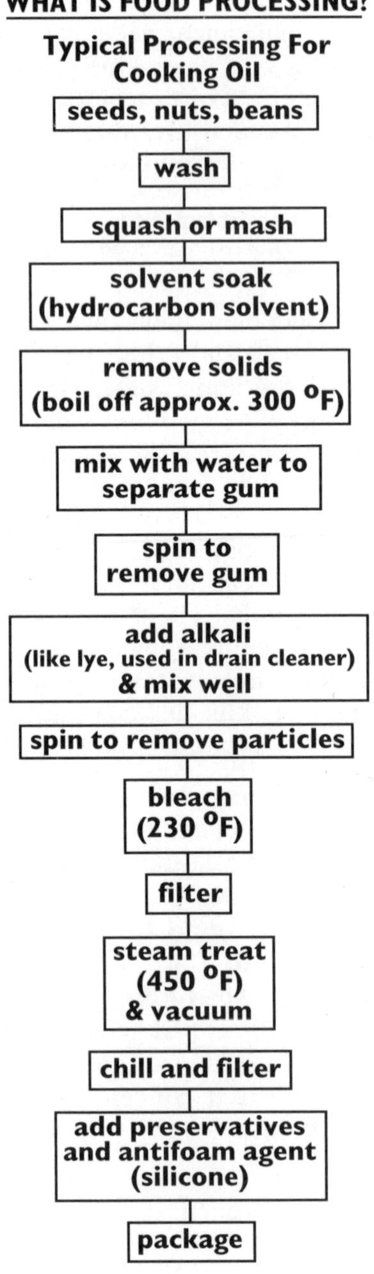
WHAT IS FOOD PROCESSING?
Typical Processing For Cooking Oil
seeds, nuts, beans
wash
squash or mash
solvent soak (hydrocarbon solvent)
remove solids (boil off approx. 300 °F)
mix with water to separate gum
spin to remove gum
add alkali (like lye, used in drain cleaner) & mix well
spin to remove particles
bleach (230 °F)
filter
steam treat (450 °F) & vacuum
chill and filter
add preservatives and antifoam agent (silicone)
package

Answers for Frequently Asked Questions

> *"... I believe there remains a general ignorance about how science 'is done....'"*
>
> James Watson – Nobel Prize-winner

Q: Will taking the Foundation of Radiant Health nutritional supplements help with any and every problem I may have?

A: The effects of the Foundation of Radiant Health are far-reaching. Many people are very surprised at the number and degree of improvements over and beyond the changes in appetite.

Q: What about the 40/30/30 carbohydrate, protein, fat diet I hear about? Is it any good?

A: The 40/30/30 diet program means getting 40-percent of calories from carbohydrate, 30-percent from fat, and 30-percent from protein. With the 40/30/30 diet, you must calculate numbers every time you eat. You learned that, structurally, we don't require any carbohydrate – our body makes glucose as long as it gets the essential nutrients it was designed to receive every day. Forty percent carbohydrate is certainly better than the 80-percent or 60-percent carbohydrate-based diets that have contributed to the epidemic in obesity and diabetes. **Nothing will take the place of solving a nutritional deficiency except eliminating the deficiency.** That's what the Foundation of Radiant Health does. Special diets are not needed.

Q: What other nutritional product would you recommend for use with basic essence?

A: An Essiac-concept detoxifying tonic is required for optimum health. We also need to supplement the nine minerals that are no longer in the soil in sufficient quantities for human nutrition. Taking a moderate vitamin supplement makes good *Life-Systems* Engineering sense. Some nutritional supplements have a long history of established effectiveness like co-enzyme Q10 and Ginkgo. What's most important is that you may find that the efficiency of many nutritional supplements increases with the addition of the Foundation of Radiant Health.

Q: How long must I wait to see results, especially the appetite reduction and cellulite reduction?

A: This depends on your personal condition. For many users, appetite reduction appears within 90 days. Others may find it takes longer, because they are so deficient and their body is more unbalanced.

A threshold level must be reached before improvements will be noticed. The hills-and-valleys of cellulite are often visibly reduced within 90 days and virtually disappear within one year. A good analogy is boiling water. We have to keep adding heat to the water until a critical level is reached. Only then do we notice steam and the water beginning to boil. Allow basic essence and the Foundation of Radiant Health program at least 90 days to start to work for you.

Q: How long will it take before I stop overeating?

A: That answer will depend on many of your personal *Life-Systems* factors. Many of us are eating too often out of habit. Such behavior will take time to change. The Foundation works on the physical, first. Then, with time, the psychological and emotional components often take care of themselves.

Q: Why could it take a while for the results to be seen? If we are so lacking in EFAs, shouldn't the results appear quickly?

A: Your body is very "smart." We postulate that, after years of deficiency, once a few EFAs arrive, your body doesn't immediately respond as if you'll keep getting EFAs continually. After a time, the body's "wisdom" signals the appestat that it can count on a continued supply. It doesn't count on this until after it gets the EFAs regularly for a period of time. Further, your body will only use a limited amount of any nutrient, regardless how much is taken. For example, if you have a deficiency of iron and take several times the RDAs of iron tablets, most of it will be eliminated, and it will still take significant time to correct the deficiency.

Q: I've noticed that my diastolic pressure (the second blood-pressure number) has gone down slightly after about 6 months of the Foundation of Radiant Health. Is this normal?

A: Yes. Basic essence makes your arteries more elastic. So, the diastolic (resting between beats) pressure may decrease a bit.

If your arteries were rigid like a straw, then your diastolic pressure would be almost equal to the higher systolic (the top number) pressure. The more flexible the arteries are, the lower the diastolic number will be. This is healthy. We want flexible arteries.

Q: I recently saw on *ABC News with Peter Jennings* that fiber (like bran) doesn't protect against colon cancer. Cancer protection was the #1 reason I ate so many carbohydrates during the past 10 years. The physicians interviewed **agreed they were wrong**, but they **still didn't change** their recommendations to eat lots of fiber (carbohydrates). The next day a newspaper article reported that the American Cancer Society says fiber "protects against 'other' cancers." Are they wrong, too? Also, will the "preventative breast removal theory" prove wrong 10 years from now? I'm outraged over the pattern of guesses by the nutrition community that are later shown to be wrong, and I may never believe another "recommendation" based on words like "some evidence," "possibly," "probably," "postulated," "believe," "likely," "tends," or "may help." Why do these mistakes keep happening?

A: Despite the best of intentions, recommendations to "eat plenty of fiber" from grains, fruits, and vegetables were not based on science. Rather, like the majority of "popular nutrition wisdom," this was based entirely on *mistaken opinion* (or flawed conclusions). I call it "fiber-fiction." The *New York Times* (January 21, 1999, page A1) reported: the **colon cancer rate *didn't* change**: ***regardless*** of type of fiber consumed, ***regardless of*** how much fatty meat or lean tofu was eaten, ***regardless*** of whether any exercise was performed, and ***regardless*** of smoking. In fact, those who ate the most vegetables got the most colon cancer! *Life-Systems* Engineers warned us of the diabetes epidemic and other diseases tied to eating excess carbohydrates for fiber. The article you referred to was on page 1 of *USA Today* (January 21, 1999). A *Life-Systems* Engineering analysis of this story and the Times leads us to 3 misleading points:

- The USA story quoted one expert who implied that, somehow, cereal provides better fiber than fiber from fruits and vegetables, or meat. He claimed that the 88,000 people in the study didn't eat enough cereal. This is *scientifically unfounded*. Fiber is fiber.

- The study's author stated: "Folic acid *probably* protects against colon cancer." If this were true, none of the fiber-eaters in the study would have gotten colon cancer, because they would have eaten leafy vegetables containing folic acid as part of their life-style diet. Some of the study's participants ate a whopping 25 grams of fiber per day — still no improvement! Therefore, this finding should have been challenged. "Probably" isn't good enough for science — certainly *not a sound basis* for recommendations.
- The author was also quoted as stating that a "high fiber diet clearly cuts heart disease risk." The study, according to these articles, does not support this recommendation. Ten years from now will we be told that this incorrect conclusion, too, was based on *mistaken opinion*?

  As you learned in *Beyond The Zone,* cause/effect relationships require rigorous testing to prove and can't be made so casually. Unfortunately, it appears that defenders of the great 20-year carbohydrate eating *experiment* will do anything to defend the *theory* that carbohydrates are wonderful, even when the facts soundly disprove it. Once again, you see that the **science** of *Life-Systems* Engineering was **right**, and virtually all the popular ***opinions*** were ***wrong***.

Q: I still find it almost unbelievable that so much of what we read and hear about nutrition is so wrong. Can you explain why this happens?

A: • In Chapter 1, I thank Professor William Siebert for **warning me that most of what is published is wrong**. This is nothing new.

• When Nobel Prize-winning physicist Richard Feynman was ready to publish his new mathematical theory, he found that it didn't agree with experimental results that were already published. He withdrew his theory from publication, but he later discovered that each publication had been ***blindly copied*** **from the same original experiment — which had been reported** ***incorrectly!*** (See pages 362-363.) Feynman's theory was consistent with the original data (not with the researchers' conclusions). Feynman went on to say that he would *never blindly accept* anyone else's results. He would *only rely on the original data*, then interpret it for himself.

- In section 43-5 of *The Feynman Lectures on Physics*, Feynman derives a complicated result and states that "… the arguments have a **subtlety** which can be **appreciated only** by a **careful and detailed** study. We shall make over the argument which led to the proper equation in a **reasonable** ***but erroneous*** way (and the [**incorrect**] way found in many textbooks!)." Feynman was proposing to show the audience how the correct argument could be distorted, or "made-over," into one that seems similar but is wrong. Even textbooks can have incorrect results. The reader must be able to analyze them.
- The distinguished biochemist Barry Sears writes in *The Anti-Aging Zone* how puzzled he is that, even after so many years, the majority of nutritionists and physicians still consider cholesterol and fat as the causes of heart disease, when the cause is so clearly tied to sugar (carbohydrates) and insulin.

  Many nutrition writers are guilty of blindly copying from one publication to another. They don't possess sufficient statistical background. Too often, nutrition researchers publish misinterpretations (half-truths) that mislead us. **Bad advice associated with credible sources gets transformed into "popular wisdom."** Mistakes are published in all scientific fields, but, after reading *Beyond The Zone*, you'll agree that no scientific field (psychology isn't included) has more inconsistencies than the "science" of nutrition. The nutrition field suffers from the same lack of critical analyses that Professor Feynman warns us against. To bring this critical analysis and accountability of results into nutrition is one of the main reasons the new field of *Life-Systems* Engineering was developed.

Q: You dispelled the myth of "increasing the metabolism" as the solution to burning more fat, because the body is <u>not</u> a heat engine, but a chemical engine. I now agree, the "heat engine" analogy is incorrect. Can you give me some insight why it is said that "fat burns in the flame of carbohydrate"? This implies that I need lots of carbohydrates to burn fat.

A: The statement is misleading. Acetyl CoA in the citric acid cycle requires oxaloacetate. Oxaloacetate *normally* comes from pyruvate (made from sugar). What you weren't told is that pyruvate also comes from amino acids (protein). See Stryer's *Biochemistry - 4th edition*, pages 612, 638.

Q: After so many years of *mis*information and *mis*leading advertising, is it possible to bring the truth about nutrition to most people?

A: No. Either they won't believe it, or they still defend their (incorrect) opinions. Whenever I get coffee, I tell the person in front of me "the truth" that "half & half" or cream is actually less fattening and healthier than milk — and it tastes better in their coffee, too. The reply is either, "I know," or "It probably is." What do they order? Coffee with nonfat milk. After 100s of times offering "the truth," I have yet to have just one of them ask me, "Why do you say that?" Yes, it is very frustrating, but if I can help just one more person to understand how their body really works, I am very pleased.

Q: Does the Foundation of Radiant Health help with hot flashes (during menopause)?

A: Yes.

Q: My appetite is greatly reduced since I started on the Foundation of Radiant Health, but I am often forced to eat late at night because I must work such long hours. Some say the digestion rate stays the same throughout the day; others say it decreases at night and that I shouldn't eat so late. Who is correct?

A: Virtually all bodily processes slow down in the evening. Lying down slows the digestive process. We could test a diabetic after he or she eats a late dinner at 11 PM compared with an early dinner at 7 PM. The blood sugar level measured at 7 AM the next morning is significantly lower after the early dinner. Late-night eating is not ideal, but processed carbohydrates late at night aggravate the situation, because that causes blood sugar levels to remain elevated while sleeping.

Q: I'm a woman, and I get slightly depressed once a month; will the Foundation of Radiant Health help?

A: PMS symptoms and related symptoms, including depression, are often reduced by a dramatic degree.

Q: The Essiac tonic discussed seems impressive. Is it as effective as the basic essence?

A: Yes, it is. The "tonic" works by minimizing the negative effects of food additives, pesticides, and so on. Basic essence *adds a positive* – "parent" EFAs. Their mechanisms are different, yet complementary. Both products together should be the foundation of your nutritional program, along with an amino acid-chelated mineral supplement.

Q: Can I still enjoy fast-foods, cakes and desserts?

A: Eat them if you still desire them. Over time, your desire for these "treats" should naturally decrease with basic essence and chelated minerals. An Essiac-concept tonic reduces the negative effects of food processing and food additives in such foods.

Q: Are you suggesting that I can eat all the fatty foods I desire and not suffer adverse effects? New studies say it's the harmful transfats we need to avoid; natural fats are fine.

A: Remember that animal fat may contain stored toxins and vegetable oils may contain pesticide residues. So, unless you are consuming a detoxifier, such as Essiac-concept tonic, you'll take in and accumulate more of these toxins. Basic essence supplies the proper levels of essential healthy oils. If the Foundation of Radiant Health is used, eating natural fat is fine. Just stay away from processed fats such as margarines, processed vegetable oils,[1] and fat "substitutes." The conclusion that natural fats, in and of themselves, aren't harmful, is based on known medical physiology. It was demonstrated a hundred years ago, and is simply being confirmed again. With the Foundation of Radiant Health, you can begin to trust your taste.

Q: It seems like more women than men are overweight. Is it because men have more muscle, so they have higher metabolisms and burn up the excess calories better?

A: Probably not. Higher metabolic activity drives us to eat more. There are numerous *Life-Systems* working cooperatively. When one thing changes, another corresponding change occurs. More muscle requires more food, so the difference may lie in the type of food men eat. The real reason for the difference may be that men aren't as diligent as women in doing what the consultants tell us. Men tend to eat more protein and natural fats than women, so they get a little more basic essence (EFAs) in their diets. Even

1 *Most commercial cooking oils are highly processed. Olive oil is an exception. Read the label.*

though low-fat and low-cholesterol diets are promoted widely, the number of steak restaurants has increased – and men order steaks more often than women do. Here's a case where it may not have paid not to listen to consultants and why the positive results in men (less obesity) were predictable.

Q: From a *Life-Systems* Engineering analysis, are you saying that all the cholesterol controversy is based on incorrect assumptions about cholesterol's role in the body? And to compound the misunderstanding, the "official" recommendations concerning cholesterol are probably based on studies of EFA-deficient people? I'm really sick and tired of advertisements claiming how good certain products (usually carbohydrates) with little cholesterol are for us.

A: You understand it well. Real-life results clearly show the fallacy of the cholesterol theory. More people than ever before eat lower cholesterol foods, yet cardiovascular disorders don't significantly decrease. Like Nobel Prize-winner Richard Feynman stated, When the results are not predicted from the theory, the theory is faulty!

Q: I have a disability, so I can't exercise much. I have gained 80 pounds over the past two years. Can I still lose this extra fat without much exercise?

A: The Foundation of Radiant Health automatically puts you in fat-burning mode, instead of fat-storing mode. You'll recall that, with the Foundation, we burn excess bodyfat three times faster than with higher carbohydrate diets. The normal exercise of just moving around is fine for most people. If you are unable to walk, the Peak Performer™, or hand weights is a good exercise aid for you and everyone who wants to maximize muscle with minimum effort.

Q: Will meditation and yoga, in addition to the Foundation of Radiant Health, help reduce stress and lower my blood-pressure?

A: Meditation, yoga, exercise, and so on are all beneficial to reduce the symptoms of stress. However, these techniques may take years of training to master or take significant time each day. Stress is external to us. The question may not be, "How do we reduce stress?" Rather, a better question is, "What is required of the body to effectively deal with stress?" A *Life-Systems* Engineering analysis shows a subtle, yet important, difference between the two questions. Nothing else will give your body the tools it needs to combat stress, at the cellular level, better than the nutrients in the Foundation of Radiant Health.

Q: Can't I have any carbohydrates?

A: Of course you can. What you must not do, though, is to make processed carbohydrates the foundation of your diet. Far too many people have. Look in the shopping cart of the person next to you at the checkout register next time you go shopping for groceries. The vast majority of grocery carts are overflowing with processed carbohydrates, to the exclusion of protein and natural fats. Look at the results of the people pushing those grocery carts. How much overweight are they?

Q: I used to take "regular" minerals, but I now understand that they aren't well utilized by the body. Many of them even compete with each other, so the efficiency is even less. Is there more information on this?

A: Yes. Minerals need to be properly chelated, that is, chemically linked to an amino acid. An excellent paper on minerals was issued by Albion Laboratories.[2]

Q: Don't I need carbohydrate drinks during my workout – especially during weight lifting?

A: No, you don't; and if bodyfat loss is important, then you certainly don't want carbohydrates before or after your workout.

Q: I've always been told I just needed to exercise more to lose my excess fat, but it never worked, no matter how much I exercised.

A: This is personal verification of the "exercise myth." Without the Foundation of Radiant Health nutrients, exercise doesn't always work as promised. This was thoroughly covered in the chapter, "Exercise: Why Sweat It?"

Q: Do I need lots of vigorous exercise to feel well?

A: No, you shouldn't. As we have seen, the Foundation of Radiant Health, along with moderate exercise offers excellent

2 *Albion Research Notes* — A Compilation of Vital Research Updates on Health Nutrition, Albion Laboratories, Clearfield, UT, Volume 6, No. 2, June 1997.

cardiovascular protection. Without basic essence and amino acid-chelated minerals the body's hunger and weight-control systems are "short-circuited," so vigorous exercise is often employed as an attempt to counteract the problems of fatigue, weight control, etc. Exercise is good for the body, but it can't make up for the real problem (lack of basic essence and minerals which your body was designed to run on). *Life-Systems* Engineering is in favor of exercise. But even if you don't have time for lots of exercise, the Foundation of Radiant Health is ideal for you.

Q: What you say about exercise makes so much sense. I tried the gym without carbohydrate-loading either before or after my workout. The difference in stamina and endurance was incredible! Less pain, less fatigue, and no extra sleep was required. Thanks ever-so-much. For years I was doing my workout very inefficiently. We need more *Life-Systems* Engineers.

A: You're welcome. Once we understand how the body is designed, it's simple to maximize its efficiency.

Q: Do we need to take extra calcium?

A: A *Life-Systems* Engineering analysis says calcium supplements are overrated. Many people take calcium to ward off osteoporosis, but osteoporosis is not caused by lack of calcium as we may have been led to believe. Whatever your reason for taking extra calcium, there are several factors involved in calcium absorption. Research shows that "the answer" isn't simply taking more and more calcium. It is in getting the most out of the calcium that is available from the food we eat! Basic essence is used by the body to make vitamin D – which increases calcium absorption, naturally. And, without other minerals that your body needs, calcium absorption is further reduced. Calcium takes up the bulk of many mineral supplements, so there isn't room in the capsule for other important minerals. This is a case of manufacturers giving the customer what they want instead of what they need.

Q: Why are there so many nutritional supplements, and why do some products have 10-50 ingredients?

A: Good question. Many nutritional supplements offer little documented effectiveness. Many supplements can't produce maximum effects if you still have a deficiency of basic essence and minerals. It is interesting that so many products include so many ingredients. If a manufacturer doesn't know what is really significant, then all they can do is to add multiple ingredients in the hope that something in the mixture works. This approach partly comes from incomplete knowledge on the part of nutritional manufacturers. But in fairness, they are supplying what the customer expects. A manufacturer may not think an ingredient is significant, yet, if it becomes a "buzz word" like chromium picolinate has become, manufacturers are pressured to add it to satisfy what the customer thinks is important.

Q: If I take basic essence, an Essiac-concept tonic, and minerals, can I still become ill?

A: Yes. Remember that our body is a very special type of "machine." If you abuse yourself consistently over a significant period of time, you will pay a price. Most people who get the common colds and flu, even while taking the Foundation of Radiant Health, find that the severity is minimized. Personally, one time at the end of a two-year period, working virtually seven days a week, I got a "head cold" (congestion). In the past, I would be so congested that I couldn't think well, and I would have required several days of bed rest. This time, there was no impairment, just a little discomfort. For most people to achieve maximum immune functioning, a year of consistent use is required.

Q: I have been using the Foundation of Radiant Health for about three months and have found that my taste for "fast-food" is decreasing. What I really liked before, I now find bland and almost tasteless. How can this be?

A: This is a common occurrence. It happened to all of our team members, too. Most "fast-food" is devoid of many nutrients other than some protein. Highly processed foods, which most fast-food restaurants serve, are short on nutritional benefit but give you a big dose of detrimental effects ... excessive processed carbohydrates from sodas, potatoes, breads, etc., and adulterated EFAs from deep-frying foods. It's amazing how hunger lets us know what is best for us, when the mechanism isn't "short-circuited."

Q: Do you see basic essence and the Foundation of Radiant Health program eliminating the new wave of appetite-suppressing drugs?

A: Yes, it has the potential to make them obsolete.

Q: When we take diet drugs, aren't we on them "for life"? I mean that, once you start taking them, you'll gain all the weight back?

A: Yes. These drugs only work while they are used. It is no natural "solution" because it only addresses the symptoms of the food cravings. They don't naturally satisfy the food cravings. That's a basic difference between "drugs" and "nutritional supplements."

Q: Now that I'm on the Foundation of Radiant Health, I notice that, during cold weather, my hands don't become dry or chap easily, the fine lines under my eyes are gone, and I heal much quicker than I used to. Are these indications that I was EFA-deficient?

A: Yes. In time, the Foundation of Radiant Health helps to improve all these conditions.

Q: I've only been on the "Foundation" a short time, yet my taste seems more keen. Most foods taste better. Does this make sense?

A: Yes, it does. The sense of taste dramatically improves, yet you eat less. Less food with better taste! What more could one ask for?

Q: My appetite has decreased so much that I now only desire to eat once a day, maybe twice. I've heard this will slow down my metabolism. Is it true?

A: No. If you aren't hungry, there is no reason to eat. Look at people who eat frequently and are severely overweight. How has "increased metabolism" from eating all the time helped them? "Increased metabolism" is a "buzz" phrase used to appeal to EFA-deficient people who constantly crave food. Some infomercials on television recommend eating four-six times a day. From a *Life-Systems* Engineering analysis, eating this often is extremely detrimental and may lead to diabetes. Our team usually eats just once or twice a day, too, and we rarely lack abundant energy or experience "sugar lows."

With EFA-deficiency, you are completely at the mercy of food; you are driven to eat all the time. The Foundation of Radiant Health gives you the dietary control that should be yours naturally. A drive to eat so frequently indicates an EFA-deficiency.

Q: This book destroys much of what has been considered "popular wisdom" and "truths" in the media. I thought I knew a lot, but after reading this, it seems like everything I "knew" was incorrect. Am I the last to get the news about the Foundation of Radiant Health?

A: Don't feel bad. There are few true experts on nutrition, since all the studies have been done with EFA-deficient (and mineral-deficient) people. Look at where we have been led. We are sicker and more overweight than ever. An entirely new approach is needed. *Life-Systems* Engineering is concerned with what works, is verified by real-life results and has a firm scientific and medical basis – not what just sounds good.

Q: Can I expect to lose more weight? or more inches?

A: Probably more inches. The Foundation of Radiant Health nutritional supplements accelerate fat loss, yet spare important muscle. Eliminating three pounds of fat is much more rewarding than dropping one pound of fat and two pounds of muscle. You'll look better, too. Many previous diet plans and programs had resulted in losing water and important muscle, giving the illusion of losing excess fat. With the Foundation, it may take a bit longer, but you lose only excess bodyfat and it won't easily come back.

Q: Instead of smoking one-and-a-half packs of cigarettes a day, I'm only smoking half a pack. Is this an unexpected benefit of the Foundation of Radiant Health?

A: Yes. Many smokers find that their habit declines over time with the Foundation of Radiant Health.

Q: Is it beneficial to take "fat absorbers" or "fat blockers" so the fat in my food won't get absorbed?

A: From a *Life-Systems* Engineering analysis, we don't find these products working as advertised. Tampering with your digestive process is ill-advised. Anyway, eating unadulterated (natural) fats and healthy essential oils won't make you fat.

Q: What do you think about "food-combining?" That is, eating acidic foods at one sitting and alkaline foods at another?

A: Here's a good example of something that sounds good, yet medical science doesn't support it. Even if you ate lots of alkaline foods (the opposite extreme of your acidic stomach), it won't significantly affect the pH of the stomach because the stomach is so highly acidic.[3]

Q: What foods are good sources of the HDL cholesterol?

A: None – that's why no foods have it listed on their labels. *This is a term referring only to the transport mechanism of cholesterol out of the cell.* **It's all the same cholesterol!**

Q: Will taking the Foundation of Radiant Health make you live longer? That is, is it good for life extension?

A: We are not concerned with this. A *Life-Systems* Engineer is concerned with: optimizing the system so you have the energy, as you were meant to have, so you are lean for life and resistant to disease. These outcomes contribute to a better quality of life. You may live longer, too, but a longer lifetime is still a secondary concern, when compared with the quality of that lifetime.

Q: I'm diabetic and have been told that oils are bad for me. Does this mean that I can't use basic essence and the Foundation of Radiant Health?

A: No. Basic essence is a balanced blend of healthy essential oils – required for life. On the contrary, it is one of the best nutritional supplements if you are diabetic or want to prevent diabetes. EFAs and minerals help the body regulate insulin.

Q: Please explain again how the body uses insulin to stimulate the conversion of excess glucose to bodyfat.

A: It's like sweeping the dust under the rug when you're in a rush to make the house look nice. (Of course, in the body, it doesn't make you look better, if anything fatter, but it keeps you alive as opposed to getting poisoned by excess sugar.)

Q: I believe that anything in moderation is OK. Why do I need to restrict processed carbohydrates?

A: First, with the Foundation of Radiant Health, there is no need to "restrict" any food. As your EFA deficiency decreases, you will

3 The pH of stomach acid is about 1.0. (Greater than a million times more acidic than water.) Acid foods are in the range of 3.0 to 6.0. "Neutral" is 7.0. Alkaline foods are above 8.0. A difference in pH of 1.0 is a factor of 10 in strength. So the stomach acid pH of 1.0 is 100 times stronger than the most acidic food (at 3.0)! Therefore, The effect of food-combining on pH and digestion is insignificant. One may even say, eating highly alkaline foods could impede digestion.

tend to desire less processed carbohydrates. The body doesn't need them, so it shouldn't crave them. Second, moderation is not always OK! How beneficial is a bit of arsenic, a tad of cyanide, or a small dose of radiation? Even in extremely small amounts, these are poisons. (Even though they could even be considered "natural"!) The lesson: some nutrients are much more significant (useful or harmful) than others.

Q: Even after reading your book, I feel that processed carbohydrates are good. I believe moderation is the key. I'll just force myself to eat less of them and I won't be overweight.

A: But you'll always be hungry! Once you start taking basic essence and the Foundation of Radiant Health, you won't want to eat so many processed carbohydrates. That is the evidence that your body's taste and hunger finally work together naturally – once the EFA-deficiency is eliminated. You said it yourself: "I'll force myself to eat less of them." With the Foundation, no self-imposed ideas about knowing what is best for your body are required. Your body was made to work correctly – automatically – and it does, with the Foundation of Radiant Health.

Q: Some "diet" doctors have told me that essential healthy oils (EFAs) won't help control weight. How do you respond to this?

A: The director of a major university hospital's obesity clinic told me the same thing. He gave his patients fish oil, a source of mainly omega 3 derivatives (not enough "parents") and it didn't work. I figured out why he might have believed that EFAs don't help with appetite fulfillment and weight control. Most physicians have limited training in nutrition, so it's understandable that many wouldn't know that a balanced blend of parent EFAs is required. Many people think that flax oil or fish oil for omega 3 is all that's needed. It has been assumed we get plenty of omega 6 from our diet. We do get an abundance of it, but the omega 6 in our diet is too adulterated to be useful. Just taking unadulterated omega 3 oils isn't enough. A wrong assumption was made which led to incorrect conclusions. Remember, this book is dedicated to providing the very best nutrition information to physicians.

Q: Experts are now saying to exercise vigorously every day. What do you think about this?

A: A *Life-Systems* Engineering analysis concludes that these people are missing an important point. Rest is required for recuperation. Physical stress is one part of the process, but constant physical exercise without proper resting isn't very beneficial. Professional bodybuilders told me that over-training (exercising without proper rest) was a significant reason for lack of progress in building muscle. With vigorous exercise every day, the body often doesn't get the rest it needs

Q: The Foundation of Radiant Health supplements have eliminated my physical cravings, but I still enjoy eating while watching television. I'm not hungry – it's just a habit. What do you suggest?

A: Many of my clients do this: Eat mixed nuts in their shells. Get a nutcracker and crack them as you eat. While the nut is in the shell, the EFAs are protected. The carbohydrate content of most nuts in their shells is low, so you won't become sluggish eating them.

Q: Is the so-called "sugar-high" really a "high"?

A: No, it is not, although too many of us think that it is. When we eat excess processed carbohydrates, the body desperately tries to remove this excess glucose (sugar). Several *Life-Systems* are called on to work extra hard. The body's reaction is not too much different than if you ate poison. Would you call that sick, sweaty feeling a "high"?

Q: Is the Foundation of Radiant Health good for my children?

A: It's exceptional! Because your children's desire for processed carbohydrates (sodas and so on) will, over time, decrease, they won't be plagued by the "sugar-highs" and corresponding "sugar-lows" all day long. The "high" and "lows" lead to lack of attention and focus during school. This reaction to processed carbohydrates can make learning very difficult. Also, serotonin is released in the brain when carbohydrates are eaten. This tends to make us drowsy and tired. How can a child learn when he or she is not alert? Because the Foundation eliminates cravings for processed carbohydrates, your children will get a double advantage: sharp attention and no "sugar-lows." You won't have to worry so much about them becoming overweight, either.

Q: ADD, or Attention Deficit Disorder, is running out of control! My child has been diagnosed, along with about a fourth of the children of the parents I am friendly with. Will the Foundation of Radiant Health help with this disorder?

A: Better than just help. It sometimes stops the disorder in its tracks – reducing or even eliminating the symptoms – sometimes within just 60-90 days.

Q: How can I tell if a nutritional supplement is really working?

A: If you aren't certain, then after using any nutritional supplement faithfully for at least 3 months, stop taking it. If you don't see or feel a difference within just a month, it may not be doing you much good. If you are taking multiple products, stop taking them one-at-a-time and see if you feel or look as well without them. For *Life-Systems* Engineers, this is a true test of effectiveness. If you only "think" and aren't positive that a particular product is beneficial, you are probably wasting your money. Vitamins, minerals, and EFAs are essential. You don't want to be short on these.

Q: Will taking more of the Foundation make it work faster?

A: Nutritional supplements often have suggested amounts based on bodyweight. If you weigh more than average, then it is usually appropriate to take proportionately more. In the body, only a certain amount of any nutrient will be utilized regardless of how much is taken. We suggest staying with the suggested amounts of Essiac-concept tonic as per the manufacturer's label, because accelerating the detoxification process could cause temporary discomforting effects. It's best to take a little longer and keep your *Life-Systems* in balance. A *Life-Systems* Engineering analysis says to be conservative. It may take a few extra weeks, but the Foundation works, because it's based on what the body needs.

Q: Isn't it too simplistic to look at just the caloric content of fats, carbohydrates, and proteins to see how many calories each contains?

A: Yes. By asking this question you have shown that you have the makings of a *Life-Systems* Engineer. It takes a certain amount of energy to break down food into its basic components. Short- and medium-chain fats, such as butter and MCT oils, are used solely as fuel. The basic essence/EFAs in natural essential healthy oils are used throughout the body. Hormone and prostaglandin regulators are made from them, and all cell membranes contain them. Proteins are broken into amino acids. Amino acids are then utilized to make enzymes, muscle, bone and other structures. Carbohydrates (sugars) don't contribute directly to anything except excess bodyfat, once the small glycogen reserves are full. Dietary carbohydrates (glucose) aren't needed for structure or important *Life-Systems* functions – your body can make glucose as needed from fats and proteins.[4] Simply comparing the amount of energy (calories) required to oxidize (break down) these substances is much too simplistic, yet it is often the only measure we hear about. This oversimplification is part of what led to the obesity epidemic in the U.S.

Q: When I went to an organic supermarket for the first time, I was amazed to find so many of the shoppers so overweight. Many of the sales help were also overweight. They didn't look healthy, either. Is there some hidden problem with "organic eating"?

A: No, that's not the problem. You have personally verified that EFA- and mineral-deficiency isn't corrected by so-called "healthy eating." I see the same obesity levels with the customers in Houston, too. Look at their shopping carts – they are typically filled with processed carbohydrates! From a *Life-Systems* Engineering analysis, only the Foundation of Radiant Health can solve our nutritional problems and reduce our cravings for processed carbohydrates, which contribute to obesity.

Q: Should I take "digestive enzymes" to get more value out of the food that I eat?

A: Unless a physician diagnoses that you have a digestive disorder, you could be wasting your money. Your body doesn't require "assistance." Enzymes will be active while in the mouth, but once they enter the stomach, they are all destroyed. Acids in your stomach break down virtually everything into basic components. Enzymes are broken down into amino acids – the building blocks of proteins. Your body produces its own enzymes from proteins. That's another reason why sufficient protein intake is important.

---

4 Although glucose plays a major role in living systems, it isn't used for structure the way natural fats and proteins are. There is little glucose in the blood. ATP (cellular energy) is generated from fatty acids, carbohydrates, and proteins. The brain uses glucose in the blood, but don't get misled into how much glucose we need. It's very little!

Q: I'm a woman in my 30's. After two weeks of taking the Foundation of Radiant Health, I noticed my appetite had decreased, especially for processed carbohydrates. I lost six pounds, and my sex drive improved. These are all positive. The funny thing is that I'm more aggressive now. Why is that?

A: What seems like more aggression may simply be more energy. You'll soon get used to this new level of vigor. Too many of us are run-down. Once we have the energy we were meant to possess, we need an outlet for it. By the way, basic essence doesn't contain hormones; it is the building block of many hormones.

Q: I am on medication prescribed by my doctor. Can I still take the Foundation of Radiant Health, and will the drug's effects be compromised?

A: The Foundation of Radiant Health is not a drug, so drug interactions do not apply, but show this book to your physician. Often drug dosages can be reduced. You can both make an informed decision, together.

Q: It seems to me that blaming cholesterol (that is, oxidized cholesterol) as the cause of cardiovascular problems is like saying: don't eat meat, because if you eat meat that has already spoiled, it will make you sick. Isn't this naive?

A: Good analogy. You are absolutely correct. The important question to answer is what caused the cholesterol to oxidize and cause problems.

Q: I know that the diet drug combination, *Phen-Fen*, was forced off the market by the FDA because of side-effects. Won't this impact the entire diet-drug industry, because everyone will be fearful of drug-induced side-effects that we aren't told about up front?

A: With the Foundation of Radiant Health, for a tremendous number of people, there is no longer a need for diet drugs.

Q: Now and then, before I started taking the Foundation, I would indulge myself on the weekend by drinking moderate amounts of alcohol. I would always get a hangover. Now, I rarely get hangovers. Why?

A: We often hear of a client's happiness about this benefit. Simply put, when your body works like the high-performance human machine it's supposed to be, its threshold for all abuse is elevated considerably. It's the same reason that, with a strengthened immune system, your frequency of becoming ill from a cold or flu decreases, too. Just remember, even the Foundation of Radiant Health can't entirely protect you against yourself.

Q: I moved 2 rooms of furniture and the next day I wasn't sore at all! I don't exercise, so I wouldn't consider myself in good physical shape. I'm amazed, because I thought I'd have to stay home from work, in bed, due to fatigue and muscle soreness. What's going on here?

A: The Foundation of Radiant Health gives the body the nutrients it is designed to run on. Now you see, first-hand, why I say we are meant to function like a high-performance Ferrari automobile, instead of the broken-down jalopy many of us feel like most of the time. We're running on the wrong fuel. Mother Nature designed us to have radiant health always. It's truly wonderful.

Q: I see lots of workers outdoors drinking sodas, eating snack cakes, chips, and all the processed carbohydrates that make you fat, yet most of these guys are relatively slim. Why?

A: They are using their muscles most of the day. As you'll recall, muscles use glucose, so people exercising a lot may eat more processed carbohydrates than the rest of us and not get fat. But they are creating problems for themselves in the future, because they continue eating processed carbohydrates. Most of us do not perform this level of physical work; we are at a desk, driving, or sitting in front of a computer. This is called "sedentary" or "sitting" work. These are the people who really need to understand how food affects us.

Q: The information you present is so complete and so well researched that it's undeniable. I still can't understand why even people with degrees in nutrition fail to understand how the body really works, so they unknowingly advise us incorrectly. Can you explain this?

A: For one thing, many nutrition books are written by people, including those with advanced degrees (even Ph.D.s), who don't understand probability and statistics well enough to correctly interpret cause-effect relationships. But they draw conclusions anyway and despite the best of intentions, may unknowingly mislead us! The STAT-SMART chapter explains how this happens so frequently. Many times, researchers and authors repeat the same information even though it may be incorrect. This is why, sometimes, what we often read and hear about a certain nutrient or nutrition subject can be WRONG. Nobel Prize-winner Richard Feynman missed publishing an important result because he relied on published information from multiple sources that was wrong. He later learned that each author copied the same incorrect source. Also, virtually no life science field asks this fundamental question: Given that a trim person has approximately 30 days' worth of stored energy in bodyfat (obese people have 60-90 days' worth), why are so many of us hungry all the time? It makes no sense. No other animal eats as frequently as we do, unless it serves another purpose. *Life-Systems* Engineering was instituted to answer such questions – a new science had to be developed – and what we uncovered was truly amazing!

Q: What do you think of the oyster shell and other "shell" nutritional supplements which supposedly cause weight loss?

A: Would you naturally eat egg or oyster shells? Our team of *Life-Systems* Engineers consider this brilliant marketing – selling a waste product from fisheries and processing plants – to unknowing consumers. Nutritionally, it makes no sense. If you wouldn't eat something as a whole food, be cautious of claims that, when it is ground up, it is OK. You wouldn't naturally eat the rind of most fruits, either, yet millions of dollars are made selling juicers. While eating an orange, even a parrot is smart enough to discard the rind and just eat the fruit. When it comes to proper nutrition, animals often appear to have more sense than humans do. Now you know better.

Q: I've lost several inches in my hips, but I've noticed my breasts seem larger. I'm delighted, but how can this be?

A: Many women are happily surprised by this effect. Your body can now produce the hormones it wanted to, but couldn't because it didn't have the raw materials. Also, *breast tissue (mostly fat) is intended to have lots of EFAs*. **With the deficiency corrected, the tissue grows.**

Q: Is coenzyme Q_{10} effective?

A: Our experience shows, that, YES, it's very effective. It is used in every cell as part of the energy production cycle (ATP in the cell's mitochondria).* Our team's personal experience shows that with the Foundation of Radiant Health, many nutritional supplements can work better.

Q: Isn't the increase in health problems directly related to more stress in today's lifestyle?

A: Settlers in the American West often died on the journey. Food distribution was poor, and medical care was marginal. Flu epidemics and disease were common killers, especially in big cities. Before cars were commonplace, you'd have to walk or ride many hours just to get to a meeting. Families would have to wake before dawn each day and not retire until late. In the early 1900s there was a good chance you wouldn't live out the day. More stress today? Our *Life-Systems* team doesn't accept that. You may feel more stressed because of the nutritional deficiencies and being exposed to more chemicals and pollution. The Foundation of Radiant Health relieves many stress-related problems. John Robinson, director of the Americans' Use of Time Project at the University of Maryland, confirms that Americans work 7-8 fewer hours per week now than in 1965! We have more leisure time, but our malnutrition negates many of the benefits.

Q: I've noticed that taking the nutritional products described as the Foundation of Radiant Health stopped my hot flashes, completely changed my eating tastes, and "calmed me down," yet I had tremendous energy. Is all this in my head?

A: No. It's not in your head and it's not a placebo effect. Our *Life-Systems* Engineering team has consistently observed the improvements in health, energy, and appearance that are experienced on the Foundation.

Q: Before starting the Foundation of Radiant Health, I would get headaches all the time. Now I hardly ever get them. Is this a coincidence?

A: No, it is not. I have a friend who routinely suffered migraine headaches. They were impacting the quality of his performance at work. Since he has started the Foundation of Radiant Health, the headaches rarely occur anymore. When you study the physiology of the body, and how the Foundation of Radiant Health nutrients positively feed it, this result is predicted.

* CoQ_{10} is derived from cholesterol. So if you have too little cholesterol, you may be short on CoQ_{10}. *Basic Medical Biochemistry*, page 51.

Q: Why is forced control required for good health? You know – we're told that everything that tastes bad, like raw broccoli, which I don't have a taste for unless there's plenty of dip with it, is particularly good for us, and food that tastes good, like steak, is particularly bad for us?

A: You've been misled. We are used to overriding our body by doing what we have been told for years – for example: we "must" eat three to six times a day; all fats, including natural fats and essential oils are "bad"; "too much protein" is unhealthy and so on. Once the Foundation of Radiant Health is implemented, your body will tell your appetite what it needs. There is no more excuse for artificially overriding the mechanisms of automatic *Life-Systems*. This is exactly the opposite of what we are used to hearing.

Q: When I go to the bathroom, I notice elimination is softer and easier than before. Is this OK?

A: Yes. Your entire digestive system becomes lubricated with the Slippery Elm Bark (in the Essiac-concept tonic), which acts like the body's natural non-stick coating, so there is less obstruction. This is the way you were meant to eliminate.

Q: What routine blood tests do you recommend?

A: I'm not a physician, but here's what I did: **1**. A *cholesterol and triglyceride (lipids) profile* prior to starting the Foundation of Radiant Health program will let you monitor your progress objectively. **2**. A *glycohemoglobin test* will show your average blood glucose levels over the past 90 days. If the number is too high, you are on your way to diabetes, so this is extremely important! Your physician can evaluate the triglyceride and glycohemoglobin readings. **3**. There is a huge increase in thyroid problems from toxic chemicals in our environment. So, once every year or two you might want to request a TSH (thyroid stimulating hormone) test from your physician. If your thyroid is damaged, there are safe, inexpensive synthetic hormones to assist it. An impaired thyroid affects all body systems and may raise your cholesterol levels, too. Unless you have a known impairment, these are my personal recommendations for the average person. Consult with your physician if you have any questions – your physician can order the appropriate tests.

Q: You mention the hidden carbohydrates in soft drinks and candy bars. Would you explain a bit more?

A: Occasionally, my office gets calls from people who aren't achieving significant fat loss. Our staff reasons that there must be hidden processed carbohydrates in what these callers are eating; they just aren't aware of it. Remember that we are all the same basic human machines – carbohydrates always go to fat, once the small glycogen reserves are filled. Most soft drinks contain more than 100 calories of processed carbohydrate (five teaspoons of sugar). Orange soda contains a surprising 220 calories of processed carbohydrate (11 teaspoons of sugar). Candy bars can easily contain 100 calories (five teaspoons of sugar) or more of processed carbohydrate. Just a few cans of soda and one candy bar a day, in addition to the carbohydrates contained in real food, can completely prevent you from burning any excess bodyfat. Humans don't require any processed carbohydrate and very little natural carbohydrate. The most common cause of not losing excess bodyfat is: EFA-deficiency and mineral-deficiency driving you to consume too many processed carbohydrates.

Q: I'm a 30-year-old man. *People* magazine (September 1997) had a disturbing cover story. It was another of the "it's OK to be fat" articles. What was disturbing was that, among the significantly obese women the editors placed a photograph of Jayne Mansfield. Ms. Mansfield had beautiful hips and was never skinny, but to place her amidst those grossly overweight women just wasn't right. The article also said that Marilyn Monroe was a size 16. This can't be true, because I recently saw an old movie of her. It seems magazines are distorting the facts to persuade us that obesity is OK. I'm sorry, call me chauvinistic, but women just shouldn't look like *sumo wrestlers*. Making excuses and even distorting the truth to justify this position is wrong. What has happened to America?

A: Your attitude proves that, without correcting the nutritional deficiencies we have spoken about, the situation is hopeless; and hopelessness is what overweight people feel. Eat the diet used to fatten a cow (grain and grass) and you will achieve the same result. It really is that simple, and that's exactly what has happened. Ranchers fatten animals by giving them grain, and without even seeing the article, I would wager that every woman in that article bases her diet on bagels, cereals, fruits, spaghetti, potatoes, rice, juice, and so on – mostly carbohydrate. The advertising has led them astray. No-fat, processed-carbohydrate foods may sound good, but biologically (and as you can see by the real-life results) they go to fat and keep you fat. My heart goes out to these misled people. The Foundation of Radiant Health nutrients are our only hope to reverse this obesity epidemic – but it does take a new understanding that many people resist.

Q: Why do carbohydrates bloat me, but fats, natural oils and proteins don't? I notice that I feel ready to "blow up," but I am very thirsty and need to drink many glasses of water after a spaghetti dinner but not with a steak dinner. Why?

A: Carbohydrates are water-soluble. They soak up all your fluid – like a sponge – driving you to drink extra water. Processed carbohydrates are, by far, the worst ones. Protein and natural fats don't do that.

Q: I suffer from allergies. Will the Foundation of Radiant Health help me?

A: Essiac-concept tonic plus Cat's Claw gives the best symptomatic relief of allergies compared with anything our team has reviewed or tried. It's in a league of its own, and it's all-natural! I can verify this, personally, because I had suffered greatly from allergies for many years.

Q: Don't Italians eat lots of pasta, and aren't they thin?

A: No, they don't eat lots of pasta; they typically eat just a small portion. Japanese, in their homeland, typically eat small portions of rice. Inaccurate "popular" knowledge is coming at us all the time and is causing great damage worldwide.

Q: The September 7, 1997, issue of *Parade* magazine featured a cover story, "How Healthy Are We?" I was shocked to find that two-thirds of the 1,752 Americans surveyed say they are in "excellent" or "good" health.

A: People often suffer delusions. If we aren't deathly ill, right now, we probably say that we are in fine health. Review the "healthy eating" test in Chapter 1 to see if you have radiant health. If you don't, it's now easy to get on the correct path.

Q: St. John's Wort has received a lot of press about its antidepressant properties. Lipoic acid has become popular, too. Would you comment on these supplements?

A: There always seems to be a new "supplement of the month." Melatonin and DHEA went through the rise/fall cycle, too. Certain nutritional supplements receive a lot of press, people purchase the products in record numbers, then sales fall off sharply as people discover that the supplement may not work as promised. Basic essence is the building block of many hormones and prostaglandins, so with basic essence entering the diet, you may not be as depressed anymore. Lipoic acid is an EFA-derivative. With basic essence, your body should generate its own lipoic acid as it needs it.

Q: Because I eat much less, I now have more personal free-time. I shop less often and spend less time cooking and cleaning up the dishes. I now only eat one main meal a day, at about six PM, and have one small snack of some nuts or cheese during the day. I don't get my previous daily sugar-low after eating each meal, so productivity at work has increased, too. I calculate a productivity increase of two hours a day. You need to mention these two important points – significant savings from decreased food costs, and increased free personal time.

A: I'm delighted that you personally discovered this. Cost and productivity savings are thoroughly described in Chapter 13.

Q: I've heard about successes of certain low-fat, high-carbohydrate eating programs. How do you explain these?

A: Success as measured over what time-frame? Recall the *Life-Systems* Engineering principle: There is a fundamental difference between reducing less harmful "negatives" compared with the benefit of adding healthy "positives." When you stop eating harmful transfatty acids, harmful pesticides and steroid residues from non-organic meat, the body responds positively. For example, the body's cholesterol levels adjust to the new conditions, but we have seen that cholesterol lowering, in and of itself, means little. With high carbohydrate diets, often cholesterol levels may temporarily decrease, but the more important and unhealthy triglycerides increase. It takes some time for the harmful effects of high carbohydrates and lack of healthy essential oils to manifest themselves. The long-term results of these programs have raised serious questions. Ann Louise Gittleman – former Director of Nutrition at the Pritikin Center, resigned, in part because of the program's shortcomings – especially in long-term clients.[5]

Q: Vitamin E "studies" keep popping up stating that increased doses of vitamin E "reduce the risk" of heart disease by half or more. I thought vitamin E is simply the "protector for EFAs." Please explain.

A: Correct. Vitamin E is used to protect the precious EFAs. If vitamin E worked as well as these studies may suggest, then few people should be suffering cardiovascular disorders, because so many of us already take mega-doses of vitamin E – just ask your local health store what the best-selling vitamins are? Read the STAT-SMART chapter so you won't be misled by miraculous sounding "studies." Vitamin E is important, but you may be better off taking moderate amounts of vitamin E along with the Foundation of Radiant Health than mega-doses of vitamin E alone.

Q: I added up all the decreases in heart-attack risk by numerous studies. If I did all the various things the studies suggest, the risk is cut by more than 100%. How can this be?

A: It can't. In the STAT–SMART chapter, you will learn that most studies incorrectly summarize their results by disregarding sample sizes. Two per 1,000 compared with one per 1,000 is not a fifty-percent increase. *It is a tenth of one-percent increase.* (0.2%– 0.1% = 0.1%)

Q: How much will the Foundation of Radiant Health performance benefits decrease if I consciously overload on processed carbohydrates?

A: You will continue to enjoy many of the health-related results, such as increased oxygen transfer for more energy, greater immunity, smoother skin, harder nails, and so on. However, you won't lose excess bodyfat or lose the carbohydrate "sugar-lows." Always remember: carbohydrates make you fat! Just two sodas a day change your body from fat-burning mode to fat-gaining mode.

5 *Beyond Pritikin*, page 23.

Q: How do you handle Chinese, Italian, and Mexican restaurants? They keep loading us up on rice, noodles, bread, beans and chips?

A: Don't eat those high carbohydrate items. At Italian restaurants, eat only a half-piece of garlic bread. When ordering the spaghetti and sausage, for example, have them hold the spaghetti. It may sound strange at first, but you will enjoy it more and cut out the carbs. At Chinese restaurants, have them hold the rice. Often they will substitute extra vegetables if you ask. Most restaurants will accommodate any reasonable request – though they may charge a bit more for the substitution. That's because rice and bread cost next to nothing, and vegetables are more expensive. While the chips in Mexican restaurants support a taste addiction for many of us, you can start by having them hold the rice and beans when you order a dinner. Try substituting cheese or guacamole. If you can't resist those high-carbohydrate items, avoid the temptation, initially, by avoiding those restaurants. Eventually, the Foundation of Radiant Health should reduce your cravings, so that you can return to those places with comfort and confidence.

Q: What supplements are best to take while traveling?

A: We find the Essiac-concept detoxifier is particularly important while traveling. Minimizing the negatives from crowded conditions and poor air quality in planes, the stress of a new climate, etc. are the initial stress factors that can lead to sickness. If you are taking a trip, make sure you take the Foundation of Radiant Health supplements – especially the tonic. (A properly formulated essiac-concept tonic, such as produced by Maximum Efficiency Products, can keep, with the cap on the bottle up to five days, if not overly heated.)

Q: If EFAs are so important, why do I keep hearing that polyunsaturated oils are so bad?

A: Most oils used in "clinical studies" are highly processed. We have already seen how important these healthy oils are to humans. The problem with these oils must lie in their processing. This is another case of not seeing the forest for the trees, and blaming the oil – instead of the true culprit – the processing!

Q: You raised an important issue in the mind-body connection section. By overloading on processed carbohydrates and keeping our sugar levels high, won't the body stay in a perpetual "fight or flight" mode? After years of this physical "conditioning," wouldn't the mind follow the body's lead and start believing the "fight-or-flight" condition is real? Could this be another reason why "stress" has become such a significant factor today?

A: YES. It's a fact that the mind can follow the body. The science of neuro-linguistic programming (NLP) makes use of this fact. Our problems with massive stress levels could be explained, in part, by this factor. See the last chapter.

Q: Does the Foundation of Radiant Health help produce growth hormone for more muscles?

A: Yes. Growth hormone is protein-based. Bodybuilding surprise: **sugar (carbohydrate) *stops* your body from producing muscle-building growth hormone**! (*Basic Medical Biochemstry*, page 702.)

Q: Would you agree that established medical research into how the body works is being masked by reams of clinical studies that are either funded by parties with a particular agenda or designed with a particular outcome in mind?

A: Congratulations! You have uncovered the heart of the problem in the health and nutrition fields — bias.

Q: I read in The *New York Times* (January 29, 1998) that the true cause of multiple sclerosis was just discovered. M.S. is now known to be a result of severed nerve cells — a completely different problem.

A: The myelin sheath speeds nerve pulses. Even without the sheath, nerve impulses are transmitted, just a bit slower, so a Life-Systems Engineering analysis would say that myelin problems couldn't be the primary cause of the disease. This is another textbook example of an assumed cause-effect relationship. The entire medical community was shocked by this new discovery. The article interviewed the acting section chief of the National Institute of Neurological Disorders and Stroke. He stated, "Every textbook article starts by saying that the most important demyelinating disease is multiple sclerosis." Dr. Richard Rudick, director of Mellen Center for Multiple Sclerosis Treatment and Research at the Cleveland Clinic Foundation, said he wrote in the current edition of a leading medical textbook (ready to go to press), "Multiple sclerosis is a demyelinating disorder that tends to spare nerve cells." The new discovery proved just the opposite. Nerve cells are destroyed, not spared. **Aren't you glad the discoveries in this book are based on already established medical research, and not conjecture!**

How the Truth ...

- "*Replacement of fat by carbohydrates has not been shown to reduce the risk of coronary disease.*"
- "Beneficial effects of high-carbohydrate diets on the risk of cancer or on body weight **have also not been substantiated**."
- [Based on 6 major studies] "A limited weight reduction is seen after people start a fat-restricted diet, but *weight loss stops after a few months,* and the **long-term net weight loss is only 0.8 to 2.6 kg.** [1.7 to 5.7 pounds]."
- "There is no good evidence that reducing total dietary fat will prevent cancer or hypertension."
- "However, long-term substitution of carbohydrate, instead, does not reduce post-prandial lipemia."

(emphasis added)

Sources: The New England Journal of Medicine, vol. 337 (August 21, 1997): Clinical Debate: Should a Low-Fat, High-Carbohydrate Diet Be Recommended for Everyone? Taken from the clinical debate by the following parties: William E. Connor, M.D; Sonja L. Connor, M.S., R.D. – Oregon Health Sciences University; Martin B. Katan, Ph.D. – Wageningen Agriculture University; Scott M. Grundy, M.D., Ph.D. – University of Texas Southwestern Medical Center; Walter C. Willett, M.D., Dr. P.H. – Harvard School of Public Health

... Becomes Distorted

Careless **language turns** ***preliminary*** **findings into facts...**

"...use words like 'prevents' and 'protects' and 'protects against' and 'lowers the risk' when they are discussing evidence that is suggestive, and hypothetical ... Authors **whose words convey more certainty than the data.**"

Source: *New York Times*, Science Section, pages D1, D6, April 25, 2000

Never Get Suckered Again – Be Stat-Smart

> *"We are suffering from a wealth of information, but a poverty of understanding what that information* ***really*** *means."*
>
> Brian Peskin — *Life-Systems* Engineer

Statistics and Clinical Studies Made Simple

To help you interpret medical and nutritional research accurately, we developed the STAT-SMART analytical method that we used to review of 3,500 medical textbooks and scientific papers.

The *Pharmacist's Letter* (the nation's premier newsletter for pharmacists) states: "Make sure you look at scientific findings with lots of healthy skepticism. We do."[1]

Most nutritional reporting is [presented as though it were] the result of "scientific studies."

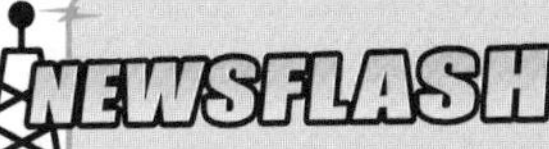

Newsweek **Magazine* refers to study results as, "Inefficient, Corrupt, and Unreliable."**

- "... trials are rife with **conflicts of interest** ...,
- ... analysis of women is **inadequate** ...,
- ... study results can be all but **useless** ..."

Life-Systems **Engineering** Analysis: Radiant Health is based on science – not biased "studies" or personal opinions.

*Source: *Newsweek*, Science & Ideas – Medicine, August 28, 2000, page 50.

When stumped as to why the real-life results weren't predicted by his physics theory, Nobel Prize-winning scientist Richard Feynman stated:

> "It turned out that all the experts had been quoting, some second or third hand, [results] from one experiment [measured inaccurately]. ... Since then I never pay any attention to anything by 'experts.' I calculate everything myself."[2] (emphasis added)

Analyzing and accurately interpreting researchers' conclusions is important for the informed consumer. Understanding some basic

1 *Pharmacist's Letter*, Vol. 12, No.5, May 1996.
2 *Richard Feynman - A Life In Science*, page 167.

methods of conducting research and reporting results will enable you to judge more accurately what the results really mean.

Tylenol brand acetaminophen is the most popular pain-killer in America. According to the manufacturer, Americans take 8 billion to 9 billion tablets of the drug per year.[3] There are many other pain-killing medications, too, besides Tylenol. We could conclude that living with pain is a natural condition of most Americans – ill-health is not only common, but is natural, or why would so many of us need a painkiller so often?

Of course, this conclusion leaves much to be desired. There are many reasons why we are in pain. It is more likely that many of our pains are caused by outside factors and it is not a natural state. Such important factors include: EFA and mineral deficiencies, along with an abundance of toxins from air, water, and food. Our body is responding to the deficiencies and toxins.

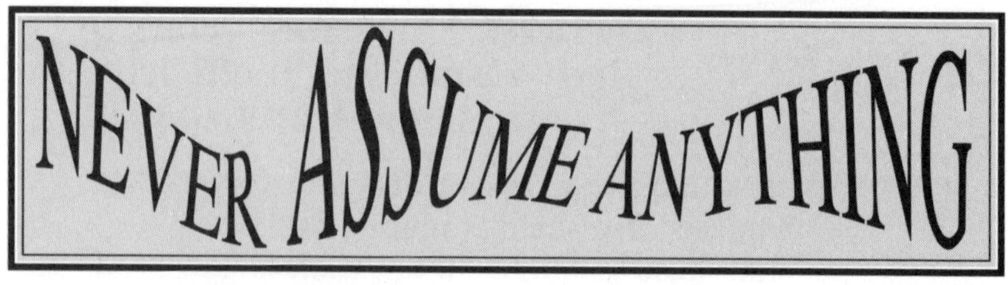

I continue to be surprised how many people try to analyze calories by grams of fat, protein, and carbohydrate. The nutritional discovery of the century – the Foundation of Radiant Health – eliminates this archaic and time-consuming method. The fat, protein, and carbohydrate contents are listed on food labels. The chart below is an example taken from a grocery store product. The real issue is how the numbers are used. Let's see how the manufacturers try to influence your choice. Of course, they count on you to make a few incorrect assumptions.

Extra helpful information:

One gram of **fat** typically contains **nine** calories.
One gram of **protein** or **carbohydrate** contains **four** calories.

3 *New York Times*, October 16, 1997, page A12.

Example: Melrose's Fried 'Tatoes

Calories: 110	Calories from Fat: 50
	% daily value
Total Fat 6gm	9 %
Total Carbohydrate 14gm	5 %
Dietary fiber 1gm	
Sugars 1gm	
Protein 1gm	4 %

The label also includes the following information: Percent daily values are based on an *assumed* diet of 2,000 calories. *Your daily values* may be higher or lower.

Let's see what this label really means.

First, don't get fooled by: "Sugars 1 gm." All digestible carbohydrates are converted to sugars in the body! Starches are made of sugar molecules, and digestion quickly breaks them into sugars. The dietary fiber does get subtracted from the total carbohydrate, because dietary fiber is not food for a human being – we cannot digest it. So the significant number for carbohydrates is (14g. minus 1g. fiber) = 13g. total digestible carbohydrate.

Every 5 grams (20 calories) of carbohydrate = one teaspoon of sugar!

Look at the fat percentage – it's only nine-percent. Sounds healthy, right? But is it really so good? At the top of the chart is "Calories from Fat: 50." To calculate the percentage of calories from fat, simply take the 50 and divide it by the total calories, which is 110. So we have 45-percent fat, not nine-percent![4] The amount of fat in any portion of this particular food by calories (not by weight) is the more meaningful measure, and it's almost half.

The distribution of total calories among fat, protein, and carbohydrate is required on the label because there is a big difference between the energy content of fat, compared to protein and carbohydrate. We need a way to compare these three on an equal basis, and the only way to do this is to convert each to calories. So where did that low nine-percent fat come from? Are they lying? Well, not exactly.

4 50 calories /110 calories = about 45-percent.

The "caloric tables" have been adjusted, allowing manufacturers to mislead you.

The federal government has established the maximum recommended daily amount (RDA) of fat at 65 grams, based on an assumed 2,000-calorie daily diet. This standard suggests that 30-percent of your food's calories should come from fat.[5] The nine-percent figure came from the grams of fat in this food divided by 65 (the assumed grams of fat to be eaten each day).[6] If this assumption is wrong, the calculations will be wrong, as well.

Some people assume they will continue to eat nine-percent fat regardless of how much they eat of Melrose's Fried 'Tatoes, because the overall fat percentage stays the same. This may be what the manufacturer hopes you'll think, but it is incorrect. One problem with this label is that all additional food for the day must contain no more fat, in order to remain at nine-percent overall.

If you ate exactly 2,000 calories' worth of this product, and no other food, you'd be at 45-percent fat.

Others multiply this nine-percent figure by the number of portions (servings). They reason: if they had three portions, and ate no more fat while consuming another 1,670 calories (2,000-330), they'd be at 27-percent fat. This reasoning is correct up to a point. Yet, it isn't a good way to calculate the various percentages if you don't eat exactly 2,000 calories every day.

If you wish to measure percentages based on calories of fat, then you must keep track (by calories of protein, fat, and carbohydrates) of each food you eat and keep a running total of type and amount of calories. At the end of the day you can add protein, fat, and carbohydrate calories separately. At that point you would know how you did that day, but what about tomorrow?

Is it productive to try to keep a total of calories and percentages of fat from what you eat? We think you will soon see it isn't.

---

5 (65 grams x 9 calories/gram)= 585 calories. 585 calories / 2,000 calories = about 30-percent.

6 Six grams/ 65 grams = nine-percent.

What is a calorie?

A calorie is a unit of heat. Heat is a form of energy. By definition, a calorie is the amount of energy required to heat one gram of water one degree Centigrade. One gram is the weight of approximately 1/4 teaspoon of water. A test chamber is used to measure how much heat is produced when burning a measured amount of material. That's OK for rating fuel for a furnace, but our bodies don't simply act as a "food furnace," so it's too simplistic to consider how much heat is generated by burning proteins, fats, or carbohydrates.

There are various opinions as to how many calories are required for daily activities. Soon you will see why we support a lower daily caloric requirement than is normally presented: once the Foundation of Radiant Health is implemented, *your body's efficiency improves dramatically.*

One of my favorite misleading calorie-related claims, from years past, is a "95-percent fat-free" ham label. One look at the piece of ham shows it has lots of visible fat – much more than five-percent fat.

Here's how the label worked. In foods with water added – ham being one of them – processors make use of the fact that water has zero calories. Our body uses water in a different way than it uses food. Also, water is relatively heavy. These two facts are an industrial food processor's dream. The fatty ham, with water added, is "95-percent fat-free" *by weight.* Processors inject water into the ham to increase the weight which *isn't counted in the fat measurement.* In this case, weight is not a valid measure of caloric content. They divide the fat's weight by the total weight of the ham including the added water. *Before the extra zero-calorie water is added, the fat accounts for at least 30-percent of the calories.*

Foods containing lots of water are usually assumed to have much lower fat contents than they actually do. For example, by calories, low-fat milk contains about 20-percent fat and regular milk is about 40-percent fat, *an even higher proportion than the ham!*

Studying the clinical studies

Acquaintances sometimes relate information from some study reported in a newspaper or a magazine and ask me what I think about it. I usually respond with: "Based on what you're telling me, I can't draw any conclusions." This is my standard answer, because publications rarely print all the conditions of the experiments that led to the stated conclusions. If a study doesn't report on a particular item, *don't make the mistake of assuming what the missing item might be.* Assumptions often lead to faulty conclusions.

Statistics are often used to sensationalize, confuse, mislead, or oversimplify.

Let's consider 13 very important problems inherent in statistical studies.

Problem #1: A proper sample is essential.

Proper "sampling" is the heart of statistics. In order to obtain perfectly accurate results, the test would have to be performed on everybody involved. Ordinarily, this is impossible. Special mathematics (statistics) have been devised to produce useful results with only a few of the people involved. Thus, we can test or survey or measure a small part (a "sample") of the total population rather than testing everybody.

With proper sampling, we need relatively few test cases (samples) to produce significant results. If the sample is large enough and properly selected, the results will be reasonably reliable – that is, the same results should be produced each time. Conversely, if either of these conditions is violated, the results will be unreliable.

Studies are frequently based on samples too small to provide reliable conclusions, or they are biased.

Some studies suffer from both defects.

Clinical studies are often performed in a sloppy manner. In 1985, the U.S. Food & Drug Administration (FDA) reviewed 441 studies on the use of radiation for preserving food. They dismissed 436 of these studies as invalid for a multitude of reasons. Only five of these studies were deemed worthy for further review![7]

7 *The Food That Would Last Forever*, Dr. Gary Gibbs, Avery Publishing Group, New York, 1993, page 16.

Problem #2: Sample size can be manipulated.

Claims can easily be phrased to make a particular product seem more impressive than it actually is. For example, a television advertisement claims that tooth whitener Brand A increases tooth brightness by 20-percent. This success rate sounds significant. But shouldn't one ask: What makes tooth whitener Brand A so much better than others? How can this claim (from an "independent certified laboratory") be made? Is the company lying? Not exactly. Maybe they just aren't telling the whole truth. It's easy to obtain this kind of result. One simple way is to manipulate the sample size.

A typical study or test focuses on measurements in a specific group – a sample. These could include people or products. Selecting the proper size of the sample is important. A statistically sound, reliable sample in this case would require about 1,000 people. In the tooth whitener case, a very small sample was used, but it was just the right size for the company to obtain the results they wanted. If, for example, groups of six "subjects" (people) each were used in a particular study, all sorts of statistically random inconsistencies could appear and be claimed as official results.

All a company has to do is use multiple samples of six test subjects each and perform the same test on each group. Sooner or later, one of the groups of six will show the result the company wants. In the above example, the desired result was: 20-percent brighter teeth (a significant percentage). Once they found a group with that result, the company could then claim that this particular tooth whitener produced brighter teeth.

What about a group of six where there is no difference in results as compared with the other brand? No problem. The company can just ignore those results.

If there are some groups which show no difference, are there also other groups which actually got worse results from this brand? Quite possibly. But there's no need to mention that, is there? This is called a "half-truth." The reported results were true, as far as stated, *but not the whole truth*. You have already seen that many erroneous conclusions based on half-truths have developed concerning our nutrition and health.

Such small group results are the basis on which many researchers release their findings. The following statement appeared in a 1996

Ms. Fitness magazine article on the oral form of the hormone DHEA: " ... In one human study with five male adults, the results showed (after 28 days with diet and physical activity remaining normal) a decrease in bodyfat without affecting muscle weight. ..." Test groups can't get much smaller than five. Also, how much bodyfat was lost? A few ounces or a few pounds? This is a key issue. Most study results are imprecisely reported in this fashion. Instead of giving actual before-and-after numbers, many articles will use relative terms such as more, less, increased, improved, decreased, etc.

We need to know the difference between a cause-effect relationship and one which occurs by association, sheer chance, or manipulation.

It should now be clear why studies are so often done with small group sizes. Sure, a smaller test costs less, but a more compelling reason to keep the sample size small is to be able to distort and control the conclusions legally.

Example:

Here's a simple test you can use to show how statistics can be misleading. Toss a coin ten times. We know that the odds of getting heads or tails are even, so you should get heads five times and tails five times, but this doesn't usually happen! If you toss the coin over five hundred times, the result will be closer to 50-percent heads and 50-percent tails. With only ten tosses, you could easily end up with five or six heads in a row, or five or six tails in a row. If this happens, you might suspect you have a different type of coin from everyone else. Nothing of the sort. You just didn't understand how random probability can affect outcomes – and most of us don't.

We're often easy prey to manipulation by numbers.

A critically important question is, **how large must a sample be to provide accurate results?** The larger the sample, the less the error. Does this mean we need a million test subjects? Not in most cases. About 1,000 subjects are required to provide a reasonably accurate conclusion for an issue such as whether aspirin eliminates your headache or not. That is, if selection of sample subjects is not biased. If the sampling is biased or prejudiced to begin with, then no number of subjects will yield correct results.

Other factors can affect the size of sample needed, as in this example:

> In the early 1950s, an experiment was conducted in the U.S. to measure the effectiveness of polio vaccination among 1,100 children. About 450 children were given the vaccine and 650 children were not given the vaccine. When a polio epidemic hit, none of the vaccinated children contracted the disease. However, neither did any of the non-vaccinated ones!
>
> The researchers failed to allow for the natural occurrence rate of the disease. The typical number of polio cases that would occur in a given number of people can be predicted from historical data. With a group this small, only two cases of polio would be expected to develop. A much larger sample (at least 6,000 subjects) was required in order to show significant results. Even the usual "1,000 subject" criterion wasn't adequate in a case like this. Since the historical data were available, this faulty result should have been anticipated and prevented by the researchers before conducting the experiment. Evidently, it wasn't. Too often, nutritional and medical research suffers from the researcher's lack of expertise in statistical interpretation. They may be in a rush (pressured by manufacturers) to prove a preferred (biased) result. Sometimes, they simply don't do their homework.

When there is a rush or a desire to prove something, results are often incorrect or misinterpreted.

Problem #3: We can get burned by bias.

If a sample group being studied is biased, or prejudiced, in any way, the result will not be accurate. It doesn't matter whether or not the researcher was aware of the prejudice. In real practice there is always a certain amount of bias or prejudice.

The double keys to reasonable accuracy are to:

a. minimize bias in the study, and

b. account for it in the conclusions.

Often, bias is either unrecognized or ignored.

That's one reason why many articles in newspapers and magazines have little real meaning.

Consider this: If most human test candidates are EFA-deficient, then would tests ignoring such bias be as valid as tests that consider such bias? No – if the deficiency affects the results, then any tests ignoring the deficiency would be less valid.

Conclusive tests to determine the extent and consequences of EFA deficiency haven't been done.

Almost everyone suffers from EFA deficiency because of modern food processing. Almost all nutritional and health studies have been performed with EFA-deficient human subjects (people) – a very significant bias. Therefore, all published nutrition and health studies involving human subjects must be questioned. Because of this bias, many of these studies could have meaningless conclusions.

Valid cause-effect conclusions can't be drawn from the many experiments which ignore EFA deficiency.

The form in which data is presented is important. In 1854, Dr. John Snow, an anesthesiologist, created statistical graphics that revealed the cause of a mysterious cholera epidemic. He correctly demonstrated, and was the first to show, that cholera was transmitted through water, not air. In contrast, with crucial data displayed in an obscure manner, the Challenger space shuttle was launched in 1986. *It blew up.* The O-ring failure should have been predicted, but the form in which the data was presented to the decision-making executives made the O-rings appear better than they were.[8] Statisticians, much like magicians, often reveal what they choose to reveal.

8 *Visual Explanations*, Edward R.Tufte, Graphics Press, Chesire, CT, 1997, page 27.

As Yale University Professor Edward Tufte states, "There are right ways and wrong ways to show data; there are displays that reveal the truth and displays that do not." It's "reader beware."

Problem #4: What is an average?

There are three (3) common types of averages: mean, median, and mode.[9] When you encounter the word, "average," you need to be aware of the three types and which one is being used; otherwise, depending on what the researcher wishes to convey, you may be completely misled.

The **(arithmetic) mean** is the total of the numbers from the samples divided by the number of samples used to get that total. This is the most commonly used type of average.

Example: There are nine bags of flour. Four bags have 1,000 insect parts per bag, three bags have 2,000 insect parts per bag, and two bags have 7,000 insect parts (the bugs really liked these two). The mean average is 24,000 parts divided by nine bags, or 2,666 insect parts per bag.[10]

This is based on a real life example. The FDA suggests maximum limits of 75 insect parts per 50 grams (3,300 parts per pound) of wheat flour.

The **median** is the value at the dividing line between the lower half and the upper half of the sample values.

Example: One-half the number of bags has 2,000 or more insect parts, and the other half has 2,000 or fewer parts. Since the dividing line is at 2,000 parts per bag, the median average is 2,000 insect parts per bag.

below the median ↕ above the median

1000 1000 1000 1000 2000 2000 2000 7000 7000

The **mode** is the value that occurs most often.

Example:

1000 1000 1000 1000 2000 2000 2000 7000 7000

The most common value (4 scores) is 1,000 insect parts per bag, thus the mode is 1,000 insect parts per bag.

9 Engineering calculations frequently use a fourth type of average: root mean square average (RMS).

10 (1,000 + 1,000 + 1,000 + 1,000 +2,000 + 2,000 + 2,000 +7,000 + 7,000) = 24,000; 24,000 ÷ 9 = 2,666.

Depending on which type of average was chosen, we could report 1,000 insect parts, 2,000 insect parts, or 2,666 insect parts per bag. The largest result is more than double the size of the smaller result. *Which average would you expect a company to report?*

Let's look at another example. The average salary of everyone in a small nutritional products distributing company might include the manager's higher salary, while the majority of employees would typically earn a much lower salary. Few, if any, employees would earn the mean salary. The lower salaried employees would be lower than this figure, and the owner's income would be much higher. The mode would probably reflect the most common entry-level salary, obviously lower than that of most employees. In this case, the median would be more representative for the "average" employee because it represents the same number of employees both above and below this figure. In average income surveys, if the mean is chosen as the average, a few wealthy individuals can shift the result upwards, making it appear that most people's income is below average.

Problem #5: The authors must account for all possibilities.

A company reported that its average employee earnings doubled over a two-year period. We could easily assume that the company doubled its hourly rate of pay. What actually happened was that half of the work force of part-time people who had been working 20 hours a week were fired, and the remaining employees (the other half) were converted to full-timers working 40 hours a week. Of course, the remaining employees made more total money (double their earnings), but they didn't increase their hourly wage – actual wages didn't go up – the company only reduced the number of employees and increased the workhours of the remaining employees. The result is far different from the original assumption of increasing the hourly pay rate. If you haven't figured it out or guessed, this company reported the *mean* as the "average."

Many years ago it was fashionable to attempt to control your breathing like a Yogi: inhale for three counts, hold your breath for three counts, and exhale for three counts. Many people read about this method in books. Some people got sick while trying to change their breathing. With biological living systems, if one thing changes, many other things also change. Too few people considered the effects on the digestive process when they changed their breathing.

If you have studied physics, you were taught that light moves in straight lines. You may be surprised to learn that this is not true. Light doesn't necessarily move in straight lines. Light has no preferred direction. We have to account for any possible direction it may go. It is only when the mathematics is worked out that we find that light appears to move in a straight line. This is an important difference.[11]

An article titled, "Slimming Herbs & Weeds" stated:

> You might think that nuts, which are high in fat, should be avoided by anyone who is trying to lose weight. But a study of more than 25,000 Seventh-Day Adventists showed that **those who ate the most nuts were the least obese**. Walnuts are our richest dietary source of serotonin, which, as mentioned earlier, helps make us feel full. Possibly they produced feelings of satiety. (emphasis added)
>
> It's important to understand, however, that Seventh-Day Adventists are vegetarians who live a much healthier lifestyle than the typical American. It's not clear that nuts would help you control your weight if you're an omnivore eating both meat and vegetables. But you might want to experiment to see if eating a handful of walnuts helps you control food cravings."[12]

At least Dr. Duke acknowledges multiple issues that could cause this effect. Unfortunately, the main reason for the walnuts satisfying the appetite so well was completely overlooked – they're full of appetite-fulfilling EFAs! I don't know of anyone eating nuts becoming sleepy. Anyone reading this article may be misled.

In the same article it is stated that "... In the end, nothing will help you to lose weight for good without a steady side-order of exercise and a low-fat, high-fiber, reduced-calorie diet."

As we will see, blanket statements such as this are often highly misleading and devoid of insight. In this case, the entire statement can be shown to be dead wrong.

---

11 *QED: The Strange Theory of Light and Matter*, Richard Feynman, Princeton University Press, 1985.

12 "Slimming Herbs & Weeds," James A. Duke, Ph.D., *Your Health*, September 2, 1997.

To solve complicated problems, we have to account for all possibilities, not just the obvious ones. Only then do we obtain correct answers to problems. *Not accounting for all possibilities* (no matter how unlikely or unexpected they may seem) *will provide limited insight and understanding*. Unknowingly following incorrect nutritional advice may be the Number One reason why Americans suffer from obesity, chronic fatigue, and ill-health.

Problem #6: The source of claims must be identified.

In their television advertisements, breath freshener brand A advertises that more dentists recommend their brand. How do the advertisers know what the dentists say? Do they conduct a survey? Not necessarily. Some companies give the dentists free samples to distribute to their patients.

> **When a dentist or physician accepts any free samples, the company counts that as a recommendation or endorsement.**

The company doesn't need to know whether patients actually got the samples. The dentist seems like a nice guy because he gives the patient something free, and the breath freshener company gets to make this claim. Does it mean their breath freshener is better?

Problem #7: We need to know the system under study.

When evaluating common cold remedies, one must know in advance that the common cold will cure itself within five to seven days whether or not the patient takes any medication. If the patient doesn't know this, then any medication taken could give the appearance of being effective.

Examples:

Let's look at this statement: "Higher blood cholesterol levels increase arterial clogging." Does this mean the presence of cholesterol itself is the problem, or is the buildup in the artery actually *caused* by something else? A *Life-Systems* Engineering analysis strongly suggests the latter explanation.

Some people think that, when they eat healthy essential oils and fat, it is immediately stored as excess bodyfat. Does this make sense? No, it doesn't make sense, and here's why. Digestion's job is to break down all food components into essential elements to be used as needed throughout the body's organs and systems. Natural fats do not just liquefy in your stomach, pass into the bloodstream as liquid fat, and end up on your thighs. Fat's essential components are used in numerous important places throughout your body. (See "Truth About Protein, Carbohydrates, and Fats.")

During my high-carb, low-fat diet and bodybuilding days, I never thought much about cause-and-effect relationships. I listened blindly to how terrible eating fat was supposed to be. On the contrary, as I learned later, fats and healthy essential oils are the most energy-efficient food we have, and our bodies need them.

There are two types of fats and oils:
1. natural fats and oils
2. chemically altered fats and oils.

Far from being a culprit, natural fats and oils are highly beneficial. In stark contrast, the chemically altered fats and oils are harmful. This is another example of the common nutritional half-truths. These half-truths can easily be used to distort information, especially when reinforced with statistics.

Problem #8: Does the measurement really mean anything?

Few researchers are willing to admit they don't know what caused an outcome. **Everyone wants an answer, and more often than not, the questioner will be given some sort of answer.**

But what is that answer worth?

Low-cholesterol and no-cholesterol foods are widely promoted, yet dietary cholesterol has virtually no influence on blood cholesterol levels – in spite of the flood of politically-correct worry about diet-cholesterol levels. The "No Cholesterol" tag is still featured prominently on food labels any time it can be claimed, even though all plant sources are cholesterol-free. Yes, most carbohydrates have no cholesterol.

A *New York Times* article discusses the oat bran fad which occurred around 1989. The fad ended when the public learned that huge amounts of oats had to be eaten to reduce the risk of heart disease. Oat bran's "remarkable" soluble fiber was largely forgotten.[13]

13 "Eating Well," Marian Burros, *New York Times,* February 26, 1997, page B8.

Shark cartilage is often sold as a supplement based on the assumption that sharks don't get cancer. First, do any fish get cancer? This question is never asked. Second, if the shark lived in polluted waters, would that change the state of its health? Maybe they don't get cancer because they don't eat processed foods or drink polluted water. And if that shark is exposed to pollution and toxins, how much of it would we get from the cartilage? Even if sharks don't get cancer, why should eating their cartilage protect us from it? Would eating Einstein's brain make you smarter? Not likely.

Many questions need to be asked before accepting a specific conclusion.

Example:

Consider the apparently simple act of weighing yourself. You have to make several decisions; otherwise, the results will be inaccurate or misinterpreted.

- You need an accurate scale: Pick a scale with a guaranteed accuracy of at least 0.2-percent over the scale's range.[14] This scale may cost as much as $60, but at least you can count on a sufficiently accurate measurement.

Each weighing should be done as close to the same conditions as possible.

- *Weigh at the same time and day:* Don't waste time taking daily weight measurements, because there are variations in bodyweight between meals and from day-to-day. You want to measure your bodyweight, not how much your last meal weighed. Pick a specific time, such as early Monday morning, before eating or drinking anything and before getting dressed.

- *Several measurements are needed over time:* Take weekly measurements over four or more consecutive weeks. This gives an accurate assessment of whether weight was gained, lost, or stayed about the same.

14 This means that, for a 200-pound measurement, you can be sure there was no more than a 0.4-pound margin of error. A 200-pound reading would indicate a weight between 199.6 pounds and 200.4 pounds.

- *Consistent input is critical:* Make sure to eat and drink the same amount at the same time each Sunday evening (or the night before your established weighing time). What has been eaten in the 12 hours before weighing needs to be relatively consistent. Even a few extra glasses of water will alter the true reading.

There is another indicator called the "body mass index" (BMI). This frequently used number doesn't take into account the individual's relative fitness level. It is based only on weight and height. The BMI measurement lumps everyone into one group, frequently giving misleading, even ridiculous, results. For example, a man or a woman who has trained in a gym will have a lot of muscle. This additional muscle weight is significant, particularly since muscle tissue weighs more than fat. Because the BMI measurement doesn't take this into account, many people involved in bodybuilding, with just six- to ten-percent bodyfat, are officially classified as "obese." Just imagine someone telling Mr. Olympia that he is overweight according to the BMI calculations.[15]

Before we decide to use weight measurement as a primary health indicator, let's answer a very important question. Is weight the best indicator of what you are after? *Muscle weighs more than fat*. If you lose bodyfat, yet gain muscle, your overall weight would decrease very little, or might even increase. Yet, you would look better. You might also weigh more when the protein you eat is more efficiently converted into muscle after eliminating your EFA and mineral deficiencies.

Some weight-loss programs stimulate loss of excess water (diuretic action), yet the faithful follower gains more bodyfat. In this case there might be no significant difference in weight, yet he or she would be fatter. Therefore, a *Life-Systems* Engineering analysis suggests that **bodyweight, by itself, is not the most useful indicator of excess fat**.

For years I had been displeased with how I looked in the mirror. After undergoing significant bodybuilding training with expert guidance, I joked that, finally, I didn't make myself sick when I looked in the mirror. Muscle mass increased, yet I never totally acquired the look I wanted because (as I only later found out) the

15 Some might argue that Mr. Olympia isn't fat, yet he is officially considered overweight. That's a personal opinion. A high BMI number implies excess bodyfat. The error is in the BMI method.

bodybuilding diet is flawed. I hadn't learned about our deficiency of EFAs (healthy essential oils) back then.

Your reflection in the mirror and a tape measure are probably the best ways to determine how you look.

Published conclusions can be, and often are, meaningless. For example, the death rate for the Navy during the Spanish-American War was nine per 1,000, yet civilians perished at the rate of 16 per 1,000 in New York City. Based on this, it appears safer to have been in the Navy during that wartime period than to have been a non-fighting citizen of New York City. But the Navy was made up of men in good health and they saw very little risky action in that war. The general population of New York City included the sick, elderly, and newborns. Each of these three groups has a high death rate. The Navy's group was much different. Consequently, the conclusion was meaningless because *the two groups didn't include the same variables*.

Problem #9: Overstated precision can be misleading.

Most people think that a 98.6 degree Fahrenheit (F) body temperature is normal. Recent tests suggest that 98.2 degrees F is more accurate. It may be that, when the tests were done to determine the average temperatures, the Centigrade scale was used, and then converted to Fahrenheit. The scientific community favors this scale.[16]

Accuracy would have been lost in two ways. First, the actual measurement was rounded up or down to the nearest degree. Second, this number was converted to Fahrenheit, and the result became the standard 98.6 degrees F we so commonly hear.[17]

Stated accuracy can be misleading. If my temperature measures 99.0 degrees F, it is probably normal. A range of temperature between 97.7 and 99.5 degrees F presents no reason for concern for most people.

---

16 There are two temperature scales commonly used by the public, so we need to be sure which units we are using: Fahrenheit or Centigrade. When you convert from one to another, the degree of accuracy automatically changes. One degree Centigrade converts to 1.6 degrees Fahrenheit, and the freezing points are 32 degrees apart (0 degrees C = 32 degrees F). Magnifications of error can take place when converting.

17 Accuracy was lost in the rounding and in the conversion to Fahrenheit.

Is 98.23651 more accurate than 98? Not necessarily. There are two main issues: What is the degree of error in the reading, and how much accuracy do you need in the situation?

To see if my car battery is still good, the mechanic uses a digital voltmeter that indicates voltage. The meter jumps from 12.59 to 12.51 to 12.54 to 12.50, and so on. (The readings fluctuate constantly.) Does that mean the voltage of the battery is changing? Not necessarily. It may be the meter that is changing. It may be that the wires aren't making a good enough connection between the battery and the meter. But, who cares? That last digit that keeps moving doesn't matter – I just need to know if the battery is good. For this application, as long as the battery is over 12.4 volts, it's fine. A reading above 12.4 volts means I can use this battery. If the reading was below 12.0 volts I know I'll need to recharge or replace it. Any greater precision doesn't matter, and could be misleading.

On the other hand, I could make a substantial study out of those readings and attempt to analyze the statistical meaning of the variations between different batteries, different manufacturers, and a host of other conditions. It might sound impressive but would actually be quite meaningless.

Overstated accuracy is meaningless, and the greatest analysis in the world can't make it better.

Problem #10: Lack of accuracy can be misleading.

The following is an example of how, too often, information is published. A newsletter printed this and cited the reference. In big bold letters, their heading reads:

> **"Vitamin C Lowers Blood Sugar in Type II Diabetics."**
> Research from Finland indicates that high doses of ascorbic acid (vitamin C) helps people with type II diabetes maintain glycemic control. A double-blind study performed at the Malmi Municipal Hospital in Helsinki found that daily doses of 2,000 mg of ascorbic acid improved both fasting blood glucose and HBA1c readings in patients with type II diabetes.[18]

This *appears* to be a great result. The question is, how well did the vitamin C actually work? This is never answered! What does "improved" mean? Was there a one-percent improvement (really

18 *Ann Nutr Metab* 1995:39(4):217-23.

insignificant), a 50-percent improvement (somewhat significant), or a 95-percent (very significant) improvement? If the results were really significant, don't you think that would be emphasized in the story? This is the type of clinical study which receives great headlines, yet is often worthless. The question of "how significant" is never addressed in the article. The vitamin C manufacturers must love this article. Vitamin C may work extremely well or it may not. *We just can't tell from what was published.*

The relevant question in statistical analysis is: *"Compared with what?"*

If I increase my automobile engine horsepower output from 120 to 125 horsepower, that's an improvement. Trouble is – you don't even notice increases of less than 10 horsepower. So maybe it's "improved," yet not to a significant degree. We must understand the requirements of the particular system under study.

Here's a misleading headline that was published in the September 1996 issue of *Redbook* magazine. "No More Stretchmarks" was the title. The article praises the benefits of Retin-A for shrinking stretchmarks. It describes a University of Michigan study in which tretinoin, considered to be the active ingredient, was found to shrink stretchmarks nine-percent in width and 15-percent in length after six months of daily use.

Far from "no more stretchmarks", the article explains that the stretchmarks only shrink a little bit. If the mark was originally six-inches long by a quarter-inch wide, it was reduced to 5.1-inches long by 0.23-inches wide. That is only a 23-percent reduction, leaving more than three quarters still visible – certainly not all that great.[19] And this took six months of treatment.

No one should call this "no more stretchmarks." The reporter may or may not have done a good job of researching this article, but the headline is highly inaccurate and misleading.

Problem #11: Conclusions can be intentionally misleading.

If someone can't prove what he wishes to prove, he may *demonstrate something else and pretend that they are the same.*

19 Six minus 5.1 = 0.9 and 0.25–0.23 = 0.02, so (1 - 0.9/6) x (1 - 0.02/.25) = 77% of the original mark remains for a 23% reduction in size or area. The reduction in length is 15%. How accurate was the width measurement? We are measuring just 2/100th of an inch difference. Are we misled again?

> A headline such as: "Brand A gargle kills 10,650 germs in 20 seconds," usually means the germs were killed in *laboratory tests performed in a test tube.*

This isn't good enough. **Will it kill as many germs in your body?** Most of us *assume* it does. We have no basis to assume such a thing because these are two completely different sets of conditions. Furthermore, is the germ that is killed in the laboratory the same type that is a problem to your body? There is an enormous variety of germs, so the chances are, it isn't. Also, if 10,650 were killed in your mouth, how many would still survive? Is the number killed significant in relation to the number remaining?

This same type of inaccuracy is commonly used with many of the over-the-counter "diet aids" that are so heavily advertised. They may perform marginally under a specific set of conditions. But more often than not, those conditions are vastly different from the normal conditions of daily living.

The fine print with many of these "miraculous" weight-loss products says that, in addition to using them, you must also eat a lot less and exercise more.[20]

Another form of deception is to present a conclusion which doesn't follow from the data.

> You may have heard how little money is made in the supermarket business: often, just a one-percent profit.

Well, the number may be true, but it isn't a valid measurement of return on investment. If it was, grocers would close their stores and put their money in the local bank. Profit isn't based just on sales. If each day, I paid $99 for products which I sold for $100, I'd make just $1 per day profit on my original investment of $99. Yet, reinvesting that original $99 each of the next 364 days, my return would amount to 369-percent on total money invested during the year, because I'd be making $1/day on a one-time $99 investment.[21]

A successful businessman usually cares much more about return on investment than he does about return on sales. Supermarkets often present profit margins as a percentage of sales so the profit seems smaller.

---

20 Does this suggest that exercise is not a particularly effective means of fat loss?

21 Profit of $1/day times 365 days = $365 profit. Divide the profit by the original investment of $99 = 369-percent true yearly profit. Would you mind this return?

> A prominent health magazine wrote that women who breast-fed babies may have less risk of hip fracture. This is according to some Australian epidemiologists who studied women over age 65. Does this conclusion make sense?

Regarding hip fracture rates, bone density is one possible factor. There are multiple conditions relating to proper bone density – for example, adequate minerals and EFAs in the diet. From a *Life-Systems* Engineering analysis, bone density isn't even the best deterrent to fracture. Bone elasticity is.

Once again, it's basic essence to the rescue! By nature of their molecular structure, EFAs increase flexibility and elasticity in all living cells: tissues, organs, and bones. A secondary factor for eliminating hip fracture might be the woman's tendency to fall – which is influenced by her balance, posture, and coordination.

To accurately make a cause-effect statement, such as "breast-feedings decrease hip fractures," one would have to perform a very complicated statistical "analysis of variance."

This type of analysis is seldom done. An analysis of variance is a mathematical way to:

1) Take into account every factor that could contribute to the outcome.

2) Figure out the importance of each factor.

3) Calculate how much each factor contributed to the result, with a calculated probability that it did.

This technique is as difficult and expensive to perform as it sounds. That's one of the reasons it is seldom done. In a study such as this, we would have expected the recipient of the breast-feeding – the baby, not the mother – to have a nutrient advantage.[22]

Certainly, breast-feeding affects Mom – there is a hormone effect, but this is only a temporary effect – it probably wouldn't support this type of long-term consequence. Should you believe any outcome of a study such as this? Absolutely not. Unless there

---

22 *Drug Topics*, July 22, 1996. This "study" was presented in a test for continuing education credits for pharmacists. It notes that breast milk contains EFAs, which *most synthetic formulas don't contain*. Deficiencies in visual acuity and neurological status often develop in children up to age 10 years who were artificially fed as infants. (It is possible that these deficiencies are never corrected, due to the almost universal EFA-destroying food processing.)

is a ream of data to go along with it, don't even waste your time. There are simply *too many unanswered questions.*

> For years, coffee has been "linked" to elevated levels of cholesterol, which supposedly increases the risk of cardiovascular problems. But a 1996 study of over 120,000 nurses found that, after researchers adjusted for cigarette smoking among coffee drinkers – regardless of how high the consumption of coffee was – there was no increase in cardiovascular risk.[23]

In this study, coffee, in and of itself, had no effect on increased cardiovascular risk. What does "adjusted for" [smoking] mean? It refers to exactly the analysis of variance we are discussing. The researchers may not have pointed out all of the possible causes of the study's results. We often hear a shocking headline, but we rarely see the headline's retraction, after it is shown to have been incorrect to begin with.

We are often misled by erroneously *assumed cause-effect relationships*. If B follows A in sequence, then most of us assume A caused B. Not necessarily. Maybe it did; maybe it didn't. (This is one way that superstitions develop.) The Latin term for such an illogical conclusion is a *non sequitur*. It simply means *the conclusion doesn't follow from the preceding statement.* Often, when one thing changes, several others change along with it. This makes accurate analysis of the stated conclusion more challenging.

Non sequiturs are used frequently to fool us into accepting false conclusions

> Researchers in Chicago concluded that sugar-coated cereal increased scholastic test performance.[24] One group was given a high-carbohydrate breakfast of a sugar-coated cereal 1/2 hour before taking an exam. Another group was given the same breakfast two hours before the exam. The reported conclusion is that sugar consumed shortly before taking an exam increases mental alertness. Let's think about this a bit.

23 *Mayo Clinic Health Letter*, July 1997, page 7.

24 An Associated Press article appearing in the *Houston Chronicle* dated October 15, 1996.

This is another illustration of a half-truth that shouldn't be overgeneralized. If increased sugar levels were a good thing, then eating sugar throughout the day would be a good thing, too. Try eating a candy bar every two hours during your eight-hour workday. You'll get sick from the sugar.

We know that you can get a sugar low within two hours after consuming excess processed carbohydrates. Could this be all that the experiment actually shows? Sugar's negative effect on human *Life-Systems* often continues even an hour or two after consumption due to the residual excess insulin.

Did the researchers compare the results of eating a no-carbohydrate meal (such as bacon and eggs) to the results of eating the cereal? Maybe that group would have had even better scores.

Published scientific "conclusions" are often just educated guesses – nothing more. There is frequently more artistry than science in deciding how to present the conclusion or deciding which statistical method to use. Many scientists know this. *Many in their audience don't.*

Not all statistical results are presented with the conscious intent to deceive, but deception occurs in at least three ways:

First, the wish to prove a desired result can cause tunnel-vision and a lack of objectivity (bias).

Second, the researcher may not know how to properly interpret his own results. Legitimate errors can occur, although before publishing, a quality peer review should eliminate the significant errors.

Third, the researcher doesn't always have control over what is printed. Magazines and newspapers want sensational news. That's how they sell their publications. It may be their editors who misinterpret, especially in writing the headline(s), or who don't present all of the researcher's qualifying comments. However, *in a medical journal the researcher has complete control over the content* (although not necessarily the headline).

It is entirely up to you to understand the limitations of what is presented.

In India, there is virtually no breast cancer. Many Indians eat no meat. They eat a lot of rice. What conclusions can we draw? Does eating meat trigger cancer? Is it a cause? Does eating rice somehow prevent cancer? These are very good questions, but they cannot be answered without additional research or more information.

We know that the body stores toxins in fat tissue. Some of those toxins are known to increase the risks of breast cancer. The toxins can come from many sources. In India, the population consumes less fat overall. Which has more influence on breast cancer prevention: the toxins (antibiotics, hormones, and steroids) in meat or the meat itself? If rice doesn't contain these toxins, eating rice wouldn't add to the toxin level. From available information, we can't say what causes the lower levels of breast cancer.

Many Indians live on the edge of starvation. This means less of all foods are consumed, including less toxins. Starving people typically eat less meat, and remember, many Indians eat little or no meat.

Another variable is whether Indian women breast-feed their babies significantly more or longer than other cultures? Has anyone studied this?

In the India breast cancer example, we can certainly guess that lack of meat in the diet, along with significant rice consumption *may be* related to a reduced risk of breast cancer. But that is all we can say. From a *Life-Systems* Engineering analysis, it's a statement devoid of deep insight. *Nor is there any indication of a cause-effect relationship here.*

An article on breast cancer, titled "Breast Cancer & Women" by Rosie Mestel, appeared in *Health* magazine.[25] There was a reference to dietary fat causing breast cancer. Here is what was said:

> "Breast cancer rates are highest in the countries with the richest diets (fats).... But **rigorous studies show the link is weak, if it exists at all**." (emphasis added)

This particular author understands and accurately reports that there is no definitive cause-effect (or causal) relationship between dietary fat intake and breast cancer. Our *Life-Systems* team would suggest the only likely causal link would be from the ingested toxins consumed in dietary fat.

25 *Health,* March 1997, pages 70-73.

Even if there were a causal relationship, would most Americans even follow an almost meatless diet? Not likely. Even though steak-eating has supposedly decreased, the number of steakhouse restaurants is at an all-time high. We don't often find Americans eating only a bowl of rice or a salad as a main dish. Nor does such a diet offer adequate nutrition.

For any statistical study to be meaningful, two things must always be presented in the conclusion:

first, the probability of the result occurring, and, *second*, the confidence level of this result.

Test conclusions must be presented in a format such as the following: "I can say with 30-percent **confidence** (certainty or sureness) that there is a 45-percent **probability** (chance or likelihood) that eating a cup of rice a day in combination with not eating beef decreases the chances of developing breast cancer by 30-percent." Is it possible that rice without beef does not decrease the chances of developing breast cancer at all? Absolutely, even with this scientific-sounding conclusion.

Unless clinical study results are reported in this form with a specific confidence level and a specific probability, we don't know the reliability of the conclusion. Aren't you worthy of having all the facts?

Are results often presented in this fashion? No, almost never in general publications and seldom in professional publications, either.

Problem #12: Conditional probability fools 'em every time!

What does a statement actually mean?
Too often, we don't look beyond the surface.

If there is an underlying factor which is assumed in a test, then the results must be properly re-calibrated. Let's look at a case where there is no trickery in obtaining a result that most readers won't initially believe could be true. This example is based on an illustration used by John Allen Paulos in his book, *A Mathematician Reads the Newspaper.*[26]

26 *A Mathematician Reads the Newspaper*, John Allen Paulos, BasicBooks, New York, 1995.

If you are frustrated by the following example, don't be concerned. I want you to see the result and understand how we can be misled by our assumptions with even the best of intentions. Statistics can't always provide an accurate conclusion or prediction. An epidemiologist and numerous people of scientific backgrounds still didn't follow the reasoning the first time they read it, either, but the reasoning is 100-percent correct.

Let's say I have a very accurate medical test. If I have Disease A, then 99-percent of the time, the test will correctly detect the disease. If I don't have Disease A, the test will also correctly tell, 99-percent of the time, that I don't have it.

The question is, if I really don't have Disease A, how often will the test say I have it when I don't?

Said another way, how often will this test give a false positive reading? How often will I needlessly be scared that I have a disease when I don't?

These figures suggest 99-percent accuracy, so I may guess that only one out of 100 times the test will be wrong. The actual answer is not one incorrect result out of 100, but an amazing 99 incorrect results out of 100! In other words, the test will almost always result in an incorrect positive diagnosis. This is a terrific example of a conditional probability.

Let's see more clearly how this works.

If we test 1,000,000 people, here's what the testing will show:

The test will show that 99 of the 100 actually sick people in this group are sick – one sick person will not be detected.[27]

The test will also show that 9,999 of the healthy people are incorrectly detected as sick.[28]

Here is where most people lose sight of the issue. **We have asked a new question** – *the number of people incorrectly tested sick*

27 To come up with this, we need to know one more bit of information. We need to know that one in 10,000 people actually have the disease (this can be accurately predicted in advance from historical data). If 1,000,000 people are tested, then 100 people are actually sick (1,000,000 tested x 1/10,000 with disease) = 100 with disease, and 1,000,000 - 100 = 999,900 actually healthy people in our test.

28 One-percent false results of 999,900 actually healthy people (1/100) x 999,900 = 9,999 false positives.

(false positive readings). The 99-percent accuracy tests didn't apply directly to this case.

To calculate the number of false positives, divide the number of healthy people tested sick (9,999) by the total of all people who tested sick either correctly or incorrectly (9,999 + 99).[29] Because we tested a large number of people (1,000,000), even a small degree of inaccuracy – just one-percent (elsewhere considered very small) – produces a large error compared with the number of people who really have the disease.

The dismaying result of our supposedly accurate test is **99-percent false (inaccurate) readings for a test that may appear 99-percent accurate**! If you are diagnosed to have a serious disease, be sure to find out the percentage of false positives associated with the diagnosis. This also underscores the importance of getting a second opinion in such cases.

This false-positive example is not just an intellectual exercise. In the late 1960s and early 1970s, Kaiser-Permanente and other HMOs attempted to institute predictive screening. Their hope was to catch a patient's medical problem before it became serious. This was a worthy goal, but the plan failed. Why? For the simple reason that even the best tests produce a significant number of errors – just like our false-positive example. The HMO would have spent a fortune treating people who didn't have anything wrong with them! The plan was cancelled.

Here's another example of a conditional probability.

> Most of us think that people live much longer today than those born in 1900. The average person born in 1900 lived to about age 50, and the average person born today now lives to approximately age 75.

The question is, does the average adult live much longer today? The answer is NO. The average adult today does not live much longer than the average adult did in 1900. There is only a six-year increase in a man's life and an eleven-year increase in a woman's life. Ten- and twenty-percent increases aren't that impressive from a *Life-System* Engineering analysis – given 95+ years of medical and technological advancements. Furthermore, we aren't talking

---

29 A group of 9,999 (healthy people tested sick)/10,098 (99 sick people tested sick + 9,999 healthy people tested sick) = 99-percent **incorrect results**.

about quality of life. These figures hide the fact that many of us are sicker but kept alive longer in hospitals, nursing homes, Alzheimer's centers, and so on.

How are we fooled into thinking modern science is significantly extending our lives? There was a condition to this question that most of us never considered – *we made an implicit assumption.* As adults, we necessarily had to survive childbirth and the infant mortality (death) rate. Back in 1900, many more newborns and infants died. If out of two births, one baby died at birth and the other baby lived to 100 years old, *the average (mean) life expectancy for those born would be 50 years: (0+100)/2.*

Because many of us mistakenly assumed the increase in life expectancy was due to people living longer, and because we neglected infant mortality, we were deceived. Today, because of better food distribution (not better food), and better hygiene, the infant mortality rate is improved. The sad truth is that science has done very little to increase the life expectancy of adults. This is verification that it is extremely difficult to correct the negative effects of a nutritional deficiency without providing the needed nutrients, no matter how many new gadgets and drugs are invented.

Making matters worse, the aged today often become institutionalized for their last days or join the growing ranks of the "walking-wounded."

> With the low-fat focus so prevalent today, has anyone asked if there are associated long-term detrimental effects from decreasing the fat content in our food and replacing it with synthetic substances? We are ingesting increasing numbers of newly developed chemical additives.

The food processors have been decreasing the fat content of many foods. This has indirectly resulted in people eating more food.

a. Many people (erroneously) think they can eat more "low fat" food without adding fat to their body.

b. EFA deficiency keeps us hungry and malnourished, while driving us to eat more.

Few dieters lose bodyfat. They tend to over-eat partly because they think that they can eat as much low- or non-fat food as they want.

Is the low-fat craze fueled in part by the assumption that low fat foods are better for you? The *politically correct assumption* is that processed carbohydrates are better than natural fats and oils. This is **factually incorrect**.

Problem #13: We can easily be misled by "experts."
(We are taught to believe them.)

Many of us have been told that excess protein damages the kidneys by placing excess stress on them. The high-carbohydrate proponents must love this myth. This conclusion was based on analyzing diabetics with high blood-glucose levels. Later, it was found that *the high blood-glucose levels caused protein to be excreted into the urine.* **It had nothing to do with the level of protein eaten!** When the same tests are performed on subjects with normal blood-glucose levels, there is no change in kidney filtration rates. Even though it's wrong, this incorrect conclusion continues to be repeated frequently.

Who determines the "official" viewpoint on nutritional information? This is important to know, because almost everyone repeats the same information.

Right or wrong, their guidelines are *assumed* to be true!

We must keep in mind that science is not immune from political and social pressures. In fact, scientists frequently tend to provide results that support the values of their society, or *those who pay the bills.*

Let's consider the reports generated by the National Institutes of Health Consensus Development Conference.

First, because it's a committee, the fifteen or so members must arrive at a consensus on what they publish. If 15 people must agree on anything, there is a high probability that whatever it is won't be too different from what the group's recommendation was the previous year – even when strong evidence is presented for a dramatic change in ideas. Expect changes, here, to come slowly.

Second, because it's a government-sponsored forum, their findings may be presented to be politically correct first, while scientific validity and accuracy rate a distant second. Let's explore this a bit further.

We have studied ten of these reports dated between 1983 and 1995. Examples of topics included: "Health Implications of Obesity" and "Treatment of Hypertriglyceridemia."

The major conclusions of these reports are, in effect:

1. they don't know what specifically causes the health problem, and
2. they don't know the cause-effect relationships among conditions relating to the reported health problem.

These two statements are often implied behind the panel's report. The words "likely," "appears to," "may," "difficult to interpret," "likely to be helpful," and "suggests" are used throughout these reports.

Several reports blame cigarette smoking as a cause of a condition although no specific reason was ever given in the report. No cause-effect relationship with smoking was presented, but the committee must have thought it was politically correct to add this caution. We all know that smoking is not healthy, but was smoking monitored in any of these studies? **Another report actually stated, "...we recommend this course of action although the data shows it doesn't work."** It's one thing to follow advice when it is based on an actual cause-effect relationship. This particular recommendation was not even supported by the published data.

One of these NIH reports called a 25-percent reduction in cardiovascular deaths a "particularly great improvement." Certainly, one less death is important, but if only one out of four is helped, that's a 75-percent failure rate for the treatment! Is there a compelling reason that, because we are dealing with people, we are allowed to call mediocre results particularly great? Apparently some in the nutritional and medical community think it's OK. In *Life-Systems* Engineering, we don't accept this low level of success as noteworthy. **If a method isn't positive for at least 80-percent of everyone, we don't consider it successful.**

Only in nutrition and pharmacological fields does a 75-percent failure rate seem to be considered excellent. Almost everywhere else this would be considered dismal.

One of the main problems with these reports may be that most of the committee members are physicians. *Physicians aren't usually scientists, but here they are asked to act as though they were.* It's not fair. *They aren't trained to be scientists.* Physicians are trained to diagnose and treat patients; scientists are not. There isn't enough school time for everyone to be trained in everything.

Let the skeptics try to explain these citings from the medical journals presented by Dr. Ali in *Rats, Drugs, and Assumptions*:

> ... Many of us, faced with someone who quotes statistics, find it difficult to distinguish whether any consequent conclusion is correct or whether we have been bamboozled...." or "... Wulff and colleagues sent a questionnaire to 250 Danish doctors (of whom 148 responded) to assess their knowledge of elementary statistical expressions ... From nine multiple choice questions, respondents produced a median response of 1.4 correct answers (85-percent wrong). ... Danish doctors who replied clearly knew little (and the 102 who did not reply may have known less). Are doctors in other countries more knowledgeable? The evidence suggests not ...." (*British Medical Journal* 294:856; 1987.)

In a paper titled, "Consensus Development at the NIH: What Went Wrong?" Itzhak Jacoby raises serious concerns about NIH procedures. At a typical conference, speakers supply the "evidence," which is then evaluated by a consensus committee which may have no personal experience regarding the topic. This committee is made up of people who aren't supposed to have an opinion on the topic. These people are chosen *specifically because they are not experts in the field.*[30]

This is the first problem with their attempting to evaluate specific conclusions. But even a real expert in the area of discussion might have a difficult time evaluating all the data in such a short period of time.

Just a day-and-a-half is spent evaluating presentations, then on the second day, the committee drafts the consensus statement. Thoroughly evaluating multiple experiments and developing accurate cause-effect conclusions can't be done that rapidly. That's one reason why the committee's findings are typically vague and

30 In such a scientific gathering, a Life-Systems Engineering perspective would require each committee member to have great personal knowledge and significant experience in the topic of discussion.

don't differ significantly from the previous ones. The findings are often kept politically correct. They often suggest continued research to answer the questions they couldn't answer, even though their study was supposed to have answered them. The conference concludes with the press publicizing the committee's conclusions. All ten reports that we reviewed, over a ten-year period, follow a similar pattern.

Perhaps the most obvious flaw in the practice is that multiple opinions of an issue may not even be presented. For example, I may say cholesterol levels above 220 are significant in causing arterial blockage, and you could say they aren't. In the 1985 meeting concerning chemotherapy for breast cancer, **the pro-chemo viewpoint had multiple representatives** presenting information. **The non-chemo alternative side had none.** The best experts are seldom invited. Only pre-selected evidence (a prejudiced selection) is heard.

In the NIH format there is little effort to organize the presentation. Speakers are presented in no apparent order as to the content of their comments. No speaker is allowed to comment on another speaker's statements or conclusions. Neither is there a provision for speakers to challenge each other's findings or to ask for clarification.

Recall how, too often, scientific and clinical studies lack sufficient detail to support their conclusions. Yet, interested parties can't ask for detail during these NIH meetings. In the absence of challenging questions, the committee would naturally be tempted to continue with the same old rubber stamp recommendations from the past.

James P. Carter, M.D., says in his book, *Racketeering In Medicine*,[31] that although organized medicine considers holistic approaches pseudo-scientific, 80-percent of all medical procedures now used in the daily practice of medicine have never been proven by scientific research studies.

> Dr. Carter goes on to say that the Office of Technology Assessment [OTA], a respected research organization for Congress, published a report stating: "**Only 10-20-percent of all medical procedures currently used in medical practice**

31 *Racketeering In Medicine*, James P. Carter, M.D., Hampton Roads Publishing Company, Inc., Hampton Roads, VA, 1992, page 6.

> **have been shown to be efficacious [effective] by controlled trial.**" (emphasis added)

That means 80-90-percent of medical procedures routinely performed are of unproven usefulness. This doesn't mean they are necessarily ineffective, but *we are given a very one-sided picture.*

The OTA further reported: *of the 10-20-percent of medical procedures actually shown to be useful, some have been based on flawed research.*

People publishing summaries of research, studies and their analysis often misinterpret the results.

An example of misinterpreted results concerns breast cancer and mammograms. The National Cancer Institute, which is part of the National Institutes of Health, and the American Cancer Society issued a joint statement saying that they agree that mammography screening of women in their 40s is beneficial and supportable with current scientific evidence.

There was little research to support this, though. In fact, **the research showed** that there was questionable value to testing. Results of the "studies" were mixed – one of them found that the death rate from breast cancer declined and *the other found it increased!*

The National Cancer Institute's director, Dr. Richard D. Klausner, said, "the data are complex, and different groups have different standards of evidence." To a *Life-Systems* Engineer this answer is unacceptable. There is only one standard – **the test either helps or it doesn't**. There was a supposed 17-percent reduction in death rate for the age-50 group, yet "it was difficult to detect with a high level of certainty." This 17-percent reduction "was derived by combining data from studies that were not truly comparable."[32] Here again is a possible misinterpretation of a clinical study.

The American people have extraordinary will power and try very hard to do what they are told, especially if it is from an authority. And this is the problem with misinformation. We mistakenly do the wrong thing over and over.

---

32 "Same Data, 3 Different Mammogram Recommendations," Gina Kolata, *New York Times* (internet edition) March 28, 1997, picked up April 1, 1997.

Here's an example of how well we are conditioned to obey authority unquestioningly. *Influence: The Psychology of Persuasion* gives the following example:

> To twenty-two separate nurses' stations in various hospital units, a researcher made an identical phone call identifying himself as a hospital physician and directed the answering nurse to give twenty milligrams of Astrogen to a specific patient. There were four reasons the nurse should not have administered this drug:
> (1) The prescription was transmitted only by telephone, a direct violation of hospital policy;
> (2) The medication was unauthorized; the drug was not on the ward's accepted drug list;
> (3) The dosage was obviously and dangerously excessive because it was stated on the container that the "maximum daily dose" was 10 milligrams. Double this maximum dose was ordered!
> (4) The so-called "physician" was someone whom the nurse had never seen, directly spoken with, met, or even spoken with on the telephone before.

Yet, in 95-percent of all calls, the nurses attempted to administer the drug before the researcher stopped them! Even against all reason, we tend to unquestionably do what the "voice of authority" requests even if it makes no sense or is dangerous.[33]

We reviewed an article, on the internet, titled "Fatty Acid," which mentioned a "Nurses' Health Study," based on 85,000 women. The study reportedly showed a positive correlation between consumption of transfatty acid (a form of distorted EFA) and increased heart disease:

1. The conclusion was that *transfatty acids accounted for virtually all the increased risk* of heart-related problems.
2. The article then went on to say that "... the total amount of fat in the diet is still more important than the contribution made by transfatty acids to heart disease."

Statement 2. in the article completely contradicts statement 1. Although an internet article without numerous references cannot

33 *Influence: The Psychology of Persuasion*, Robert B. Cialdini, Ph.D., William Morrow and Company, New York, 1993, pages 224-225.

always be relied on, this one illustrates a common type of inconsistent logic we have seen throughout these statistical reports.

Nutritional advice is frequently based on clinical studies and statistical analysis. It is crucial for you to know the truth about how research is conducted, summarized, and presented.

In the book, *Fats that Heal: Fats that Kill*, Udo Erasmus states: "Don't trust the 'experts' too much. They have an annoying tendency to generalize from the limited to the infinite. There is some truth to what they find, but their information must be kept in context."[34]

In *Rats, Drugs, and Assumptions*, by Majid Ali, M.D., the doctor cites two examples of studies reported in the prestigious *New England Journal of Medicine*. The first study called a mere 0.19-percent (approximately 1/5 of one-percent) reduction in the rate of heart attacks with a certain drug, a "44-percent reduction in risk" (*New England J Med* 321:129; 1989).

The second study presented an actual 1.4-percent reduction in the rate of heart attack as a "34-percent risk reduction" (*New England J Med* 317:1241; 1987).

How can this be? Did the journal lie? Well, not exactly. *Just because the reader assumes a clinical journal will be accurate with statistics doesn't make it so.* Here's how Dr. Ali's proper application of statistical measurement uncovered the deception:

The first study was the basis for the "aspirin-a-day" prescription for preventing heart attack from myocardial infarction (restricted blood flow which causes a shortage of oxygen to the heart).

In this study there were about 255 heart attacks per 100,000 people[35] taking the drug compared with about 440 per 100,000 not taking the drug.[36] It's reported that one hundred forty-five (145) fewer people had heart attacks taking the drug, but what does this really mean?

34 *Fats That Heal, Fats that Kill*, Udo Erasmus, Alive Books, Burnaby, BC, Canada, 1993, page 314.

35 There were far fewer than 100,000 people in the study. This was an interpolated result.

36 *Rats, Drugs, and Assumptions*, Majid Ali, M.D., Life Span Press, Denville, NJ, 1995, pages 96-102.

We must realize that the number of heart attacks in the no-drug group was extremely small to begin with – just 0.44-percent (4.4 attacks per thousand).

With the drug there is a 0.25-percent (2.5 per thousand) chance of heart attack, and without the drug there is a slightly larger 0.44-percent chance. The two figures (percentages) are then subtracted. So the drug is just 0.19-percent effective. Not 19-percent, not one-percent, but *less than one fourth* of one-percent. This is insignificant from a statistical analysis.

Why not use (0.44-0.25)/0.44 = about 43-percent as the measurement? After all, isn't this the formula for percent of decrease? Simple – you don't take a percentage of a percentage. It just doesn't give a meaningful result. Never has, and never will.[37] The difference between one-percent (one out of a hundred) and two-percent (two out of a hundred) is one-percent (one out of a hundred). It's not one out of two or 50-percent. You subtract the two results. The authors of *Basic Medical Biochemistry* (page 109) understand this concept.

Don't feel bad if you missed this. Even *Consumer Reports On Health* reported the forty-percent figure in 1997. So did the *New York Times*, also in 1997.[38] This study was conducted back in 1988. The journalists either failed to research the actual data themselves, simply repeating the incorrectly reported summary, or they didn't understand how to correctly interpret the data.

Based on these mis-stated summaries, many nutrition books rave about how great aspirin is in preventing heart attacks and strokes. *The aspirin group got more strokes.* This fact did not get a headline. Either way, they are giving you the wrong idea of aspirin's effectiveness based on this study.

This repeating of one publication by another is how incorrect information sweeps across the country. In this example, even nine years later, the results are still being incorrectly reported! Can everybody be wrong? YES. Now you see why *Life-Systems* Engineers dislike careless reporting so intensely.

---

37 Nor can you simply take the difference as a percentage of the drug vs. non-drug death rates expressed as a percent (440-255)/440 = 33-percent. This doesn't take sample size into account. If we could use this method, then, 440 deaths out of 440 people would be no different than 440 deaths out of 100,000 people. Of course, it is much different.

38 "Study Finds Apparent Trigger Of Heart Attacks And Strokes," *New York Times*, April 3, 1997, A13.

The entire field of probability and statistics is based on understanding sample size.

Most studies ignore the sample size. A new "technical term," called, "endpoints," was even created to make it appear legitimate.

The second study actually showed that raising HDL cholesterol and simultaneously lowering LDL cholesterol with a drug was not at all effective for stopping coronary heart disease.

In this case, there were 56 heart attacks (about 27 per 1,000 people) in the drug test group and 84 heart attacks (about 42 per 1,000 people) in the non-drug group. There were 2,000 patients in each group. This was a terrible result. The group taking the drug suffered more deaths from coronary heart disease during the five-year period of measurement! The effectiveness is 4.2-percent minus 2.7-percent = 1.5-percent decrease in heart attacks with the drug. Although the drug may have helped a little, it certainly wasn't very effective.

A small fortune is often spent by pharmaceutical companies to develop, test, and approve their creations. They want the drug dispensed by physicians. So that results such as this aren't in full and obvious view of the reader, studies often either bury the raw data in the middle of a lengthy article, never include the raw data at all, or talk about something sounding similar yet altogether different! The journals often manipulate the data.

The physicians, because they are so busy, may often read only the headline, and we, the poor patients, pay a heavy price being subjected to costly, and often ineffective, or possibly harmful medications.

What patient would be satisfied with just a one- or two-percent improvement from an expensive drug that may even cause severe side-effects? Almost no one – no matter how desperate!

Nowadays, slanted articles are routinely purchased, often without the magazine editors even knowing it. "The practice of buying editorials reflects the growing influence of the pharmaceutical industry on medical care."[39] Some physicians reading these

39 *New England Journal of Medicine* 331:674; 1994.

publications don't know that they are being duped. Do they lose out? Yes, a little. But you and I surely do – paying for costly drugs with possible harmful side-effects and questionable benefit.

Here's an example of a classic use of "experts." Many years ago a major candy bar manufacturer claimed that eating their candy bars was better for you than eating apples. Given the information in this chapter, you may now be in a position to figure out the method used along with its techniques of deception.

1. A "scientific clinical study" was done showing that eating apples is bad for your teeth. This is easy to establish because, if left for a few days, apple stuck between your teeth will feed the bacteria that forms the plaque, causing erosion of enamel.
2. Chocolate dissolves in saliva, so any chocolate on the teeth doesn't last for long.
3. The lack of nutritional value in the candy bar was ignored.
4. Arrangements were made for a retired physician to give a stamp of approval to the desired conclusion.
5. The story was released to selected newspapers, magazines, radio and television stations as a *news item*. The word was spread across America efficiently, and without the expense of a big advertising campaign.

Although this type of conclusion seems absurd, the conclusion went unchallenged for quite a while. It caught everyone off guard. It was finally stopped when it was discovered that the candy bar manufacturer financed the study.

Proper analysis of cause-effect relationships isn't limited to nutrition. Here's a cooking example you may find useful.

Cooking in a cast iron pan is superior to cooking in aluminum or stainless steel pans. It is a well-established fact that a heavy cast iron pan is superior for pan grilling and frying – especially frying chicken, hamburgers and pork chops.

But why is it better? Most people will say that, because cast iron is so heavy, it retains the heat better, so the oil stays hotter when the food is placed in it.

This is incorrect. Heat is constantly supplied to any pan by the burner. As long as the same amount of oil is used in each pan, once the oil is brought to proper temperature, there can't be a significant difference in the amount of heat. The reason for the superiority is the *higher radiant heat emission* from the cast iron. The molecular structure of cast iron causes the heat waves to be more efficiently transferred into the food. Other metals don't have as high *radiant* heating ability.

If I didn't take this fact into account, I might conclude that we should make stainless steel or aluminum pans thicker. That wouldn't help at all. The heat transfer superiority comes from the material itself.

I'm not the only one perturbed over the sloppiness, erroneous product claims, and misleading conclusions. In the July 1996 issue of *Cosmetics & Toiletries* magazine, Ken Klein, president of Cosmetec Laboratories, Inc., addresses this topic.

> Q: What problems crop up because of marketing's love affair with jargon?
>
> A: We scientists need to make sure marketing keeps at least some semblance of scientific truth in the package copy.
>
> "**Natural**" may be the most overused/misused word in our business ... From this chemist's perspective, *anything made from the first 92 elements in the periodic table is natural.*
>
> **Fragrance-free:** What does this mean? Nothing! The word "fragrance" has been replaced by the names of individual fragrance ingredients.
>
> **Hypoallergenic:** This claim implies greater mildness and safety than usual, but the FDA says that hypoallergenic means whatever the marketer wants it to mean. How is that for meaningless? (FDA web page http:\\\www.fda.gov).

Are studies based on rats and mice meaningful?

Life-Systems Engineering recognizes the vast metabolic differences between animals and humans. Our answer is that one must be extremely cautious when applying animal results to humans, as we saw in the widely publicized case of the leptin receptor. **Animals had one result; people had the opposite!**

Two highly distinguished physicians, Dr. Neal D. Bernard (President of the Physicians Committee for Responsible Medicine) and Dr. Stephen R. Kaufman (Co-chair of the Medical Research

Modernization Committee) published an article titled, "Animal Research Is Wasteful and Misleading." [40]

> Many of the apparent anomalies seen in animal experiments, however, merely reflect the unique biology of the species being studied, the unnatural means by which the disease was induced or the stressful environment of the laboratory. Such irregularities are irrelevant to human pathology, and testing hypotheses derived from these observations wastes considerable time and money.
>
> ...Evolutionary pressures have resulted in innumerable, subtle, but significant differences between species.... A stimulus applied to one particular organ system perturbs the animal's overall physiological functioning in a myriad of ways.... Such uncertainty severely undermines the extrapolation of animal data to other species, including humans.
>
> ...Important medical advances have been delayed because of misleading results derived from animal experiments. David Wiebers and his colleagues at the Mayo Clinic, writing in the journal *Stroke* in 1990, described a study showing that, of the 25 compounds that reduced damage from ischemic stroke [caused by lack of blood to the brain] in rodents, cats, and other animals, none proved efficacious in human trials.
>
> ...David Salsburg of Pfizer Central Research has noted that, of 19 chemicals known to cause cancer in humans when ingested, only seven caused cancer in rats and mice using the standards set by the National Cancer Institute.
>
> ...Indeed, many substances that appeared safe in animal studies and received approval from the U.S. Food and Drug Administration for use in humans later proved dangerous to people.... The antiviral drug fialuridine seemed safe in animal trials yet caused liver failure in seven of fifteen humans taking the drug (five of these patients died as a result) ....
>
> These frightening mistakes are not mere anecdotes. The U.S. General Accounting Office reviewed 198 of the 209 new drugs marketed between 1976 and 1985 and found that **54-percent had "serious postapproval risks" not predicted by animal tests or limited human trials....**

40 "Animal Research Is Wasteful and Misleading," Neal D. Bernard, M.D. and Stephen R. Kaufman, M.D., *Scientific America*, internet version, April 1997.

> Research into the causes of birth defects has relied heavily on animal experiments, but these have typically proved to be embarrassingly poor predictors of what can happen in humans....
>
> Animal "models" are, at best, analogous to human conditions, but no theory can be proved or refuted by analogy. Thus, **it makes no logical sense to base a theory about humans using animals**. Nevertheless, *when scientists debate the validity of competing theories in medicine and biology, they often cite animal studies as evidence*. (emphasis added)

In the late 1950s and 1960s, even thalidomide didn't produce the number and severity of birth defects in animals as it did in humans.

Producing *Life-Systems* results requires a new understanding

One of the reasons that Thomas Edison, holder of more than 1,000 patents (including the electric light), was so successful was his lack of regard for popular opinion. He possessed a never-ending drive to discover what worked – regardless of what others thought. Even though he possessed no formal education, **Edison relentlessly chided his college-educated colleagues that their schooling had led them to see only "that which they were taught to look for.**" He felt many of nature's greatest secrets could be too easily overlooked because of narrow-mindedness.[41]

Modern science is often too occupied with control. This focus may work well in non-living systems; however, living systems don't always obey the same rules as non-living systems. In living systems, Mother Nature has provided natural, automatic control mechanisms. (They are not meant to be tampered with.)

Life-Systems Engineering principles are consistent with Mr. Edison's philosophy. Here's an example of how far we have fallen from reality in our desire to find a drug-related solution to our obesity problem.

"Look at the larger picture of infectious agents' causing chronic diseases," said Dr. Benjamin Caballero of Johns Hopkins University. He was referring to recent discoveries that viruses and bacteria may contribute to heart disease, some cancers and ulcers.

---

41 "Unlocking the Legacies of the Edison Archives," Seth Shulman, *MIT's Technology Review*, February/March, 1997, pages 42-51.

"I have no reason to believe obesity would be any different," he said.[42] But is he looking in the wrong place? He doesn't indicate that he is aware of any virus or bacteria directly leading to obesity.

Analysis Example:

Here's an article from *Bottom Line - Personal,* dated August 1, 1997. The article is based on the study of Walter Willett, M.D., at Harvard.[43] It reads, *"Risk of diabetes is lowered by eating a high-fiber diet."* It goes on to state that "Women who ate plenty of fiber-rich cereals, whole-grain breads, beans and brown rice were less likely to develop adult-onset diabetes. Those who consumed more sugars and processed starches – such as colas, white bread, white rice, and potatoes – were at greater risk. Another study has found a similar effect in men. In the body, these high-risk foods are converted to glucose, which raises blood sugar. This, in turn, causes a release of insulin. Over time, the body is unable to produce enough insulin, thus triggering diabetes."

Insulin and diabetes have been fully explored in this book. However, we now understand enough about statistical studies and their findings to ask serious questions. When a magazine provides only a summary of research, it's impossible to tell whether the magazine was accurate or inaccurate about what the researcher stated and whether the researcher was accurate in analyzing the findings.

Let's look at this from a *Life-Systems* Engineering perspective:

1. We are only given the relative words "less likely," and "greater risk." No absolute numbers are stated. A red flag should immediately signal you not to automatically believe everything the article concludes. In a study such as this, levels of significance are very important.

2. Based on the article, the reader may get the mistaken impression that complex carbohydrates are not broken down into glucose – stimulating insulin. All carbohydrates, when digested, are converted to glucose by the body.

42 "Virus May Raise Chance of Obesity for Some," *New York Times*, April 8, 1997, page B10.

43 Dr. Willett is professor of epidemiology and nutrition, Harvard School of Public Health, Boston. The article is based on his study of 65,000 women, published in the *Journal of the American Medical Association.*

3. What exactly are these "fiber-rich" foods listed in the article (cereals, whole-grain breads, beans and brown rice) – It's never discussed. Although they contain complex carbohydrates, the reader may get the impression that they are something else.
4. How much carbohydrate was consumed before diabetes was triggered?
5. How long did it take for diabetes to commence?
6. We can't keep people in controlled environments, so we should ask, "What other factors and foods, along with the fiber differences, were involved in triggering the diabetes?"
7. What does "plenty" of high-fiber mean – four ounces a day, half-pound a day or even more?
8. What timespan was used in this study? It is never addressed.
9. Think about how difficult it would be to record 65,000 people's food choices. Do you believe what people said they ate? Why should you? How were their choices recorded? Again, very important information is lacking.

Should you believe everything that an abbreviated article such as this concludes? No *Life-Systems* Engineer would, because *too many important pieces of information are left unanswered.* Generally, articles unaccompanied by the actual raw data and not specifically telling the reader the *assumptions* used, can't be relied on for any conclusions.

The article *looked* impressive. It was found in a national newsletter and based on a Harvard physician's studies. The M.D. has an impressive position at a prestigious university. And it was based on 65,000 people – a huge number. Do any of these make the newsletter's summary more reliable? No, not at all. In fact, as we're beginning to see, from a *Life-Systems* Engineering perspective, the newsletter's or physician's conclusions may not make sense.

Diabetes may be induced by overloading on any carbohydrates – simple or complex.

Always remember,

> **"... Theories, no matter how pertinent, cannot eradicate the existence of facts."**
> Jean Martin Charcot

Richard Feynman, a Nobel prize-winning physicist, in his November 1964 "Messenger Lectures" at Cornell University, provides us with some useful guidelines.

Anyone involved in presenting research conclusions should be required to read the following passage no less than three times.

> The most reasonable possibilities often turn out not to be the situation. If science is to progress, what we need is the ability to experiment, honesty in reporting results – the results must be reported without somebody saying what they would like the results to have been – and finally – an important thing – the intelligence to interpret the results.
>
> An important point about this intelligence is that *it should not be sure, ahead of time, what must be*. It can be prejudiced and say, "That is very unlikely; I do not like that." Prejudice is different from absolute certainty. Then we compare the result of the computation to nature, with experiment, or experience, compare it directly with observation, to see if it works. If it disagrees with [our] experiment, it is wrong. In that simple statement is the key to science.
>
> ... It does not make any difference how beautiful your guess is. It does not make any difference how smart you are, who made the guess, or what his name is – **if it disagrees with experiment it is wrong**. That is all there is to it.
>
> It is truc that one has to check a little to make sure that it is not wrong, because whoever did the experiment may have reported incorrectly ...
>
> ... There is always the possibility of proving any definite theory wrong; but notice, you can never prove it right. It is simply not wrong.
>
> ... Physics and chemistry cannot distinguish between natural beet sugar molecules and synthesized sugar molecules made

from carbon dioxide and water. Sugar is a complicated molecule. If you make exactly the same arrangement except substituting left as right, then for a phenomenon not involving life, they are precisely the same. Living creatures find a difference. Remarkably, bacteria eat one kind, the natural variety – but not the other.

Simple bacteria know the difference between the natural beet sugar and the man-made creation.

... It is scientific only to say what is more likely and what is less likely, and not to be *proving all the time* the possible and the impossible."

... **Living creatures don't always obey the same laws as inanimate things**."

"For a successful technology, reality must take precedence over public relations, for **Nature cannot be fooled**." [44] – Richard Feynman, Nobel Prize-winner

"*The point is to get it right*, not to win the case, not to sweep under the rug all the assorted puzzles and inconsistencies that frequently occur in collections of data."[45] An article titled "Damned Liars and Expert Witnesses," discusses the difficulty of ensuring that those who provide the data don't have hidden agendas.[46]

Doesn't this sum up perfectly why the results of the great carbohydrate experiment have been so catastrophic? *Mother Nature cannot be fooled.* By learning how she works, and **cooperating with her**, we can accomplish desired results. This is the definition of *Life-Systems* Engineering. If Professor Feynman were alive today, he'd probably give the new field a gold star.

Before publishing their studies, nutritional researchers should understand these concepts that Dr. Feynman stated. When you see the next wonder product or diet program promoted, you'll know better what questions to ask before automatically jumping on the bandwagon.

---

44 *Visual Explanations*, page 53.
45 *Visual Explanations*, page 32.
46 "Damned Liars and Expert Witnesses," Paul Meier, *Journal of the American Statistical Association*, 81 (1986), pages 269-276. Also see "*Statisticians Econometricians, and Adversary Proceedings*," Franklin M. Fisher, pages 277-286.

The STAT-SMART analytical tool, for understanding studies.

This is a summary of the primary STAT-SMART aspects that will help you analyze published conclusions for yourself.

1. Does the conclusion make any logical or scientific sense?
2. Does the evidence support a cause-effect relationship? That is, does the evidence support the given conclusion?
3. Does the conclusion account for all possible factors that could influence the conclusion?
4. Does the statistical information given include the sample size and selection of the sample tested? A test based on only ten people probably won't mean much, unless all of them got the same results.
5. Does the conclusion include the sample size or does it disregard the sample size? Just publishing the "end-points" in its stated effectiveness is misleading. Recall, the difference between one-percent and two-percent is not 50-percent, as suggested by the *endpoint method.* The actual difference is only one-percent!
6. Will the proposed solution cause other unforeseen problems? (ie., in the process of "curing" disease A, disease B was induced)
7. How many of the original study's participants dropped out because of bad side-effects? Were they included in the "failure rate?" Allowing failures to drop out before the study is complete and not counting them as failures is misleading.
8. Did the study *really* measure what you *thought* was measured? For example, women are routinely diagnosed with breast cancer tumors when there are only scattered non-malignant abnormal cells (no continuous tumorous cells growing together). "Ductal carcinoma in situ" (DCIS) is *mis*used to imply a woman has breast tumors when she doesn't. Therefore, the "cure rate" is drastically inflated because there was no disease to "cure" to begin with! This fact comes from wrong conclusions based on mamograms.
9. Does real life experience confirm the result?

Surprise:

Dr.William Campbell Douglass' *Second Opinion* newsletter warned us that the PSA prostate cancer test was wrong 2/3 of the time (66% FALSE POSITIVEs). You don't have prostate cancer, but the test says that you do have prostate cancer. The test was SUPPOSED to reduce prostate cancer rates by 69%.

However, a re-evaluation of the PSA test by physicians at the European Institute of Oncology paints a different picture!*

* *Dr. William Campbell Douglass' Second Opinion*, Vol. IX, No.3, March 1999.

Ref. *Lancet*, 1998; 351:1563.

Surprise! Carbohydrates are aldehyde or *ketone* compounds...[47]

Some members of the medical community refuse to acknowledge established medical research showing the critical importance of ketones throughout the body. They continue propagating the high carbohydrate theory in spite of its detrimental effects. This is an excellent example of inadequate understanding of how the body works.

You Need To Know This:

Your body needs the ketones produced from running on your own bodyfat.

They are normal and important.

For example, your heart and kidneys prefer ketones to glucose! So do your skeletal muscles. It may take a few weeks for your body to adjust to running on the fuel Mother Nature designed – your own bodyfat – instead of being forced to run on sugar (carbohydrates).

Sources: *Protein Power* – Michael Eades, M.D. and Mary Dan Eades M.D., referring to *Biochemistry* (fourth edition), Dr. Lubert Stryer, Professor of Biochemistry, Stanford University, *Biochemistry* – Dr. Donald Voet and Dr. Judith Voet; *Textbook of Medical Physiology* (ninth edition)

Typically, before ketosis (leading to ketoacidosis), low blood pH could ever become a problem, your respiration would substantially increase to almost double your normal breathing rate, in an effort to stabilize blood pH (make it more alkaline). Only after *3-4 days of virtually complete starvation* (fasting) do ketones become significant. *Even after 5 weeks* of starvation, blood glucose levels only drop to 65 mg/dl! (normal is 70-90 mg/dl). In addition, your renal rystem "kicks in" to stabilize your system. There are 3 *Life-Systems* at work: respiratory, circulatory buffer system, and the renal (excretory) system. Often, there is a lack of insight into how the various *Life-Systems* work together. Sufficient salt is required for the circulatory buffer system to work properly — lack of salt means lack of sodium bicarbonate ($NaHCO_3$) — a fundamental *Life-System* component that Mother Nature requires.*

47 *Biochemistry*, page 463.

* *Body Fluids And Electrolytes*, pages 93, 99; *Basic Medical Biochemistry,* page 369.

Three Rs of Radiant Living

Radiant Health

Your doorway to living *Beyond The Zone* will swing wide open with 7 simple keys to Radiant Health. You feel good, and you feel good about yourself, too. This allows you to build powerful relationships.

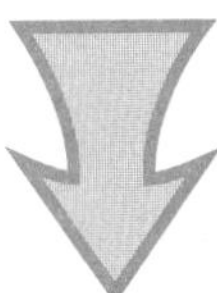

Relationships

When you radiate positive energy, you maximize your ability to attract and sustain loving relationships. Loving relationships are the foundation of our emotional needs. Without loving relationships our attention is continually distracted away from other goals, such as building a better income. With established loving relationships you are empowered to concentrate on generating abundant revenue.

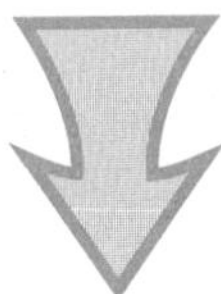

Revenue

Radiating positive energy enhances your career. Money is packaged energy. The more energy you have, the more money you can generate.

When Marcus Conyers asks people across the country, "What do you want out of life?" more than 95% of people say, "I just want to be happy."

These three R's can be the fast track on your road to sustained happiness. When you have radiant health, you have boundless energy, your body is lean, and you feel good about yourself. You radiate a positive energy that is very attractive to the people around you, including the opposite gender. This boundless energy can be channeled into the second R, your relationships.

When you're brimming with boundless energy, your mood will tend to be more positive, making you more attractive and fun to be around. Nobody enjoys a low-energy "nega-holic."

Think about it. When do you snap at the people you care about? That's right – it's when your energy level is low. When single people achieve radiant health, they find themselves becoming much more attractive to others, because the unconscious mind is looking to select companions who are healthy.

You have seen this yourself. Some people walk into a room and radiate a positive energy that immediately attracts attention. People want to be around them. When you are enjoying radiant health, and you are already in a relationship, you'll have more energy to share with your partner, which in turn will boost the quality of your relationship. This leads to the third R, revenue.

When you have boundless energy, and your relationships are going well, what happens to your ability to perform at work? That's right, it's dramatically increased.

And in business, positive energy is more than a terrific advantage, it's almost everything! For example, if you walk into a store intending to buy a pair of jeans, and you already know what size, style, color, and price you plan to buy. As you go to select your jeans, you notice that the sales people in the store have negative attitudes. What would you do? Marcus has asked this question in his seminars, and thousands of people have responded in the same way. Most would walk out of that store.

He then asks them, "Do you ever walk into a store not intending to buy anything, but the personnel are so positive and energized, that you walk out with loads of stuff? Once again, thousands of hands went up in agreement.

When it comes to a job interview, research shows that, very often, you are hired or not hired within the first few minutes of starting the interview. Largely, it's the level of positive energy you project that will determine whether you are hired. As Marcus works with organizations around the world, the first training he does is to teach people skills for sustaining positive energy. This is the single most important factor at succeeding in business and generating more revenue for you and your company.

Those individuals he's worked with, earning over $200,000 per year, consistently display one attribute more than any other – their ability to sustain positive energy.

When you are drawing on a strong foundation of radiant health, there is no limit in terms of the revenue that you can generate.

> "Your future can improve dramatically once you have radiant health – because radiant living is based on having radiant health first. The Seven Keys To Radiant Health are the basis for improving your relationships and your revenue, too."
>
> Marcus Conyers - Peak Performance Consultant

> **"Health is a state of complete physical, mental, and social well-being and not merely the absence of disease or infirmity."**
>
> World Health Organization

Imagine being lean for life, brimming with boundless energy, able to accelerate through your day with laser-sharp concentration and a steel-trap memory.

This is what life is like when you combine peak performance and radiant health. This is living *Beyond The Zone*. This state of peak enjoyment is sustained when you run on your body's ideal fuel – your own bodyfat, made possible when you:

- Nourish your body with nutrients it can't make itself, including healthy oils and minerals.
- Detoxify yourself with Essiac-concept tonic.
- Focus your mind on what's useful, positive, and healthy.

There are seven keys that help unlock your natural ability to experience radiant health. These seven keys helped Marcus to: lose more than 20 pounds of excess bodyfat in 10 weeks, give him the energy to consistently work 60-hour or more work weeks – conducting 150 seminars for thousands of people, co-writing two books, and appearing on numerous television and radio shows – all with plenty of energy left over for an active social life. He no longer suffers from exhaustion, food cravings or excess weight.

No less important, these seven keys are easy to use and they can increase the pleasure and quality of your life.

7 Keys to Radiant Health

Reduce

consumption of processed carbohydrates and sugar.

Add

healthy essential oils and essential minerals to your diet.

Detoxify

your system by removing the toxins.

Inspire

more of your thoughts to be healthy, positive and useful.

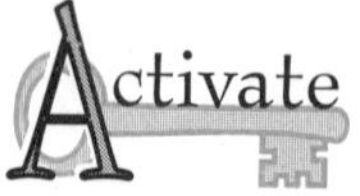

Activate

new ways to provide enjoyable, moderate exercise.

Nourish

your body with high quality protein, along with with fresh fruits and vegetables, in addition to essential oils and minerals.

Take Timeout

for relaxation each day to reduce the effects of stress.

SR

Minimize consumption of processed carbohydrates and sugar.

"No carbohydrate is required in the diet .... It has been shown experimentally that human beings can survive for months on a diet of meat and fats."

Phillip Bondy, M.D., Chairman, Department of Internal Medicine, Yale University

Despite this fact, sugar consumption has increased from 4 pounds per person annually in 1750 to 160 pounds per person annually by 1990. (Source: University of Iowa)

Excess carbohydrates are converted to fat and stop you from accessing your body's best fuel – your own bodyfat. (Source: Textbook of Medical Physiology)

Excess carbohydrates reduce your brain's capacity to think and concentrate. Your brain uses 2/3 of the circulating glucose. Insulin quickly pulls sugar out of your bloodstream, and stores it as fat. Your brain, sensing a resulting energy shortage, sends the neurotransmitter signal to "*Eat More Now.*"

Many business professionals feel drowsy after a typical lunch. Dr. Judith Wurtman, of M.I.T., showed that excessive carbohydrates lower performance.

Excess carbohydrates prevent release of your Fat-Mobilizing Hormone, glucagon. Without this fat-mobilizing hormone, you crave even more carbohydrates, adding more bodyfat.

Action:

- Cut back on the soda. Each cola has from 5 to 10 teaspoons of sugar. Your body doesn't want sugar swings. Artificially sweetened drinks zap your brain, making you hungry.
- Cut back on candy and other sweets.
- Back off from bagels, bread, chips, rice and pasta. A bagel is equivalent to 6 teaspoons of sugar. A serving of pasta or rice is often equivalent to 8 teaspoons of sugar.
- Curb the cravings by adding the right nutrients.

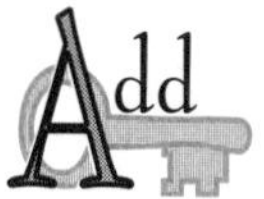

Include healthy essential oils and essential minerals in your diet.

Sixty-six percent of people die from just two conditions that involve fatty degeneration:

Cardiovascular disease – 43.8%
Cancer – 22.4%.

95% of Americans are deficient in essential oils – EFAs.
(Source: Fats That Heal, Fats That Kill)

Adding EFAs maximizes your protection against these two biggest killers.

EFAs deliver the essential nutrition you need, so carbohydrate cravings are curbed.

As you cut back on carbohydrates, you start tapping into your body's best fuel – your own bodyfat – giving you boundless energy and permanent fat loss.

Boost your brain power with EFAs. You actually think faster. EFAs make up a large proportion of your brain's white matter, so the myelin sheath increases the speed of messages inside your brain.

Add an essential mineral supplement. Your body can't make minerals, and your food no longer contains many of them in the amounts or the form your body requires. Bioavailable minerals are vital to radiant health.

Action:

- Take basic essence/EFAs 2-3 times a day.
- Take essential bioavailable minerals every day.

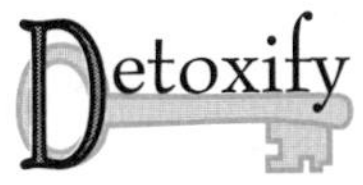

Remove toxins from your system.

Over 600,000 tons of pollutants are released every year.

Toxins disrupt proper body functions and place severe stress on numerous life-systems. This often results in ill-health and fatigue. You can't have boundless energy when toxins are zapping your energy reserves. Low energy puts a damper on your love life, too.

Municipal water supplies are often contaminated – they are not continually tested for all chemicals. Purified water is good insurance against ingesting pollutants from your water supplies.

Make sure you get enough rest each night. This helps your body remove toxins, too. You'll probably need less sleep once your body is detoxified.

President Kennedy's physician, Dr. Charles Brusch, prescribed Essiac-concept tonic to combat the negative effects of toxins. Dr. Brusch also used it himself. (Source: The Essiac Report)

The air we breathe, the water we drink, and the food we eat often contain toxins.

Your body stores toxins in its fat.

Toxins stored in fat inhibit your body's natural fat-burning process.

The best nutrition and the best supplements in the world are not enough to ensure optimum health, without a daily detoxifier.

Action:

- Take Essiac-concept tonic every day.
- Drink purified water.
- Get adequate sleep each night.

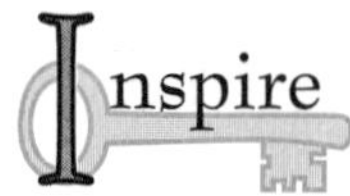

Direct more of your thoughts to be healthy, positive, and useful.

"If you want something different, you've got to do something different. What are you going to do differently today to make a positive difference in your life?"

(Russell J. Martino, President, Insight International)

You have approximately 4,000 thoughts each day. (Source: University of Minnesota) How many of those are healthy and positive?

Each thought you have has a biochemical consequence. Motivational speaker Les Brown estimates, from his research, that more than 80% of most people's self-talk is negative. 80% of 4,000 = 3,200 negative thoughts each day!

In a long-term study of Harvard graduates, optimism stood out as the primary determinant of health beginning at age 45 and continuing the next 20 years. (Source: Learned Optimism)

Low energy is a leading cause of negativity. Boost your energy level with healthy oils, minerals, and detoxification.

After 20 years of research, on over 1.1 million people, researchers have identified **4 keys to happiness**:

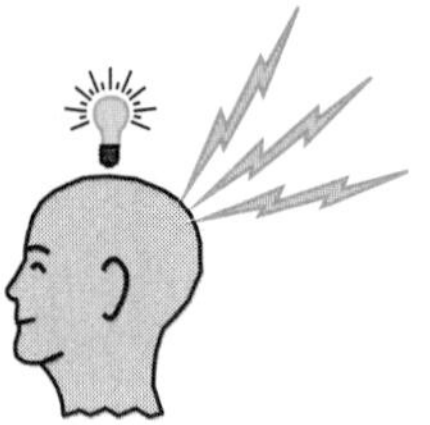

Radiant Health

High self-esteem

Feeling in control

Positive attitude

Action:

- Ask yourself positive questions daily. Two of Marcus' favorites are: WIN? What's Important Now? And what's UP? What's Useful and Positive?
- Repeat positive affirmations every day. For example, "I am now lean for life, brimming with boundless energy. I now have laser-sharp concentration and a steel- trap memory."

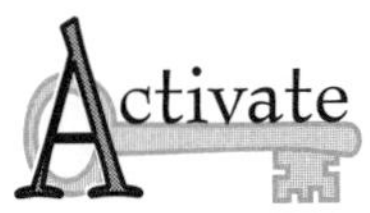

Increase enjoyable activities
that provide moderate exercise.

Moderate exercise, such as walking, can give health benefits equivalent to hours of aerobics and exercises.
(Source: Harvard Alumni Study)

The "no-pain, no-gain" myth has prevented millions of people from enjoying moderate exercise. While jogging with Stu Middleman, world record-holder for running 1,000 miles in eleven days, Marcus asked him, "What do you do when it starts to hurt?" Middleman's answer? "I slow down, because I made a mistake."

Maximum health benefits from exercise come from consistency, so you must enjoy the exercise you choose. Walking is an excellent form of exercise, as are simple things, like working around the house and yard – all of which have some level of aerobic activity.

Possibly, the best overall workout can be achieved with simple rebounding (using a small trampoline) with weights. The equipment is low-cost, takes little time, can be done year-round, and is a lot of fun, especially with your favorite music.

Using isometric exercise, putting the force of one muscle group against another, you can tone lean muscle and release more of the fat-mobilizing hormone. This takes only a few minutes per day.

Action:

- Find a mode of exercise you actively enjoy.
- Walk more often. Every little bit counts.
- Check out more information on rebounding and simple isometric exercises, with the PEAK PERFORMER.™

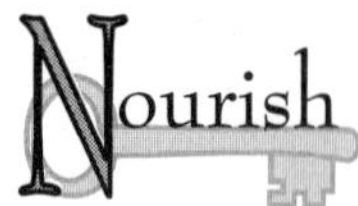

Eat plenty of high quality protein with fresh fruits and vegetables, in addition to essential oils and minerals.

"According to the studies of prominent fat researchers like Drs. William Connor, Donald Rudin, David Horrobin, Barry Sears, Udo Erasmus, and Edward Siguel, essential fats [EFAs] have proven effective in controlling, preventing, and reversing a number of disease conditions."

(Source: Beyond Pritikin)

Begin with the essentials and enjoy the enjoyables. Begin each day with essential oils, minerals, and Essiac-concept tonic. Then add high-quality dietary protein, fresh fruit and vegetables, with bread and pasta added only occasionally. Enjoy the pleasure of eating without guilt.

Ensure you get good quality sources of protein each day, including fish, eggs, meat, and vegetarian sources like cheese. This will activate your body's primary fuel – your own bodyfat.

Enjoy a healthy food balance among the healthy foods your body needs – plenty of protein, healthy oils and natural fats – but very little of the processed carbohydrates that it doesn't need.

Action:

- Begin each day with essential nutrition.
- Eat in a healthy, balanced way.
- Enjoy what you eat.

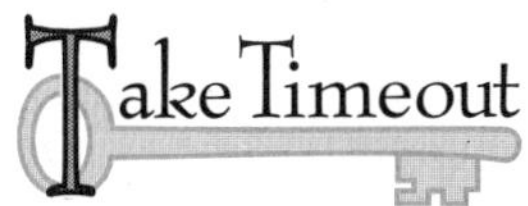

Reduce the effects of stress by taking time out for relaxation each day.

"60-90% of all doctor's office visits are stress-related...."
Herbert Benson, M.D. – Harvard Medical School

Your body's best antidote to the "fight or flight" response is relaxation, as detailed by Herbert Benson, M.D., in his book, *The Relaxation Response*.

One simple way to get relaxed is to take a "virtual vacation." This can be done in only a few minutes:

Sit in a quiet place.

Imagine a perfect vacation spot that you've been to or you'd like to go to.

Imagine it in all 5 senses. For example, if you like the beach, feel the sand beneath your feet and the sun upon your shoulders. Hear the sound of birds calling or the waves washing up on the shore. Smell and taste the salt on your lips. Smell the mouth-watering aromas from the nearby cafe.

Your brain doesn't always distinguish between what you experience and what you vividly imagine.

Get a good night's rest each night.

The Foundation of Radiant Health nutrients improves the quality of your sleep and gives you the extra energy to enjoy your personal time.

Action:

- Read *The Relaxation Respons*e, by Dr. Herbert Benson. Listen to Marcus Conyers' "Virtual Vacation Tape."
- Get the best bed you can afford. You spend more time in it than you spend in your car.
- Take time out for yourself each day. As Dr. Stephen Covey would say, "Sharpen the saw."

Introducing:

The

Radiant Health Sphere of Nutrition

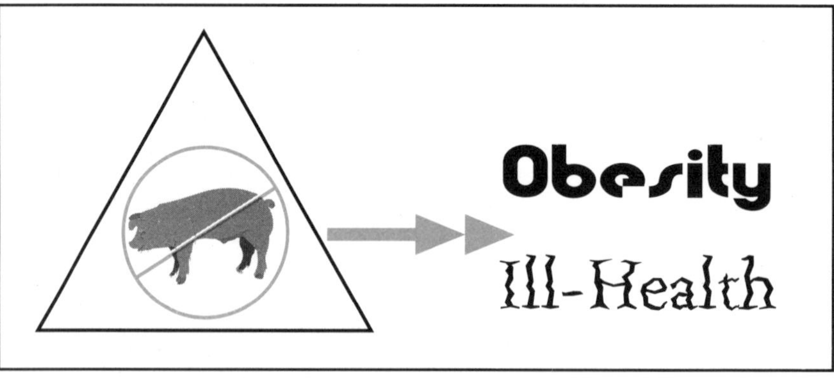

The USDA pyramid is the feedlot diet. It's what they feed hogs to fatten them. It's not appropriate for people.*

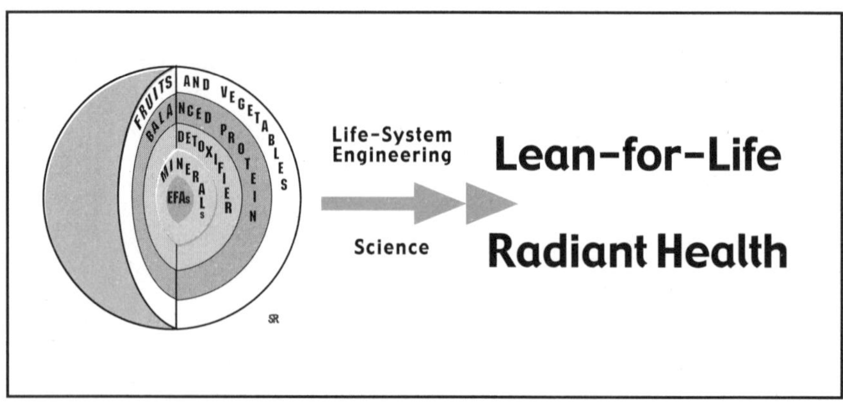

* *Self* magazine, March 1997.

Bibliography

Out of print:

Calories Don't Count, Herman Taller, M.D., Simon & Schuster, New York, 1961.

Gayelord Hauser's Treasury of Secrets, Gayelord Hauser, Farrar, Straus and Company, New York, 1963.

Martinis and Whipped Cream, Sidney Petrie, Parker Publishing, West Nyack, NY, 1966.

Magic Minerals, Carlson Wade, Parker Publishing, West Nyack, NY, 1967.

Available:

Bowes & Church's Food Values of Portions Commonly Used, Jean A. T. Pennington, Ph.D., R.D., Lippincott, New York, 1997.

Dr. Bernstein's Diabetes Solution, Richard Bernstein, M.D., Little, Brown, and Company, New York, 1997.

Enter the Zone, Barry Sears, Ph.D., HarperCollins Publishers, New York, 1995.

Exploding The Gene Myth, Ruth Hubbard, Ph.D., Beacon Press, Boston, 1993.

Fats That Can Save Your Life, Robert Erdmann, Ph.D., and Meirion Jones, Bioscience Publishing, Port Orchard, WA, 1995.

Fats that Heal, Fats that Kill (second edition), Udo Erasmus, Alive Books, Burnaby, BC, Canada, 1993.

Food That Would Last Forever, (The), Gary Gibbs, Ph.D., Avery Publishing Group, New York, 1993.

Mathematician Reads the Newspaper, (A), John Allen Paulos, Ph.D., BasicBooks, New York, 1995.

Molecular Biology of The Cell (third edition), Bruce Alberts, Ph.D.; Dennis Bray, Ph.D.; Julian Lewis, Ph.D.; Martin Raff, M.D.; Keith Roberts, Ph.D.; James D. Watson, Ph.D., Garland Publishing, New York, 1994.

Nutrition For Fitness & Sport (fourth edition), Melvin H. Williams, Ph.D., Wm. C. Brown Communications, Dubuque, IA, 1995.

Physiology Coloring Book, (The), Wynn Kapit, Robert I. Macey, Esamail Meisami, HarperCollins Publishers, New York, 1987.

Prostaglandins in the Cardiovascular System, Birkhauser Publishing, Basel, Switzerland, 1992.

Prostaglandins and Control of Vascular Smooth Muscle Cell Proliferation, edited by Karsten Schor, M.D., and Peter Ney, Ph.D., Birkhauser Publishing, Basel, Switzerland, 1996.

Protein Power, Michael Eades, M.D., Mary Dan Eades, M.D., Dell Publishing, New York, 1996.

Rats, Drugs, and Assumptions, Majid Ali, M.D., Life Span Press, Denville, NJ, 1995.

Roles of Amino Acid Chelates in Animal Nutrition, (The), H. DeWayne Ashmead, Ph.D., Noyes Publications, Park Ridge, NJ, 1993.

Sunlight, Zane R. Kime, M.D., World Health Publications, Penryn, CA, 1980.

Textbook of Medical Physiology (ninth edition), Arthur C. Guyton, M.D.; John E. Hall, Ph.D., W.B. Saunders Company, Philadelphia, 1996.

Your Body Knows Best, Ann Louise Gittleman, Simon & Schuster, New York, 1996.

Visual Explanations, Edward R. Tufte, Ph.D., Graphics Press, Cheshire, CT, 1997.

WARNING, LADIES: Most Recommendations for Hysterectomy Found Inappropriate!

Based on data collected by 9 medical groups reviewing the cases of 497 women – **76%** of the hysterectomies were **not appropriate treatment!**

Why? They noted "... failure to try **alternative treatments** ***before*** hysterectomy."

Source: *Obstet Gynecol* 2000;95:199-205

***Life-Systems* Engineering analysis:** Radiant Health is a woman's best friend when it comes to shielding against disease.

Expanding Impact – Custom Programs

After reading this book, you can now clearly see how easy it is to activate the many benefits of radiant health. Let's look ahead and consider the value of spreading radiant health into all aspects of our lives, and the lives of those around us.

You can be Beyond The Zone

The power to change your life is more solidly in your own hands than ever before. By acting on the information in this book, you will attain a new level of performance, awareness, and just plain feeling good – all the time.

Imagine what it will be like when you are seldom, if ever, "too tired." When you feel really good, accomplishment comes easily and naturally. With increased mental focus, it is easier to get things done.

Obviously, you're sincere in your desire for better health. Until now, there has been confusion regarding what to do and what not to do, to achieve better health.

The Nobel Prize-winning discoveries in this book clarify the confusion and illuminate the path to radiant health.

There is no better time to start on the road to radiant health than right now.

See Appendix B for full information on sources of products.

Spiritual Power from Beyond The Zone

Your body is your transformer – your connection – between the spiritual and physical. When the body is not operating at its very best, the spiritual connection suffers. By contrast, when your body is working with peak performance, your spiritual connection greatly improves.

Imagine how high your spirit can soar when your body is glowing with new-found radiant health. The Foundation of Radiant Health can help answer two prayers:

1. As you achieve higher energy, become lean for life, and enjoy better overall health, your energy and focus for spiritual growth increases.
2. The Foundation of Radiant Health can also play a role in providing additional funding for your spiritual organization.

Physicians working Beyond The Zone

The Foundation of Radiant Health is the ideal cornerstone of preventative medicine. As a doctor, your focus can shift more from treating symptoms to maintaining good health.

This shift in perspective gives doctors the opportunity to concentrate on methods of maintaining health, building stronger relationships with patients, and expanding more into preventative medicine.

Nutrition Counselors helping others live Beyond The Zone

Of all the people who read this book, the greatest responsibility rests with the persons to whom the public turns for nutritional guidance and answers – Nutrition Counselors. They are in an ideal position to share this information and make maximum impact, with the greatest number of people in the shortest period of time!

With the Nobel Prize-winning research detailed in this book, you will be equipped with a new level of understanding, far surpassing other programs and products. *Knowing how the body works, so that we can work with it to achieve truly radiant health*, is positively the most exciting nutritional development of this century.

The results will speak for themselves; your clients will benefit from a professional who can objectively guide them through the stages of improvement.

Health Care Organizations & HMOs move Beyond The Zone

Dramatically improve the fiscal health of your HMO. Healthy clients equals contained costs for HMOs. The Foundation of Radiant Health puts operating costs on a diet.

Healthier members mean less expense per member with fewer routine treatments. Members can look forward to fewer catastrophic illnesses, with increased immunity to disease, unparalleled cardiovascular protection and cancer prevention. Faster recuperation from surgical procedures means shorter hospital stays.

When the health of members improves, operating costs plunge while revenue remains constant. This means more profit. Lower costs also allow more competitive rates, which lead to more business, leading to even more profit.

Cost analysis have demonstrated that every $1 spent on prevention saves $4 to $6 in treatment costs! Until now, we haven't known how to make prevention work consistently in a way that makes a big difference in containing health care costs. Now we do, with the Foundation of Radiant Health.

Business Beyond The Zone

Imagine you and your employees brimming with energy, full of enthusiasm, and operating at peak performance levels all day long.

When your employees are living Beyond The Zone, they will have higher energy and better health, which means greater productivity, better attitude, and fewer sick days.

The average company loses 20% of its customers each year because of poor customer service. Imagine the increase in customer retention when your customer service representatives feel great every day, all day long.

Business managers can look forward to lower health care costs, too – especially important for self-insured groups.

How would you like your company to experience:

Healthier employees with better attitudes
Lower operating costs
Greater productivity
A reputation for genuinely caring about employees.

Education Beyond The Zone

Imagine classrooms around the nation filled with calm, attentive students, eager to learn. Imagine an environment ideal for teaching.

Teachers, when you are operating Beyond The Zone, you will feel better and work more effectively. When your students are Beyond The Zone, they will bring to your classroom less disruptive behavior, more focus and attention and fewer discipline problems. You will have an improved learning atmosphere.

Eliminate sugar lows leading to lack of attention. Enjoy natural calmness that makes studying easier. Laser-sharp concentration results in higher test scores and better performance.

A Nation Beyond The Zone

As a nation, we are weakened by fatigue, poor health, stress and lack of focus. The Department of Health and Human Services, in the U.S., states that a staggering 13.6% of our GNP is spent on health care – almost one-seventh of the total output. An average of $3,759 was spent on health care for every American in 1996. And it's getting worse each year.

Greater personal energy and sharper mental focus overcome apathy and decline. A nation Beyond The Zone can potentially save billions of dollars in health care expenditures as it maximizes protection against cardiovascular disease, cancer and infections. Reduce food requirements nationwide, and increase personal productivity.

Now imagine our entire nation filled with people enjoying the luxury of radiant health: more smiles, more accomplishments, more energy, all leading to a new level of vibrancy and achievement. As radiant health spreads from coast-to-coast, it will make our great nation an even better place to live and raise our families.

Just think of all the wonderful things we can achieve with the entire nation filled with radiant health.

A World View Beyond The Zone

According to the World Health Organization's 1996 report, heart-disease, cancer, and infection are the top killers in virtually every nation. And their casualties keep increasing. How much of the world's GNP goes toward health care?

How much of the fighting and quarreling between peoples and nations is related to hunger and poor health? What kind of world might we have if everyone was operating with all the benefits of radiant health?

How much more easily could we all work together with better mental clarity and focus?

Food supplies become more abundant when overall appetites are reduced by 30-50 percent.

In short, our entire world can benefit greatly as it starts operating Beyond The Zone.

Radiant Health Supplements and Products

Radiant Health:

For Radiant Health products, endorsed by Life-Systems Engineer Brian Peskin, contact:

United States:

Maximum Efficiency Products
2020 Naomi Street
Houston, Texas 77054
USA
Toll-free: 888-432-0001
Tel: 713-796-2431
Fax: 713-796-9770
Web site:
www.radianthealth.org

UK and Europe:

The Best of Health
Strathclyde Medical Park, Unit 7,
Mallard Way,
Bellshire, Lanarkshire ML4 3BF
SCOTLAND
Tel: +44 (0) 1698 740777
Fax: +44 (0) 1698 740222
Web site:
www.thebest-ofhealth.com

What you receive when you order direct:

A Special Starter Package includes: a one-month supply of the three Radiant Health nutritional supplements – **Basic Essence** healthy essential oils (EFAs), **Mineral Essence** bioavailable minerals, and **Herbal Essence** Essiac-concept tonic, plus the highly acclaimed four-hour audio series "Low-Fat and Other Lies," the Conyers Crave-O-Meter to chart your progress in decreased food cravings, a 1-year subscription to *Radiant Health News*, an exclusive "behind the scenes" audio tape interview with *Life-Systems* Scientist Brian Scott Peskin, and the "Professor Peskin Unleashed" CD with information even the nutritionists don't know. This package is greater than a $295 value, but is available for $149.95 (plus shipping).

Be sure to visit their Web site at **www.radianthealth.org**. The site is loaded with information you can use on health and nutrition. The site features a "Frequently Asked Questions" section and an opportunity to e-mail your individual questions.

Like to attend a live seminar?

There's no better way to experience the thrill of living Beyond The Zone than attending one of our live seminars. Call Maximum Efficiency Products at (713) 796-2431. They conduct wonderful Beyond The Zone Seminars.

Especially for Physicians

The following services are available for physicians:

Maximum Efficiency News for Physicians reviews current developments in nutrition and is published three times a year. Our team of Life-Systems Engineers sorts through and analyzes current information, so you can quickly and easily keep abreast of the latest in nutrition research. If you want to stay current in nutrition-related information for your patients, this newsletter is for you.

Custom Seminars, designed for your special concerns. We can accommodate group sizes from half-a-dozen to hundreds.

Foundation of Radiant Health supplements are available in convenient monthly unit packaging.

Learn more about how this nutritional discovery of the century – the Foundation of Radiant Health – can help your patients and your practice. Direct inquiries to: "Physician Support."

For Nutrition Counselors

Maximum Efficiency Products equips you with the means of helping your clients achieve higher level results and to move them confidently forward to enjoying their own radiant health.

If you'd like to deepen your knowledge and understanding about the *Life-Systems* Engineering approach to radiant health, the *Life-Systems* Counselor Program may be for you.

After successfully completing the requirements for this prestigious program, you are awarded a certificate granting specific rights and privileges.

To learn more, direct inquiries to the *Life-Systems* Counselor Program at Maximum Efficiency Products.

Health Care Organizations and HMOs

Trial programs are available, so you can quickly and cost-effectively demonstrate how Beyond The Zone technology will add to your health care organization's bottom line. You'll have happier, healthier members, too.

Business

Pilot programs are available to quickly and cost-effectively prove to yourself how Beyond The Zone technology can boost your organization's effectiveness and the bottom line.

Education

Introductory programs are available to efficiently demonstrate how Beyond The Zone technology can add to your school's performance and better test scores.

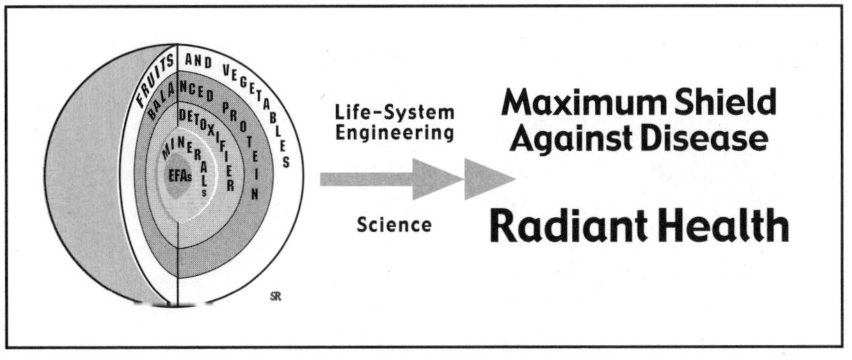

Now you actually can think smarter

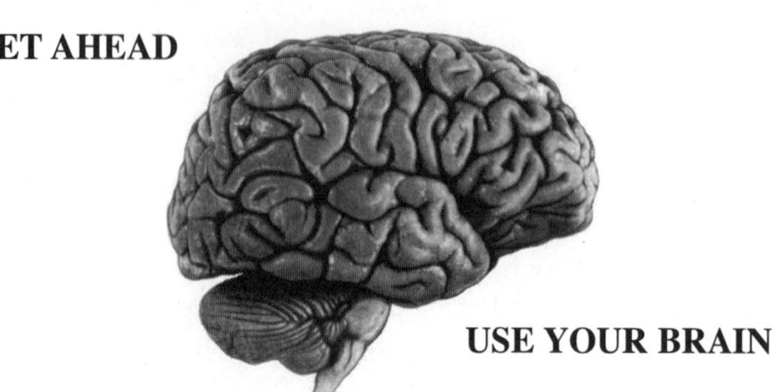

Learn a toolbox of strategies that will transform your brain's unlimited potential into the results you want in your personal and professional life.

To arrange for a Marcus Conyers (co-author) keynote or workshop for your organization contact:
Maximum Efficiency Products +(713) 796-2431

For his TAPES, BOOKS, and PRODUCTS contact:
www.brainsmart.com

WARNING! You Haven't Been Told:

"There is a **progressively higher risk of death** (over 40% greater) as glucose tolerance worsens, and **the risk is independent of [other] established risk factors** for cardiovascular (heart) disease. ... **higher death rates** even for those with milder forms of glucose intolerance, **which may or may not turn into diabetes.**"

***Life-Systems* Engineering Analysis:** Impaired cell membranes and an overworked pancreas caused by the great 25-year carbohydrate eating *experiment* can kill you even if you aren't yet a diabetic! **If you don't want a heart attack then it's critically important to keep blood sugar levels controlled.**

Source: American Diabetes Association's 59th Annual Scientific Sessions, June 1999, Frederick L. Brancati, MD, NHANESII

Additional Resources

Sources of Other Miscellaneous Products

Toasted Onion crackers, *Tree of Life*® brand: a delicious snack cracker. A few of them go a long way, too. Fifteen of these bite-size crackers are equivalent to just 2 teaspoons of sugar. They're great with cheese. Ask your health market to carry this brand.

Salt, *Flower of the Ocean*™: Most salt is commercial grade for use in chemical industries. In our opinion, *Flower of the Ocean*™ is the world's finest salt. It's naturally harvested and imported from France. It is 85% sodium chloride, compared with 99% sodium chloride in commercial or industrial salt. It's available from Grain & Salt Society. The salt is about $14.50/ half-pound. Their telephone is (800) TOP-SALT. You can also order this delicious salt from Maximum Efficiency Products, at a discount with your Foundation of Radiant Health order.

Black Pepper, *Talamanca*: Most pepper is irradiated, fumigated, and chemically treated. This one isn't; these peppercorns are only washed quickly in water and dried. This is a delicious pepper. It comes in 2 oz. bags, from Brugger Brothers, at (305) 949-2264. They also sell an excellent pepper mill. With your Foundation of Radiant Health order, Maximum Efficiency Products can supply you this fine pepper at a discount.

Cast iron cookware, *Wagner's 1891*™ brand: This is a fine brand and can be found in many hardware and specialty stores.

Ghee: Chefs also call ghee "clarified butter." My cooking teachers told me about clarified butter, and I've enjoyed it for years. It is exceptional to cook in. Ghee is butter that has been gently simmered until all the water is evaporated. Then the milk solids are skimmed off. What's left is a golden oil that is resistant to even high heat, because it is naturally saturated. *Purity Farms* brand ghee from Sedalia, Colorado is made from organic milk, so there aren't any residues to worry about. Ask for it at your cooking, sauteeing, and frying, ghee is great (substitute 1/2 tsp. ghee for each 1 tsp. of butter in any recipe).

Chocolates, *Chocolates To Die For!* They use all-natural, fresh, hand-made, "clean" chocolates imported from Belgium. Unlike most chocolates, these contain no preservatives and no hydrogenated oils. They are available at most Whole Food Markets, gourmet shops throughout the country, and directly from 1-888-BEL-CHOC. **My personal favorite is their White (Gran Marnier) "Manon" made with heavy cream.** Just 1 or 2 of these will completely satisfy any craving you may get. They are wonderful for parties.

Chemical-free meats, Welsh Family Farm can ship chemical-free "Oregon Tilth Certified" standard meats to you. Their beef tenderloins are superb for that special occasion, and their chuck roasts are perfect for grinding your own hamburger (like I do). They offer a full line of steaks, chicken, turkey, and pork products. They are located in Iowa. (319) 535-7318, e-mail: wfof@ptel.net

Elevated Insulin [from carbohydrates] Levels Associated with Impaired Blood Clotting Function

"Elevated levels of fasting insulin [from carbohydrates] are *associated with* impairment of the bodily system that helps prevent blood clots from blocking blood vessels."

"These findings *suggest* a mechanism for the observed increased risk for CVD (**cardiovascular disease**) associated *with* hyperinsulinemia (insulin resistance)."

Source: *Journal of the American Medical Association*, 2000;283:221-228

***Life-Systems* Engineering Analysis:** Have you wondered why heart disease keeps increasing yet dietary fat and cholesterol consumption has decreased over the past 30 years? We ordinarily avoid terms such as "suggest" and "associated with." However, in this case they are appropriate. America, and now Europe, are on a crash course with massive increases in insulin resistance and accompanying heart disease because of the great 25-year carbohydrate eating *experiment!*

Further Reading

Ageless Body, Timeless Mind, Deepak Chopra, M.D., Crown Publishers, New York, 1993.

Best & Taylor's Physiological Basis of Medical Practice (12th edition), John B. West, M.D., Williams & Wilkins, Baltimore, MD, 1990.

Biochemistry of Exercise & Training, Ron Maughan, Michael Gleeson and Paul L. Greenhaff, Oxford University Press, New York, 1997

Biochemistry of Lipids, Lipoproteins, and Membranes, D.E. Vance; J. Vance, Elsevier Science Publishers, Amsterdam, The Netherlands, 1991.

Doctors Vitamin and Mineral Encyclopedia, (The), Sheldon Saul Hindler, M.D., Ph.D., Simon & Schuster, New York, 1990.

Dr. Atkins' New Diet Revolution, Avon Books, New York, 1992.

Eight Weeks To Optimum Health, Andrew Weil, M.D., Alfred A. Knopf, New York, 1997.

Essential Fatty Acids in Health and Disease, Edward N. Siguel, M.D., Ph.D., Nutrek Press, Brookline, MA, 1994.

Essential Medical Physiology (second edition), Leonard R. Johnson, Ph.D., Lippincott-Raven Publishers, Philadelphia, 1998.

Handbook of Essential Fatty Acid Biology, Shlomo Yehuda; David Mostofsky, Humana Press, Totawa, NJ, 1997.

Harper's Biochemistry (24th edition), Robert Murray, M.D., Ph.D.; Daryl Grammer, M.D.; Peter Mayes, Ph.D., D.Sc.; Victor Rodwell, Ph.D., Appleton & Lange, Stamford, CT, 1996.

Healing Mind, Healthy Woman, Alice D. Domar, Ph.D, Dell Publishing, New York, 1996.

Omega Plan, (The), Artemis P. Simopoulos, M.D., HarperCollins Publishers, New York, 1998.

Optimum Health, Stephen T. Sinatra, Dell Publishing, New York, 1998.

Relaxation Response, (The), Herbert Benson, M.D., Avon Books, New York, 1990.

Richard Feynman, A Life In Science, John Gribbin and Mary Gribbin, Penguin Books, New York, 1997.

Smart Fats: How Dietary Fats and Oils Affect Mental, Physical and Emotional Intelligence, Michael A. Schmidt, Ph.D., Frog, Ltd., North Atlantic Books, P.O.B. 12327, Berkeley, CA, 1996.

The Thin You Within You, Abraham J. Twerski, M.D., St. Martin's Press, New York, 1997.

Timeless Healing, Herbert Benson, M.D., Simon & Schuster, New York, 1996.

2 Fiber Studies Find No Benefit for the Colon

"Well, here we are. There's not a shred of [cancer fighting] evidence from these trials."

Dr. Gilbert Omenn stated "... the surprising results [no cancer protection] showed the need to **rigorously put belief systems to the test**, especially when you are making recommendations to literally hundreds of millions of people"

" ... it is time to **abandon the idea** that fiber can help prevent colon cancer."

Dr. David S. Alberts, director of cancer prevention at the University of Arizona's Cancer Center, said, "I think we **have definitely disproved the fiber hypothesis** for colon cancer."

Source: *New York Times*, page 1, April 20, 2000.

Life-Systems **Engineering analysis:** Radiant Health is not based on "beliefs or what may sound good." This finding is old news to the *Life-Systems* Engineers who told you about "fiber-fiction" 6 years earlier!

Red Wine Increases Antioxidents In Blood But <u>Does Not Influence</u> LDL Oxidation

Red wine shown worthless in protecting against oxidation of lipoproteins.

Source: *American Journal of Clinical Nutrition*, 2000;71:67-74.

Life-Systems **Engineering analysis:** Were you drinking lots of red wine to help keep your "arteries clean"? Sorry, you were **misled again.**

Why haven't we been told?

Acknowledgements

This book would not have been made possible without the help of my associates, family, and friends. I wish to particularly thank:

Debra Peskin, my wife. Her sacrifices while encouraging me during the thousands of hours devoted to research, hypothesis testing, cause-effect analysis, writing and revising is deeply appreciated. Without her support this book would not be here. As a registered pharmacist, she offered valuable technical expertise and real-life observations of people in daily struggles to find working solutions anchored in modern science. Debra was the first to discover how EFAs can give you the energy to work even a 12-hour day without becoming overly tired.

Stephen Ruback, *Life-Systems* Engineer and my chief associate, for the thousands of hours spent analyzing the cause-effect relationships detailed in this book; for his many wonderful illustrations used to present these discoveries; his appealing cover design, and to the countless hours spent crafting and fine-tuning the exacting language and easy to read layout used to present the discoveries in this book. He is a uniquely multi-talented scientist.

Marcus Conyers, Peak Performance Consultant and my co-author, for his writing, research, for naming the book, and for making the book "BRAINSMART" and especially easy to read and understand. In short, taking PH.D.-level science and making it understandable to everyone. In my opinion, he's one of the world's top specialists on how your brain naturally assimilates information. His contributions were an important part of making this book easy to understand.

Robert and Marilyn Peskin, my parents, for allowing me, as a child, the never-ending opportunity to keep asking "why?"

Carlene, **Renda**, **Deloris**, and **Christina**, my wonderful staff, for their dedication to this project, and outstanding competence in assisting our many clients so effectively. Without their help, this book could not have been completed.

Howard Stephen Berg, the *world's fastest reader*, for teaching me the techniques that enabled me to read and absorb thousands upon thousands of pages of scientific and medical material faster than ever before.

David Zell, for his insight into the nature of cause-effect relationships, and ability to get to the "heart of the matter" quickly.

Russell J. Martino, for his immeasurable assistance in formalizing the information so it could be presented in a credible, yet not overly scientific way.

Wayne McGinty, my lead editor, for his relentless enthusiasm to undergo revision-after-revision, making the information crystal clear and understandable – a difficult mission.

Stephen Peskin, my brother, for making the comment, "Obesity is from just eating too many calories...." I felt there was much more to it, and with that "spark," the long search he inspired triggered a whole chain of new discoveries and connections that otherwise might have remained hidden.

Marge Hallan, for her relentless altruistic efforts making the discoveries in this book known around the world!

Prenatal PCB Exposure Affects Weight, Height

"Children exposed to environmental compounds PCBs and DDE before birth tend to be [abnormally] taller and weigh more [not good]. ... These things are ubiquitous [found everywhere] in the environment."

Source: *Journal of Pediatrics* 2000;136.

***Life-Systems* Engineering analysis:** Women need to protect their developing children with a daily detoxifier.

Index

C

D

E

F

I

J

K

L

N

O

P

Q

R

S

T

U

V

W

X

Y

Z

Three Important Papers

Men, Women and Children NEED TO KNOW...

(I thank Professor Michael A. Schmidt for bringing much of this information to my attention.)

Understanding the critical value of basic essence EFAs – particularly in brain development – is important to everyone. But because of the increased nutritional requirements, pregnant and nursing mothers need to be especially aware of their importance. Likewise, do the mothers of school-age children need to know the importance of **basic essence** EFAs.

For the reasons discussed in the book, *Peak Performance, Radiant Health*, the "Stat-Smart" chapter, I rarely place much confidence in studies. However, there are 3 exceptions:

1. A study can be conclusive in proving a "negative." If I theorize that fiber prevents colon cancer and then I give 1,000 people plenty of fiber, but they still get colon cancer in the same proportions as the general population, then clearly, the theory's premise was false. This fiber protection *theory* actually was *dis*proven in 1999.

2. A study that is <u>not</u> funded by a pharmaceutical, food, or nutrition company will be <u>much</u> <u>more</u> <u>credible</u> than an industry-funded study, because the researcher has less financial bias.

3. A study exploring or verifying established basic science - such as medicinal biochemistry - will be much more credible than a study designed to test a specific practical application - such as the effect that eating cereal has on the test scores of students.

Based on studies which meet these high standards, the following information reinforces the science presented in *Peak Performance, Radiant Health.*

• Did you know that animals consuming <u>reduced</u> amounts of <u>EFAs</u> over just 3 generations experienced an actual <u>reduction</u> in <u>brain</u> cells (smaller brains) and deficiency of omega 3 and omega 6 in the brain by the 3rd generation?[1]

---

1 Sinclair, A.J., Crawford, M.A., "The effect of a low fat maternal diet on neonatal rats," *Br J Nutr*, 1973, 29:127-137.

***Life-Systems* Engineering analysis:** As with animals, the human brain needs certain raw material from the diet - it can't make healthy brain or nerve cells without the 2 **E**ssential **F**atty **A**cids (EFAs) that I refer to, together, as "**basic essence**." Without adequate and proportioned supplies of basic essence, the brains of each succeeding generation of children become progressively more and more damaged!

Basic essence is typically removed or chemically altered by modern food processing, so we can predict that most parents and most children will be deficient in **basic essence**.

• Did you know that brain synapses (nerve cell connections) have a higher concentration of basic essence-derived DHA (docosahexaenoic acid) than almost any other tissue in the body?[2] You may recall, from *Peak Performance, Radiant Health*, that *myelin* (the insulating sheath around the nerve that speeds up the transmission) formation is critical to the development of the brain in children. As you learned in *Peak Performance, Radiant Health*, myelin production is also increased with **basic essence** EFAs.

• Scientists studied the brains of people with multiple sclerosis (MS) and compared them to the brains of healthy people. They found low levels of DHA in the brains of the MS people, low levels of omega 3 (one of the 2 "parent" basic essence structures) in the blood, and almost no omega 3 stored in the adipose (fat) tissue.[3]

Multiple sclerosis is a medical condition characterized by nerve destruction.

***Life-Systems* Engineering analysis:** The structure of the brain **absolutely requires** the basic essence-derived DHA. The body normally makes all the DHA it needs when it has an adequate supply of omega 3. It is a logical conclusion that, to develop proper nerve integrity and maximum brain abilities, you need to ensure that you obtain enough "parent" omega 3.

---

2 Bazan, N.G. "Supply of n-3 polyunsaturated fatty acids and their significance in the central nervous system," Ref: Wurtman, *Nutrition and the Brain*, Vol. 8, New York: Raven Press, Ltd., 1990:2.

3 Nightingale, S, et al. "Red blood cells and adipose tissue fatty acids in active and inactive multiple sclerosis," *Acta Neurol Scand*, 1990, 82:43-50.

• Did you know that animals consuming inadequate basic essence couldn't learn well? Rats were subjected to a life-threatening situation and had to learn an avoidance behavior in order to survive.

With sufficient basic essence, these test animals showed a **100% success** response against a life-threatening situation. **Without** basic essence, **only 40% success** - even after the 20th attempt to learn the required behavior![4]

Life-Systems **Engineering analysis:**

> ***Less basic essence = reduced learning ability!***

This is in animals. Imagine how much more important **basic essence** is to a human being, with a much bigger brain. Does your child have a learning-related problem? Now you have identified one of the prime suspects.

• Did you know: Purdue University found that children with attention deficit (ADD) and hyperactivity (ADHD) had lower levels of basic essence omega 3 and DHA in their blood?[5]

Is your child overly aggressive? Supplementation with DHA, a natural **basic essence**-derivative, often makes a significant improvement in students.[6] This is yet another confirmation of the predictive value of the science of *Peak Performance, Radiant Health.*

• Hydrogenated (processed) cooking oils were patented in 1911.* These oils contain little basic essence; the process changes the EFAs into harmful *trans*fats. More and more foods contain these hydrogenated oils: check the label on your margarine, cake mix, peanut butter, popcorn, cookies, and so on.

* Such oil is no longer food; it is a man-made invention.

---

4 Yokota, A. "Relationship of polyunsaturated fatty acid composition and learning ability in the rat," *Nippon Saniujinka Clakkadji* (in Japanese), 1993, 45:15-22.

5 Stevens, L.J., Burgess, J. "Omega 3 fatty acids in boys with behavior, learning, and health problems," *Physiology Behavior*, 1996, 59(4-5):915-920.

6 Hamazaki, T., et al., "The effects docosahexaenoic acid on aggression in young adults," *J Clin Invest*, 1996, 97:1129-1134.

Our children are now at least the 3rd generation since 1911 (see bottom of p. 471 and top of p. 472). Could this lack of unprocessed basic essence in today's diet explain the catastrophic increases in ADD, ADHD, other classroom-related learning disabilities, and violence and aggression in today's children?

***Life-Systems* Engineering analysis: Absolutely.** The Purdue study is more confirmation of learning-related problems linked directly to a **basic essence** deficiency.

Insufficient basic essence = lowered learning ability!

• It is now known that there are certain critical windows of development during which nerve cells and their connections MUST grow and become myelinated (that is, covered with myelin). These connections set the stage for potential intelligence and physical (body) control ability. The efficiency of brain connections is also impaired by a deficiency of **basic essence**. (See discussion of multiple sclerosis.)

• It is a well-known "basic" physiology fact that, if you can't see well, then you can't read well, either. It is now known that the retina (the "sensing" part of the eye) has the highest concentration of DHA (a **basic essence** derivative) of any tissue in the body – even higher than in brain synapses (see discussion above). Experiments show that, when **basic essence** is lacking in the diet, the levels of critical APTase (the chemical communicator) in the nerve endings fall by about half! After only 4 weeks of this malnutrition, dramatic changes take place in the retina. **It takes as much as 10 times more light to make the eye respond!**[7]

***Life-Systems* Engineering analysis:** If you don't have enough basic essence, then expect vision-related problems, which lead to vision-related learning problems.[8, 9]

---

7 Bourre', J.M., *Brainfood*, Little Brown, and Company, 1993, pages 56, 208-209.

8 Bazan, N.G., Gordon, W.C., Rodriguez de Turco, E.B., "The uptake, metabolism, and conservation of docosahexaenoic acid (22:6n-3) in brain and retina alterations in liver and retinal 22:6 metabolism during inherited progressive retinal degeneration," Sinclair, A., Gibson, R., eds., *Essential Fatty Acids and Eicosanoids*, Champaign, Ill: American Oil Chemists' Society, 1992, pages 107-115.

9 Birch, E.E., Birch, D.G., Hoffman, D.R., Uauy, R., "Dietary essential fatty acid supply and visual acuity development," *Invest Ophthalmol Vis Sci*, 1992, 33(11):3242-53.

• Many nutritional supplements are made available to increase blood flow to the brain, and with good reason - almost 1/5th of your heart's capacity is used to provide blood flow to the brain.

The brain receives almost 25 times more blood flow, on a pound-for-pound basis, than a muscular tissue such as an arm or a leg.[10] Any restriction in blood supply weakens brain function. As you learned in *Peak Performance, Radiant Health*, **basic essence (especially the "parent" omega 6 component) is the body's *natural* nutrient to increase blood flow** and, at the same time, decrease high blood pressure.

***Life-Systems* Engineering analysis:** Is it any wonder, then, that younger and younger children are developing clogged arteries and heart disease, they are developing learning disorders in unprecedented numbers, **and they can't learn** - and **nothing seems to help?**

• Did you know that students performed better when their sugar intake was reduced and food additives were removed? From 1979 through1983, one million (1,000,000) school children in 803 public

Parents - please make sure your children get their basic essence, so they'll be healthier!

schools in New York City were put on a diet free of food additives and with reduced sugar. Those schools' rankings increased to become the best ever — from 12.9% of the students performing 2 or more grades below proper level to just 4.9% performing poorly! The entire school system posted an increase of 15.7 percentage points.[11]

***Life-Systems* Engineering analysis:** Imagine the potential compounded results when a modest nutrition program, such as this one, is coupled with a **Radiant Health** supplementation program!

---

10 Bourre', J.M., *Brainfood*, 208-209. (Based on work of neuroscientist Nicholas Bazan.)

11 Schoenthaler, Stephen, et al., "The impact of a Low Food Additive and Sucrose Diet on Academic Performance in 803 New York City Public Schools," *Intl J of Biosocial Res*, 8(2), 1986, pages 185-195.

• Do you think that you are "eating healthy"? Have you even adopted a vegetarian diet?

***Life-Systems* Engineering analysis:** the book, *Peak Performance, Radiant Health*, clearly explains, scientifically, why vegetarianism is inappropriate nutrition for a human being. Real-life results of physicians found that long-term vegetarians were especially low in DHA (a basic-essence derivative).

Because they didn't eat meat, vegetarians didn't obtain the DHA that meat and fish provide. Children of vegetarians were deficient, too – but much more so – they had just a third (1/3) of the level of their mothers who ate vegetables and meat![12, 13, 14]

Here's a significant question: Do all the adulterated, damaged oils and fats (hydrogenated oils and *trans*fats) from fast-food restaurants, most supermarkets, and processed foods simply increase the deficiency of basic essence or is the problem even worse? Do they actually replace good EFAs in the brain, organs, and cells - even crossing the placenta to affect the developing baby? **You won't like this answer :** The damaged fats and oils REPLACE the natural ones - especially in the brain!

They also find their way into the heart, liver, myelin sheath (nerves), retina (eye), sciatic nerve, and blood vessels. The greater the **basic essence** deficiency, the greater the damage to the body! If the tissue doesn't have enough of the exact required nutrient, the next "closest fitting" EFA-derivative is used instead - and it doesn't work like the required one.[15, 16, 17]

---

12 Argen, et al., "Essential fatty acid composition of erythrocyte, platelet, and serum lipids in strict vegetarians," *Lipids* 1995, 30(4):365-69.

13 Reddy, S., Sanders, T.A.B., Obeid, O., "The influence of maternal vegetarian diet on essential fatty acid status of the newborn," *Eur J Clin Nutr*, 1994, 48:358-68.

14 Reddy, S., Sanders, T.A.B., "The influence of a vegetarian diet on the fatty acid composition of milk and the essential fatty acid status of the infant." *J Pediatr*, 1992, 120:S71-77.

15 Dopeshwarkar, G.A. *Nutrition and Brain Development*, Plenum Press, 1981, pages 70-73.

16 Grandgirad, A., Bourre', J.M., Julliard, F., et al., "Incorporation of trans long-chain n-3 polyunsaturated fatty acid in rat brain structure and retina," *Lipids*, 1994, 29(4):251-258.

17 Peterson, J., Opstvedt, J., "Trans fatty acids: Fatty acid composition of lipids of the brain and other organs in suckling piglets," *Lipids*, 1992, 27(10):761-69.

A pregnant woman requires **basic essence** for her developing child. Pregnancy places considerable extra stress on the body, which leads to an even worse **basic essence** deficiency for mom. During pregnancy, her **basic essence** levels are reduced (the child takes it), as compared to non-pregnant women, and this condition persists even after her pregnancy unless the deficiency is remedied.

***Life-Systems* Engineering analysis:** For the healthiest child, you must begin to correct the basic essence deficiency at least 6 months before conception. With **basic essence** deficiency, both you AND your child suffer - perhaps permanently.[18, 19]

Pregnant women - please make sure you have sufficient basic essence, so your newborns aren't brain-deficient!

Are you angry that results such as these, conclusively showing the *real-life* results of **basic essence** deficiency, aren't publicized to the general public? You have every right to be outraged! The majority of these studies were published - mainly in limited-circulation professional journals - in the early 1990s. Popular health and nutrition magazines keep touting: take lots of vitamins and calcium, don't eat fat, eat lots of carbohydrates, and exercise extensively. **Could it be that almost everyone is repeating the wrong advice?**

Yes, they are, and now *Peak Performance, Radiant Health* gives you the established medical science that predicts the *real-life* results of these and other studies. Isn't it time that you put the power of *Life-Systems* Engineering science to work for you instead of trusting popular opinion?

---

18 Van Jaarsveld, P.J., et al., "The essential fatty acid status of women from a community with low socioeconomic status," *Med Sci Res*, 1994, 22:719-21.

19 Holman, R.T., Johnson, S.B., Ogburn, P.L., "Deficiency of essential fatty acids and membrane fluidity during pregnancy and lactation," *Proc Nat Acad Sci*, 1991, 88:4835-4839.

Polycystic Ovary Disorder

Why are so many young women developing facial hair and male sexual characteristics, endometriosis, and fibroid tumors?

The "great carbohydrate eating *experiment*" is a root cause of this epidemic, too. Let's review what some current medical textbooks have to say.

"Excessive **insulin** secretion occupies a **central role** in expression of the *polycystic ovary syndrome*. Thus, receptors for insulin and insulin-like growth factor 1 have been identified in the ovary, and their stimulation sensitizes the ovary to stimulation by gonadotrophins ... hypersecretion of **insulin inhibits** hepatic synthesis of sex hormone binding globulin which, particularly in obese patients, results in an apparent disparity between circulating testerone concentrations and the degree of hirsutism [excessive hair in women - particularly on the face]...."[1]

"An association exists **between PCOD** [polycystic ovary disorder] or hyperthecosis, virilization, acanthosis nigricans, and **insulin resistance**; in the ovary, insulin may interact via the insulin-like growth factor receptors to **enhance androgen [male]** synthesis in insulin-resistant states."[2]

***Life-Systems* Engineering analysis:** Both of these medical textbook references are a "mouthful," yet they specifically state the basis of the problem. Once again, we find that excess insulin is causing grave damage. *Insulin* is produced by the body in response to eating or drinking carbohydrate. Although any woman can suffer from these symptoms, a young woman's delicate testosterone-estrogen-progesterone balance is upset, so that overtime, subsequent sexual development is impaired - perhaps permanently.

---

1 Internet Search site: http://commodore.perry.pps.pgh.pa.us/~odonnell/pco.html. (ref.: *Oxford Textbook of Medicine* - 3rd edition, Oxford University Press, 1996.

2 Internet Search site: http://commodore.perry.pps.pgh.pa.us/~odonnell/pco.html. (ref.: *Harrison's Principles of Internal Medicine* -13th edition (on CD ROM).

Could this explain precisely why so many of today's young women are developing:

- a "blocky" (no feminine curves) figure,
- excess facial hair (moustaches),
- problems with menstrual periods,
- endometriosis,
- aggressiveness, and
- obesity.

As you learned in *Peak Performance, Radiant Health:*

1. Lack of the healthy essential oils (basic essence) will impair sexual hormone development.

2. Lack of basic essence also contributes to a defective cell membrane. A defective cell membrane directly contributes to *insulin resistance*. Insulin resistance keeps the blood insulin level elevated, and this is now known to cause extensive damage.

3. Many hormones are made from proteins. With the "great carbohydrate eating *experiment*," are you certain that your child is getting enough protein?

It is unfortunate that this information is known and published in medical textbooks, yet not distributed to the general public. Dr. John R. Lee, a physician specializing in women's hormonal requirements, is distressed by the prescribing of estrogen (estradiol supplementation) even when progesterone is low: he says this makes no sense. Dr. Lee says that estrogen should always be taken with progesterone and that women routinely require only 1/4 - 1/2 of the "recommended estrogen dosages." (John R. Lee, M.D. *Medical Newsletter*, Nov. 1998). Provera is a trade name for a progesterone drug.

***Life-Systems* Engineering analysis:** Even after menopause, the hormone androstenedione is converted into estrone and ultimately into estradiol. The question that MUST be asked is, "did Mother Nature intend for women to become deficient in estrogen and become diseased because of it after menopause?" This speculation doesn't make sense, but it does make sense that problems would arise if there was a "basic essence" deficiency. ***Life-Systems* Engineering concludes** that this is the real problem - not a "supposedly" natural estrogen deficiency suffered by all American women. Dr. Lee agrees. For your information: natural estrogen is produced by the body in 3 forms. From the most potent to the weakest, they are: estradiol, estrone, and estriol. Does the "estrogen" prescribed consist of the exact ratios Mother Nature chooses? No. You only get 1 component instead of the 3 that Mother Nature uses. And we wonder why we continue to become sicker and sicker ....

If you are taking estrogen supplementation, it is interesting to note that common symptoms of estrogen overdosing are:

- Fibroid development[3]
- Weight gain
- Water retention
- Headaches
- Anxiety.

Dr. John Lee has an excellent section in his book, about women and their hormones, that American women can't afford to be without. It's available from your local health store. The title is: *"What Your Doctor May Not Tell You About Menopause."*

3 It is known that estrogen dominance stimulates the growth of fibroid tumors. With the *natural* decline of estrogen during menopause, fibroids shrink.

The Truth About Ketones and Ketosis

There is almost as much *mis*information regarding the health threat from ketones and ketosis (leading to metabolic acidosis) as there is *mis*information regarding the benefits from eating carbohydrates. **The following is based entirely on the world's leading medical textbooks including: *Textbook of Medical Physiology, Basic Medical Biochemistry, Biochemistry* (Stryer's 4th edition), and *Essentials of Biochemistry.***

Unfortunately, we all have been *un*knowing victims of a massive experiment – the *"great carbohydrate eating experiment"* – forcing us to endure a diet proper to fattening a cow but not proper for a human. For the past 25 years, we Americans have been told to make carbohydrates the basis of our diet - currently publicized as the "Food Pyramid." Starting in the late 1950s, the "Four Basic Food Groups" model showed us that we should eat "balanced" portions of bread/cereal, fruits/vegetables, dairy, and meat. The first 3 of these groups are almost all carbohydrate. In the 90s, the "Food Pyramid" model officially replaced the older model. The base of this model, the largest food group, is bread/cereal, with other carbohydrates still making up most of the rest. **This is in contrast to the diets proven successful for hundreds of years** - eating more proteins and natural fats with less carbohydrates - the diet of our parents and grandparents, and of most Americans before 1975. They told us not to eat too many potatoes, not to eat too much pie, and not to have too much cereal. Did mom tell you, "Now don't eat that junk food - I'm fixing you a good meal, and that will 'spoil' your appetite"? She was at least partially right.

What was the result of this experiment? **Unprecedented levels of obesity and diabetes have occurred *during the exact time-frame of this experiment.*** Heart disease and strokes have *not decreased* during this time-frame. We are victims, and we have every right to be upset. You also have a right to find out who perpetrated this *experiment* on us and what their motivation might have been. More than 25% of our children are now obese and more than 55% of adult Americans are certified obese.

Surprise #1 - Carbohydrates are either aldehyde or ketone compounds. ***Life-Systems* Engineering analysis:** Even the carbohydrates we are told are so good for us are loaded with the building blocks of ketone bodies. **Carbohydrates directly generate a problematic insulin-response; ketones don't.**

Surprise #2 - Biochemically, **ketones** are the **#1 preferred** fuel of the following organs: the skeletal muscles, the heart, and the liver. ***Life-Systems* Engineering analysis:** These organs don't want sugar (carbohydrate). Are we doing great damage by not giving these vital organs the fuel which Mother Nature designed them to run on?

Surprise #3 - Ketones are *natural* products of fat-burning. When bodyfat is oxidized, ketones are produced. ***Life-Systems* Engineering analysis:** Unless you want to keep all the excess bodyfat you have, you don't want to stop generating ketones.

Surprise #4 - We have been led to believe that the medical condition called "ketosis" (leading to metabolic acidosis - low blood pH) happens very quickly. This is *in*correct. Only after *3-5 days of virtually complete starvation* (fasting) do ketones in the body become significant. You will learn in the book, *Peak Performance, Radiant Health*, that our bodies have been compromised. Our bodies have been **forced** to try **to adapt** and run primarily on carbohydrates. You will learn why carbohydrates are not designed by Mother Nature to be our primary food.

The great 25-year carbohydrate eating *experiment* was instituted with no scientific basis. It was founded on *biased opinion* with no underlying established medical science. Contrary to popular *mis*information, running on ketones is the body's preferred and most efficient state, and the leading biochemistry and physiology textbooks support this fact. ***Life-Systems* Engineering analysis:** We have been *mis*led into believing what the body's preferred natural state and its proper fuel are. We have been tricked into forcing our bodies to run on a diet of harmful sugar (carbohydrates). Mother Nature never intended this, and the *real-life* results are terrible.

Surprise #5 - We've even been *mis*advised to eat numerous times a day. As a result of frequently eating foods improper to a human being, we have become accustomed to cravings. But we know that many religious sects *fast* for prolonged periods of time (days to weeks) and have safely done so for thousands of years. ***Life-Systems* Engineering analysis: *Real-life* results** and Mother Nature's time-tested wisdom offer more valuable guidance than the most popular suggestions by those defending biased positions. **The diabetes epidemic is accelerated by this bad advice.**

Surprise #6 - We have been told that ketosis will cannibalize our muscle tissue. (That's why eating enough protein is so important!) Actually, after just 3-5 days of fasting, our body requires only 1/3 the amount of glucose it has been forced to tolerate during the 25-year "carbohydrate eating *experiment*." Even now, you could eat **less than 1/2 of a bagel a day (for carbohydrate "requirement") and maintain superb health**. The brain and nervous system start to use ketones, because they finally get them. Our muscle is spared. ***Life-Systems* Engineering analysis:** If you have spent much time in a gym, then you know how difficult it is to add muscle. Do you really think that Mother Nature would allow that precious muscle to be quickly wasted? *Peak Performance, Radiant Health,* clearly details how a widespread but unrecognized nutrition deficiency is at the core of our problem, and it has nothing to do with ketosis.

Surprise #7 - Protein and ketones are NOT "hard" on the kidneys and liver. Protein can't even enter the kidney directly. Most of the supposedly harmful nitrogen from the protein is converted to urea in the liver and excreted by the kidneys (a normal process). The carbons are oxidized to make carbon dioxide and water. The **ketones are used as primary fuel by the kidneys, skeletal muscles, and heart**.

Surprise #8 - Carbohydrates, not protein, are hard on the kidneys. High blood glucose levels place excessive stress on the kidneys. That is why **diabetes is the single greatest cause of kidney failure in the U.S.** Too many nutritionists and physicians continue to "parrot" outdated misinformation.

Surprise #9 - Ammonia generated as a natural byproduct from digesting protein is NOT harmful. Before carbon skeletons of amino acids can be oxidized, the nitrogen must be removed. Ammonia is formed and converted to urea, which is nontoxic, water-soluble, and **readily excreted in the urine**.

Surprise #10 - If you perform a Medline Internet search on "kidney, high-protein diet," you will find article-after-article attesting to the scientific FACT that a high-protein diet is not harmful (to any normal person.) An example found is: "The concomitant increase of renal net acid excretion and maximum renal acid excretion capacity in periods of high protein intake appears to be a **highly effective response of the kidney** to a specific food **intake leaving a large renal surplus** capacity for an additional renal acid load." ***Life-Systems* Engineering (L.S.E.) translation:** The body's natural *life-systems* perform perfectly as Mother Nature intended. In contrast to the body's protein response, its carbohydrate response is strongly associated with renal (kidney) failure. This *L.S.E.* analysis is consistent with medical textbooks and established human biochemistry.

Surprise #11 - Have you heard the unfounded claim that excess protein "leaches" calcium from the bone and causes osteoporosis? Then why does the *Textbook of Medical Physiology* state, "... **protein** functions in the brush borders of these cells to **transport calcium into the cell** cytoplasm.... **The rate of calcium absorption** seems to be **directly proportional to the quantity of this calcium-binding protein**." ***Life-systems* Engineering analysis:** Calcium is transported via protein. Along with the protein, the calcium is actually going into the cell - not being taken away! You need to *understand* what you are doing with your health. Furthermore, most Americans get plenty of calcium in their food. There is no fundamental "calcium deficiency." However, **grains** (cereals) contain *phytates* that **render minerals, including calcium, ineffective!**

Surprise #12 - Mother Nature designed 3 *Life-Systems* to prevent any of the so-called "problems" with which the high-carbohydrate promoters continue to scare us: respiratory system, circulatory buffer system, and renal (excretory) system. Often, there is a lack of insight by nutritionists into how the various *Life-Systems* work together:

• Before ketosis COULD EVER BECOME A PROBLEM (in an extreme case, ketosis could lead to ketoacidosis - whereby low blood pH would cause severe complications), your respiration would have to increase to almost double your normal rate. **Has this ever happened?**

• Sufficient salt is required for the circulatory buffer system to work properly - lack of salt means lack of sodium bicarbonate ($NaHCO_3$). Could Americans' obsession with reducing dietary salt be the real reason that this critical *Life-System* is compromised and unable to do its job? *Peak Performance, Radiant Health* clearly details how important salt is to proper functioning. (Also, it *doesn't* raise blood pressure like we have been *mis*led to believe.)

• Our renal system responds further to stabilize our system.

Surprise # 13 - If a nutritionist tells you that the traditional diet for a person with kidney malfunction is low protein, **you need to resist this advice**. This paper discusses nutrition for healthy people, not ones with already diseased kidneys. Protein does not cause kidney failure (high carbohydrates are the likely culprit). As you will learn in *Peak Performance, Radiant Health,* a normally functioning kidney REPELS excess protein in the blood. If the kidney doesn't work, it *may* make sense to restrict protein levels. However, as *Diabetes Forecast* (Jan. 2000) states, "Other [health care] teams don't use it [low-protein diets] even after almost total (Stage 5) kidney failure (requiring dialysis)." Don't get misled.

Note # 1: Only a Type I, insulin-dependent, diabetic who has no access to insulin (virtually no one) could possibly have a problem with eating protein. **But that diabetic would have a life-threatening problem eating carbohydrates** without the insulin to protect him from excess blood sugar.

Note #2: "Following the ingestion of a high protein meal, the gut and liver utilize most of the absorbed amino acids.... The liver takes up 60-70% of the amino acids in the portal vein. **These amino acids, for the most part, are converted to glucose [sugar] – to fuel its own energy of digestion – they don't get used for bodily structure."***

---

* *Basic Medical Biochemistry - A Clinical Approach*

That's one reason why we need to **eat more protein** than many nutritionists recommend. The majority of dietary protein fuels its own digestion!

Note #3: Anyone suggesting you take the result of a "rat" study and automatically apply it to a human being is misleading you. More often than not, a rat's physiology **doesn't correlate directly** with a human being's physiology. ***Life-Systems* Engineering translation:** People aren't rats! Never automatically rely on an animal study to "prove" anything about how the item under study applies to a human being. The best scientists and physicians never do. Critical analysis must be used to determine when a proper analogy to a human being may be made.

Note #4: If you exercise by running, you produce lots of "extra" carbon dioxide - a waste product, because respiration increases. If you eat more protein, you automatically produce more ammonia. If you insist that "extra" ammonia is "bad," then following the same logic, you must say that exercise, causing "excess" carbon dioxide is "bad," too. Don't get mislead by illogical information.

Note #5: "Addition of carbohydrates (glucose) to proteins [auto-glycosylation] happens spontaneously (without aid of enzymes) in proportion to additional carbohydrates – **ketone**-derivatives are produced."* The more carbohydrates you eat, the more they auto-oxidize, and more ketone derivatives are *automatically* produced!

***Even after 5 weeks* of complete starvation, (but drinking water), blood glucose levels in the average, healthy adult only drop to 65 mg/dl (normal is 70-90 mg/dl). From burning our excess bodyfat, we *still* get all the sugar we require - and it's right out of the *Textbook of Medical Physiology*!**

Again, the preceding is based almost entirely on the world's leading medical textbooks including: *Textbook of Medical Physiology, Basic Medical Biochemistry, Biochemistry* (*Stryer's 4th edition*), and *Essentials of Biochemistry.*

---

* *Basic Medical Biochemistry - A Clinical Approach*

Why Believe Me?

• First, I am a scientist by training - not another nutrition writer who merely parrots outdated ideas. I go directly to the world's foremost scientific sources, and I perform my own direct research. Massachusetts Institute of Technology's (MIT - my alma mater) course description of their program in Bioengineering and Environmental Health states, "Each course applies principles of chemistry, biology, and engineering to issues of human health." Isn't it comforting to know that these are the same scientific principles on which I founded *Life-Systems* Engineering in 1993. The book ***Peak Performance, Radiant Health,*** and the related discovery of **Radiant Health** are the products of my far-reaching discoveries of proven facts and principles, **based on science - not opinion**.

• Second, I am professor emeritus (1998) of the endowed *Life-Systems* Engineering Chair, College of Pharmacy and Health Sciences at Texas Southern University, Houston, Texas. There, I taught our nation's up-and-coming pharmacists and physicians **current** nutrition information - not parroting outdated information disproved 25-50 years ago.

• Third, physicians, pharmacists, exercise physiologists, and clinical nutritionists both nationwide and internationally are applauding the outstanding *real-life* success of my discoveries in their patients' treatment.

For the first time, you can rest **assured** that the nutrition information you get will be **accurate**, **unbiased**, and completely **scientific**.

Scientifically, we aren't "all different." Quite the contrary. We really are much more alike than we are different ...

"Humans have perhaps 80,000 genes, and we are 99.9 percent identical."

Source: *Newsweek*, page 53, April 10, 2000.

***Life-Systems* Engineering analysis:** Radiant Health works so well because, contrary to popular opinion, we **aren't all different** – we all have **the same nutritional needs.**

The Solution To Modern Health Problems...

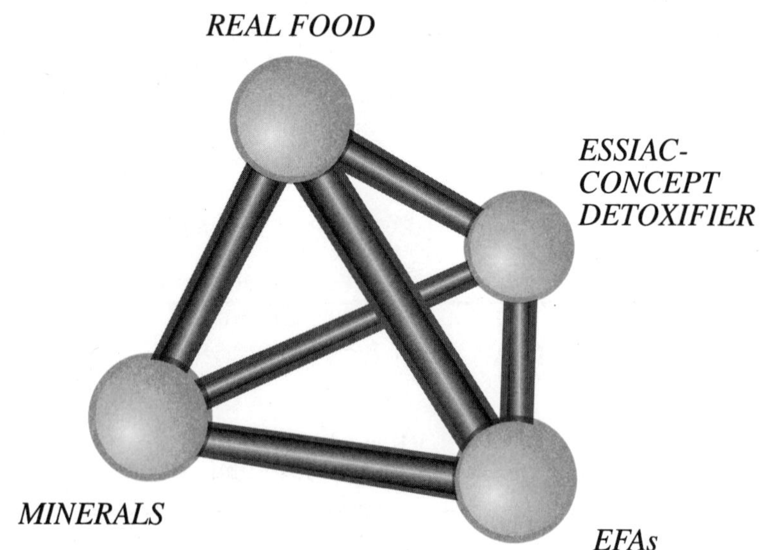

Radiant Health

The discoveries in this book will allow you to enjoy the pleasure of eating again. Your taste and appetite for certain foods will automatically change — expect a decrease in your craving for processed carbohydrates. Americans have exceptional willpower, so don't stop eating all of them at once — just minimize them — otherwise, you change your system balance too rapidly.

Women, because of your generally strong willpower in following what you thought was correct – the great 25-year carbohydrate eating experiment – you may require an additional 90 days (6 months total) of Radiant Health to re-balance your hormones. **Please be patient; your improved health is worth it!**

The Best Chocolate Pudding

4-6 ounces bittersweet chocolate
3 cups heavy cream (whipping cream)
1/3 cup sugar
1 cup whole milk (do not use low-fat milk)
4 egg yolks
1 tablespoon *un*salted butter, cut into 4 pieces
chopped or diced almonds (optional – but luscious!!!)

1. Melt the chocolate (a double boiler works best because it is very gentle).
2. In a medium saucepan, heat the cream, milk, and sugar over medium heat until warm (not hot).
3. Whisk the egg yolks together until smooth.
4. Slowly whisk the cream mixture into the yolks. Stir over medium heat about 8 minutes until the mixture coats the back of a spoon (a wooden spoon works best).
5. Strain the egg/cream mixture to remove any small egg particles (optional).
6. Whisk the cream mixture into the melted chocolate and mix until the chocolate has blended well. Stir in the butter.
7. Pour into bowls and chill at least 4 hours for best texture and flavor.

Top with whipped cream:
1 cup heavy (or whipping) cream
1 1/2 tsp. vanilla extract (Tahitian vanilla is great to use, but any vanilla extract will do)
1 tsp sugar (optional)

1. Pour all ingredients into a mixing bowl.
2. Beat with an electric beater on low for a few seconds and increase speed to medium and beat for a few more seconds. Finish off by increasing speed to high until mixture is fluffy.

– Enjoy!

***Chocolate** - There are many varieties of chocolate available. The higher the chocolate percentage, the higher the purity (e.g. 73% bittersweet dark chocolate is much less sweet than 45% milk chocolate). A few fine brands are: El-Ray (73%), Scharffenberger (70%), and Valhrona (from France). Soon I'll introduce my own brand that will be 76%. It will be luscious; look for it soon!*

COMING **— January 2001**

The cookbook of the century!

Rapid Recipes for Radiant Health

Why Don't People Question *Marginal* Results Posing as "Significant Improvements"?

After 5 years of completing an **extremely difficult to follow, low-fat, low cholesterol diet,** and doing **lots of exercise**, here are the results: "Among the **20 patients who completed** the program in 5 years, the **average decrease** in participants' artery blockages **after a year** was **4.5%** and after 5 years it was 12.5%."*

***Life-Systems* Engineering analysis:** Even if this result is to be believed – you'll learn the questions to ask in the "Never Get Suckered Again – Be Stat-Smart" chapter – the results measured by *Life-Systems* Engineering standards are **not nearly significant enough.** (If the blockage was originally 50% it was reduced to 47.75% after one year; 43.75% after 5 years.)

Given the **Stanford University School of Medicine** (2000) **results of <u>carbohydrate's</u> <u>direct</u> correlation with <u>poor blood</u> chemistry [bad],** one must ask: **Is it only the extensive exercise component (always required** with the high-carbohydrate, low-fat diets) **that provides anything positive?**

**U.S. News & World Report*, pages 56-60, July 12, 1999.

We Knew It Back Then; Why Don't We Know It Now?

In Ancient Greece, Plato wrote what was apparently common knowledge – that fruit "stimulates" the appetite, making us hungry, and that oil (basic essence) is essential:

"...as well as the woodland kind which gives us **meat** and drink **and oil together**, the ***fruit*** of trees that ministers to our pleasure and merriment and is so hard to preserve, and that we serve as a welcome dessert to a jaded man ***to charm away his satiety***."*

***Life-Systems* Engineering analysis:** It appears that, in the 4th century B.C., the significance of meat and oil to fulfill the appetite was understood. It was also understood that fruit makes us hungry again! Why did we lose this ancient wisdom?

The UK and Europe Aren't Listening Either

The world's leading universities and physicians know the truth about proper nutrition for peak performance and radiant health, but few have listened in the US. It appears that few have listened in the UK and Europe, also.

"Association of serum IgA antibodies to milk antigens with severe atherosclerosis"

A study published in 1989 showed a **very strong association** between (processed) **milk and atherosclerosis** (arterial disease). XO (xanthine oxidase) levels were significantly elevated in the milk drinkers who had advanced arterial disease.**

***Life-Systems* Engineering analysis:** This was a scientifically sound study because of the development of advanced analytical techniques that weren't available with similar studies performed in the 1970s. As you will learn in *Peak Performance, Radiant Health*, the XO issue was raised for processed milk and suspected to contribute to heart disease many years ago. Why haven't we listened instead of believing advertising campaigns?

Why haven't these findings been made public?

**Gateway To Atlantis*, Andrew Collins, page 59, Headline Book Publishing, London, 2000. Source: Plato's *Critias*, pages 115a-115b, 4th century B.C.

***Atherosclerosis*, 1989;77:251-256, (researched at the University of Bologna, Italy, Elsevier Scientific Publishers Ireland, Ltd.)

Most Patients <u>Do Not</u> Achieve Target LDL Cholesterol Levels

Based on information from over 4,000 patients of 900 physicians:

With drug therapy, only 39% lowered their LDL to "target" level – not a dramatic improvement considering there was a 34% decrease with those on nondrug therapy.*

***Life-Systems* Engineering analysis:** Two points must be raised: **First, the drugs were *only* 5% more effective than nondrug methods** (exercise, etc.). This is far short of the 80% effectiveness that Life-Systems Engineering methods try to maintain. Second, even with drugs to force the body's metabolism to artificially alter itself, the "target" still can't be met! Therefore, does the "target" level of LDL we are told to meet make sense? Is it arbitrary?

<u>Are we looking for results in the wrong place?</u>

Study Disproves Soy as an Aid in Fighting Hot Flashes

Soy has been widely promoted to assist women in everything from decreasing hot flashes to decreasing cancer risks. Forget the decrease in hot flashes... The Mayo Clinic recently found that cancer survivors who took soy pills did not experience any noticeable decrease of hot flashes. "Despite optimistic hopes that this soy phytoestrogen product would alleviate hot flashes, the scientific data from this study demonstrated that it did not help. ... For now, we have to move on and find things that work for patients..."**

***Life-Systems* Engineering analysis:**

We have an enormous body of **science** that **tells us what works.**

<u>It's called *Radiant Health*, and it's here today.</u>

**Archives of Internal Medicine*, 2000;160:459-467

***Journal of Oncology*, Feb. 29, 2000, Medscape Wire (Internet edition)

Radiant Health Comes to the UK and Europe

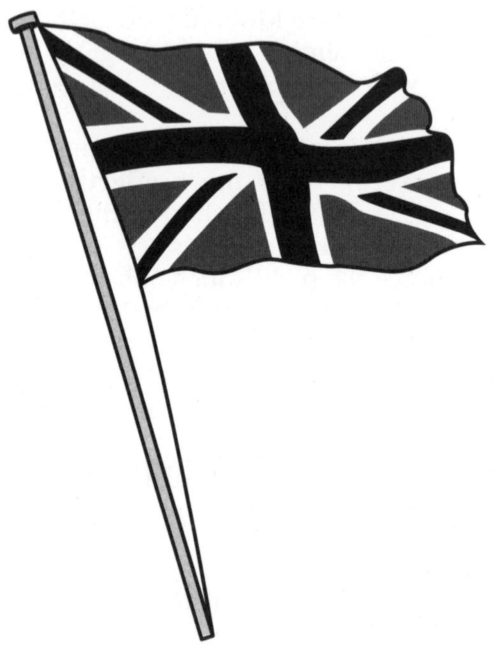

For enquiries from the UK and Europe:

For the full line of Radiant Health products, please contact the exclusive distributor, our sister company, **The Best of Health**, headquartered in:

Strathclyde Medical Park, Unit 7
Mallard Way
Bellshill, Lanarkshire, ML4 3BF
SCOTLAND
Tel: +44 (0)1698 740777
Fax: +44 (0)1698 740222
Web site: www.thebest-ofhealth.com